The Nervous System and the Heart

The Nervous System and the Heart

Edited by

Gert J. Ter Horst, PhD

University of Groningen, Groningen, The Netherlands

Foreword by

Douglas P. Zipes, MD

Krannert Institute of Cardiology, Indiana University School of Medicine, Indianapolis, IN

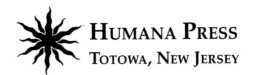
HUMANA PRESS
TOTOWA, NEW JERSEY

B S

© 2000 Humana Press Inc.
999 Riverview Drive, Suite 208
Totowa, New Jersey 07512

This publication is printed on acid-free paper. ∞
ANSI Z39.48-1984 (American Standards Institute) Permanence of Paper for Printed Library Materials.

Cover design by Patricia F. Cleary.

Due diligence has been taken by the publishers, editors, and authors of this book to assure the accuracy of the information published and to describe generally accepted practices. The contributors herein have carefully checked to ensure that the drug selections and dosages set forth in this text are accurate and in accord with the standards accepted at the time of publication. Notwithstanding, as new research, changes in government regulations, and knowledge from clinical experience relating to drug therapy and drug reactions constantly occurs, the reader is advised to check the product information provided by the manufacturer of each drug for any change in dosages or for additional warnings and contraindications. This is of utmost importance when the recommended drug herein is a new or infrequently used drug. It is the responsibility of the treating physician to determine dosages and treatment strategies for individual patients. Further, it is the responsibility of the health care provider to ascertain the Food and Drug Administration status of each drug or device used in their clinical practice. The publisher, editors, and authors are not responsible for errors or omissions or for any consequences from the application of the information presented in this book and make no warranty, express or implied, with respect to the contents in this publication

Cover illustration taken from Figure 2B in Chapter 1 of this book. They are photomicrographs showing immunoreactivity for the general neural marker protein gene product 9.5. Scale bar = 50 µm.

For additional copies, pricing for bulk purchases, and/or information about other Humana titles, contact Humana at the above address or at any of the following numbers: Tel.: 973-256-1699; Fax: 973-256-8314; E-mail: humana@humanapr.com, or visit our Website: http://humanapress.com

Printed in the United States of America. 10 9 8 7 6 5 4 3 2 1

Library of Congress Cataloging in Publication Data

Main entry under title:

The nervous system and the heart/edited by Gert J. Ter Horst.
        p.   cm.—
    Includes index.
    ISBN 0-89603-693-6 (alk. paper)
    1. Heart–Innervation. 2. Nervous system, Vasomotor. I. Ter Horst, Gert J.
    [DNLM: 1. Heart—physiology. 2. Autonomic Nervous System—physiology. 3. Heart—innervation. 4. Neurosecretory Systems—physiology. 5. Pain—physiopathology. WG 202 N4565 2000]
    QP113.4N47 2000
    612.1'78—dc21
    DNLM/DLC
    for Library of Congress   99-25404
                                                                 CIP

5-9-03

Foreword

The heart is an amazing organ, capable of maintaining rhythmic contractions autonomously when transplanted to a new body or even in a Langendorff preparation. However, for optimal function, electrical and contractile performances need to be modulated. This is the role played by the autonomic nervous system. Carrying information to and from the heart, neural activity profoundly affects cardiac function. Although the study of head–heart interactions has been the focus of research for many years, there is still so much to learn. *The Nervous System and the Heart*, ably edited by Gert J. Ter Horst, brings together the state-of-the-art knowledge on autonomic control of the heart, hypothalamo–pituitary–adrenal modulation, heart pain, modulation by humoral factors, and the relationship between cognitive/neuropsychiatric disorders and heart disease. The importance of these interactions cannot be overstressed, not only for understanding cardiac function and physiology, but also for its impact on sudden cardiac death.

Many years ago at an international symposium, my presentation followed that of a basic scientist who had begun to unravel the function of the adenylate cyclase system in the cell. Intimidated by such shining science, I started my presentation with a "low tech" example by showing the electrocardiogram of a patient who spontaneously developed ventricular fibrillation five days after an unremarkable recovery from a myocardial infarction seconds after he was told that his mother had just died. Although the importance of knowing the intricacies of the adenylate cyclase system is unquestioned, one must also study an intact organism with functioning neural pathways to understand head–heart interactions that can explain why (and how) this patient developed ventricular fibrillation. A more contemporary example of neural modulation involves the recent observation of increased cardiovascular mortality during winter months in adults. Close inspection of the literature reveals that this increased winter mortality occurs in infants and dogs as well, whether in the northern or southern hemispheres of the world, in mild winter (e.g., Los Angeles) or more severe climates (e.g., Canada).

The common denominator from all these studies appears to be not the stress of the cold or the holidays (Thanksgiving in the United States, Christmas, and New Year's), but the shorter days of winter. The likely mediator of decreased daylight is the suprachiasmic nucleus and its modulation of a host of cardiovascular processes. Understanding such head–heart interactions may lead to increased understanding in neural control of the heart and new approaches to reducing cardiovascular mortality. The information in *The Nervous System and the Heart* will be invaluable in this quest.

Douglas P. Zipes, MD

Preface

The heart and the brain are very intimately related, much more so than any other two organs in our bodies, and they rely strongly on each other. The heart guarantees an optimal blood supply to the brain to meet the brain's high oxygen and glucose needs. The activities of the various components of the heart are controlled by dedicated brain circuitry in order to achieve an optimal functioning of this complicated pump in all conditions. Not only biologically, but also psychologically, the heart is associated with the brain. We all know that our cognitive abilities reside within the central nervous system, but we can find many examples of the association of the heart with these human capabilities. There is, however, a logical explanation for this brain–heart projection. Emotional situations—love, hate, rage, anxiety, and so on—all generate alterations of heart rate and blood pressure. We sense this rapid change in our physiology and, as any conditioning stimulus in experimental animals, we associate this immediately with the emotional experience, leading to overestimation of heart rate effects in our daily lives.

The basic mechanisms of heart–brain interaction are shown in Fig. 1. Apart from afferent and efferent nerve fibers, various humoral factors contribute to the communication between the heart and the brain. On the efferent side, this communication is achieved by the sympathetic and parasympathetic nerve supply of the heart, and by the hypothalamo–pituitary–adrenal system. The afferent side is composed of sensory nerve fibers that relay cardiovascular information to the central nervous system via the vagus and sympathetic nerves. Humoral factors are also involved. Angiotensin and mediators of inflammation are typical examples of humoral factors that can alter cardiovascular functions via the brain.

Although it is well established that automaticity in the heart is intrinsic to the various pacemaker tissues, heart rate and rhythm are very much under the control of the autonomic nervous system. The

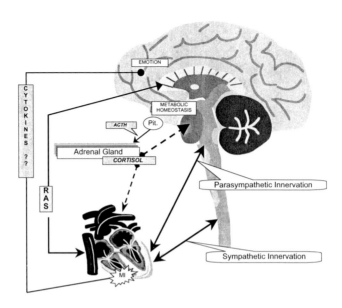

Fig. 1. Schematic illustration of mechanisms of heart–brain interaction presented in *The Nervous System and the Heart*. The parasympathetic vagus and the sympathetic nerves, respectively, contain the autonomic efferent and sensory afferent fibers of the heart. Humoral factors participating in heart–brain interaction involve the hypothalamo–pituitary–adrenal system, the RAS, and, possibly, the cytokines. Abbreviations: MI = myocardial infarction; ACTH = adrenal corticotropic hormone; Pit. = pituitary.

autonomic innervation generates immediate alterations of heart rate, force of contraction, and coronary blood flow during emotional situations. Parasympathetic activity slows heart rate (bradycardia) and conduction, and decreases the force of contraction. Sympathetic activation has the opposite effect. The fine tuning of sympathetic and parasympathetic activity is achieved by nervous circuitry in the brain stem and spinal cord that integrate feedback from baroreceptor activity and respiration as well as commands from higher limbic structures involved in maintenance of metabolic homeostasis. The nerve supply of the heart is discussed in **Chapter 1,** which addresses the innervation of the various parts of the pig heart, and the location and biochemistry of the autonomic ganglia. Nervous circuitry controlling cardiac activity as part of emotional expression is the topic of **Chapter 2.** The anatomical substrate(s) of cardiac diurnal rhythms is presented in **Chapter 3,** which describes the connections between the suprachiasmatic nucleus of the hypothalamus—the location of the biological clock cells—and the heart. Since the central nervous system has considerable effects on cardiovascular activity, it has become clear that dysfunction of the brain may underlie cardiac disease pathogenesis. **Chapters 4** and **5** discuss the cardiovascular effects of neuropathological conditions in patients and experimental animals, respectively. These studies supply a neurobiological basis for the occurrence of cardiac arrhythmias and for sudden death during stressful emotional conditions.

The effects of (chronic) stress are not mediated solely by the autonomic nervous system, but involve neurohumoral factors, in particular the adrenal corticosteroids. Stress is associated with increased sympathetic activity and activation of the hypothalamo–pituitary–adrenal system. Release of corticosteroid hormones into the circulation has an effect in both the heart and the brain. These highly lipophilic hormones penetrate the blood–brain barrier (BBB) to bind the cytoplasmic mineralo- and glucocorticoid receptors, which are differentially expressed regionally in the central nervous system (CNS). After binding cortisol (human) or corticosterone (in animals), the receptor–ligand complex migrates to the nucleus to bind to the promoter regions of selective genes. Expression of these selective genes affects the cellular biochemistry—for instance, at the membrane receptor, second messenger, or transmitter level—and subsequently, neuronal and circuit activity. Biochemical alterations may be long lasting and reset the autonomic tone in favor of the sympathetic drive, which eventually may lead to development of cardiac disease as a consequence of chronic hypertension and/or arteriosclerosis. Very limited information is available on the effects of corticosteroids on the heart. Mineralo- and glucocorticoid receptors have been identified in the myocardium, but whether or not chronic activation of these receptors has adverse effects has not been studied in depth. **Chapter 6** reviews our current knowledge of the role of corticosteroids in both the cardiovascular control circuitry and the myocardium.

The neurobiological foundation of heart pain (angina pectoris) is the topic of Part III, which describes the cardiac nociceptive system, and the pain pathways. Myocardial ischemia resulting from coronary vasospasms or arteriosclerosis is considered the main cause of angina pectoris. These ischemic conditions trigger the formation and release of noxious compounds that activate the cardiac nociceptors. Adenosine, bradykinin, lactate, serotonin, prostaglandins, and many other substances are released as part of a so-called "ischemic cascade." **Chapter 7** presents current knowledge regarding the activation of cardiac nociceptive systems in angina pectoris. It discusses the biochemical aspects and the various clinical manifestations of angina pectoris, including silent ischemia and syndrome X.

Neuroanatomical Fos–protein expression studies in animals do supply information at the cellular level about the structures and pathways involved. Fos is a member of the so-called immediate early gene protein family that is selectively expressed in nerve cells between one to six hours after the activation, and is used for characterization of neuronal network architecture, for example, in the study of pain transmission. However, validated animal heart–pain models are needed to use this Fos imaging successfully. Few such models are available, and most are handicapped by the need that they be conducted on anesthetized animals because of local animal welfare regulations. All anesthetics affect the transmission of pain information and thus distort the patterns of Fos–protein induction in the central nervous system, which reduces their value. Visceral pain-processing systems were analyzed with Fos induction in conscious rats treated with intravenous infusion of noxious compounds like 5-HT (serotonin) and intraperitoneal injections of formalin solutions. **Chapter 8** describes these investigations and presents an overview of central visceral and heart–pain processing pathways, the potential role of the vagus nerve, and the anatomical basis of referred pain. Neurophysiological studies described in **Chapter 9** substantiate the anatomical findings and supply additional information about the possible role of the afferent vagal nerve fibers in cardiac pain processing. It is demonstrated that cardiac vagal afferent fibers can modulate neuronal activity in the upper cervical spinal cord levels, which implicates these spinal areas in visceral pain modulation. Patient studies, conducted to elucidate the neurobiological substrate(s) of angina pectoris and syndrome X, are described in **Chapter 10.** Using alterations of regional cerebral blood flow during the attack, as measured in patients with Positron Emission Tomography (PET scan), it was established that these forms of heart pain are processed by different neuronal circuitries in the forebrain. The forebrain activity pattern of syndrome X patients resembles that of psychiatric patients suffering anxiety disorders.

Neuroendocrine mechanisms participating in the regulation of cardiovascular functions are discussed in Part II. Neuroendocrine regulation implies that the CNS controls the release of humoral factors involved as part of the flight-or-fight response pattern. However, many other humoral factors, for which the release is not controlled by the CNS, affect the functioning of the heart. Such substances may generate cardiovascular effects through modulation of brain circuitry activity, or alternatively by modulation of myocardial contractile function, coronary blood flow, or both. Typical examples of humoral factors that can fulfill such roles are angiotensin and the mediators of inflammation (discussed in Part IV). Angiotensin II is the active component of the renin–angiotensin system (RAS) and one of the most important humoral factors involved in the regulation of body fluid and cardiovascular homeostasis. Renin, the precursor of angiotensin II is released by the juxtaglomerular kidney cells in response to decreased blood pressure, cardiac output, or total blood volume, and during reduced peripheral resistance, and after norepinephrine secretion by sympathetic nerve fibers. After its production, angiotensin II activates membrane-associated receptors both in the periphery and in the CNS to initiate the physiological responses. All components of the RAS system have been identified in the central nervous system. Centrally mediated cardiovascular actions of the RAS, the receptors and regions involved, and clinical aspects are discussed in **Chapter 11.** The role of the RAS in cardiovascular regulation was recognized several years ago, but only recently has evidence been provided that mediators of inflammation may contribute to the development of neuropsychiatric disease after myocardial infarction.

Mediators of inflammation, such as the proinflammatory cytokines, tumor necrosis factor alpha (TNFα), and interleukin-1 (IL-1), generate a fever response via the central nervous system, and the hypothalamic thermostat cells in particular. However, it is not known how these cytokines penetrate the BBB. Regions lacking a barrier like the hypothalamic lamina terminalis (OVLT), the subfornical organ, and the area postrema all could transmit signals to the hypothalamus about an altered cytokine expression in the blood. Alternatively, it has been demonstrated that vagal afferent fibers can mediate a cytokine response. Both these routes of cytokine signal transduction somehow influence central autonomic processing, either primarily at the level of the hypothalamus, or in the visceral–caudal part of the nucleus of the solitary tract. The visceral sensory area relays the information to regions participating in cardiovascular regulation at all levels of the neuraxis, including the autonomic tone circuitry in the brainstem in a bottom-up fashion. The hypothalamic route of admission represents a top-down effect in these same areas. The admission routes of cytokine signal transduction are not reciprocally exclusive, and most likely act simultaneously to alter metabolic homeostasis during infections. Elevated plasma cytokine levels have been found after myocardial infarction (MI). In animal studies, MI led to selective BBB leakage within the cardiovascular control regions of the forebrain, in particular the anterior cingulate cortex. This selective BBB leakage pattern could be mimicked with intravenous administration of recombinant TNFα, but not with recombinant interleukin-1β. The role of cytokines in cardiovascular regulation and the process of arteriosclerotic plaque formation are presented in **Chapter 12.** The authors hypothesize that cerebralendo-thelial leakage in emotional circuitry, as, for instance, in the cingulate cortex, may underlie the process of development of a neuropsychiatric disease in MI patients. A large group of MI patients suffer depression and anxiety disorders for long periods after their recovery. Moreover, these patients have an increased risk of mortality, as was observed in epidemiological investigations. Occurrence of mood disorders in heart disease patients is discussed in **Chapter 13.** This chapter illustrates once more that the heart and brain are indeed tightly connected. Brain circuitry dysfunction not only is a cause of heart disease, as was demonstrated in **Chapters 4** and **5,** but reciprocally, heart disease also affects brain circuitry function and may lead (eventually) to the occurrence of comorbid neuropsychiatric symptoms.

Gert J. Ter Horst, PhD

Contents

Contributors

ROBERT H. ANDERSON • *Department of Paediatrics, The National Heart and Lung Institute, Imperial College of Science, Technology, and Medicine, London, UK*

RICHARD BANDLER • *Department of Anatomy and Histology, University of Sydney, Sydney, Australia*

BÉLA BOHUS • *Department of Animal Physiology, University of Groningen, Haren, The Netherlands*

RUUD M. BUIJS • *Nederlands Instituut voor Hersenonderzoek, Amsterdam, The Netherlands*

DAVID F. CECHETTO • *Department of Anatomy and Cell Biology, University of Western Ontario, London, Ontario, Canada*

COLIN I. CLEMENT • *Department of Anatomy and Histology, University of Sydney, Sydney, Australia*

SIMON J. CRICK • *The National Heart and Lung Institute, Imperial College of Science, Technology, and Medicine, London, UK*

JAIPEI DAI • *Nederlands Instituut voor Hersenonderzoek, Amsterdam, The Netherlands*

MIKE J. L. DEJONGSTE • *Department of Cardiology, University and Academic Hospital Groningen, Groningen, The Netherlands*

HANS A. DEN BOER • *Department of Biological Psychiatry, University and Academic Hospital Groningen, Groningen, The Netherlands*

BJÖRN E. ERIKSSON • *Department of Cardiology, Karolinska Institute, Huddinge Hospital, Huddinge, Sweden*

ROBERT D. FOREMAN • *Department of Physiology, University of Oklahoma Health Sciences Center, Oklahoma City, OK*

HANNELE HAVANKA • *Department of Neurology, University of Oulu, Oulu, Finland*

MICHAEL L. H. J. HERMES • *Nederlands Instituut voor Hersenonderzoek, Amsterdam, The Netherlands*

ANDRIES KALSBEEK • *Nederlands Instituut voor Hersenonderzoek, Amsterdam, The Netherlands*

KEVIN A. KEAY • *Department of Anatomy and Histology, University of Sydney, Sydney, Australia*

JUHA T. KORPELAINEN • *Department of Neurology, University of Oulu, Oulu, Finland*

S. MICHIEL KORTE • *Department of Animal Physiology, University of Groningen, Haren, The Netherlands*

VILHO V. MYLLYLÄ • *Department of Neurology, University of Oulu, Oulu, Finland*

LAWRENCE P. REAGAN • *Laboratory of Neuroendocrinology, The Rockefeller University, New York, NY*

STUART D. ROSEN • *Medical Research Council Unit, Imperial College School of Medicine, Hammersmith Hospital, London, UK*

ANNE SAARI • *Department of Neurology, University of Oulu, Oulu, Finland*

FRANK SCHEER • *Nederlands Instituut voor Hersenonderzoek, Amsterdam, The Netherlands*

MARY N. SHEPPARD • *The National Heart and Lung Institute, Imperial College of Science, Technology, and Medicine, London, UK*

CHRISTER SYLVÉN • *Department of Cardiology, Karolinska Institute, Huddinge Hospital, Huddinge, Sweden*

GERT J. TER HORST • *Department of Psychiatry, University of Groningen, Groningen, The Netherlands*

UOLEVI TOLONEN • *Department of Neurology, University of Oulu, Oulu, Finland*

DORIEN M. TULNER • *Department of Biological Psychiatry, University and Academic Hospital Groningen, Groningen, The Netherlands*

PART I

Autonomic Control

CHAPTER 1

Neural Supply of the Heart

Simon J. Crick, Mary N. Sheppard
and Robert H. Anderson

1. Introduction: Cardiac Innervation

The heart receives an extrinsic efferent (sympathetic and parasympathetic) and afferent innervation, as well as possessing an intrinsic (intracardiac) nerve supply. This intrinsic nervous system interacts with efferent nerve fibers in a complex fashion to help maintain adequate cardiac output. Intrinsic neurones also receive afferent inputs from mechano-sensory and chemosensory nerve endings located in cardiovascular and pulmonary tissues, together with afferent fibers from centrally located neurones. The importance of the intrinsic nervous system is often overlooked. It is now thought that this system may even function as a "mini-brain" within the heart, where incoming neural information is processed and integrated, with the final outcome being an effective "fine-tuning" of cardiac dynamics. A description of all aspects of cardiac neuroanatomy will be reviewed, based on an account of the individual neural components, and their interaction with each other. Noradrenaline (NA) and acetylcholine (ACh) are the predominant "classical" transmitters utilized by the mammalian heart. Nevertheless, many other types of neurotransmitter or neuromodulator have been localized to cardiac nerves, many of which, but not all, have

From: *The Nervous System and the Heart*
Ed: G. J. Ter Horst © Humana Press Inc.

been found to coexist with either NA or ACh in the same nerve fibers. This review will characterize the plenitude of neurotransmitters and neuromodulators to be found in the mammalian heart, together with a brief account of their putative effects on cardiac dynamics. Finally, we will discuss the denervated cardiac transplant and its prospects for reinnervation.

2. Anatomy of Cardiac Innervation

From a neuroanatomical standpoint, the heart is a complex organ. Despite the fact that it is composed of predominantly muscular and fibrous tissue, a significant proportion of the heart (up to 30% of the volume of some cardiac tissues) contains neural tissue (1,2). This is no more than expected, considering that cardiac functional dynamics must be controlled in a rapid and effective manner in order to serve the circulatory requirements of the body. This can only be achieved by the integrated action of the autonomic nervous system. The heart receives an extrinsic nerve supply, originating from extracardiac ganglia with axonal inputs from central neurones. It also possesses an intrinsic nervous system, originating from intrinsic cardiac ganglia. The parasympathetic efferent preganglionic neurones are located in the medulla and project axons to the heart via the pneumogastric (vagus) nerves. Sympathetic efferent neurones are localized in paravertebral ganglia, such as the stellate, and project axons via mediastinal nerves to the heart. Central cardiac control is now thought to occur by the action of longitudinally arranged parallel pathways involving the forebrain, brain stem, and spinal cord (3–6). The extrinsic innervation, traveling in the cardiac branches of the vagal and sympathetic trunks, enters the base of the heart to form a complex interconnecting network of mixed nerves called the cardiac plexus. A proportion of the fibers within the cardiac plexus then interacts with neurones of the intrinsic nervous system, an interplay that can sometimes be neglected (7–9). Other nerve fibers of the cardiac plexus, mainly efferent postganglionic sympathetic and parasympathetic fibers, bypass the intracardiac ganglia and travel to innervate various cardiac tissues directly. Postganglionic nerve fibers are capable of simultaneously innervating several types of cardiac tissue and/or a number of anatomically diverse cardiac regions. For example, branches of the same efferent postganglionic nerve can innervate both the endocardium and the adjacent myocardium. This type of branching nerve fiber possesses numerous varicosities. It is these terminal swellings that, in effect, represent the neuroeffector junction of the majority of cardiac nerve fibers. They are structurally different than the fixed neuromuscular junctions, or synapses, observed in skeletal muscle. The extensive branching of nerve fibers means that terminal varicosities are at variable distances from the cells they innervate, such as bundles of cardiac myocytes, which are electrically coupled with each other and have a diffuse distribution of receptors (10). The heart also possesses afferent connections, which arise from sensory endings localized throughout the atria, ventricles, and great vessels. The cardiopulmonary region possesses such numerous sensory "receptors," strictly sensory nerve terminals, from which afferent nerve fibers travel to the central nervous system either in the vagus or in sympathetic nerves to their cell bodies in either the spinal cord or brainstem. The overall arrangement of the neural connections to and within the heart is illustrated in Fig. 1.

2.1. Efferent (Extrinsic) Innervation

Efferent sympathetic nerve fibers, which are primarily noradrenergic, originate from the cell bodies of the paravertebral chain. These come from the superior, middle, and inferior cervical ganglions of the sympathetic trunk, together with the upper five ganglions of the thoracic segment of the trunk, but chiefly from the stellate ganglion. They represent postganglionic fibers within the cardiac plexus (11,12). The number and location of sympathetic neurones in these extrinsic ganglia exhibit significant variation within mammalian species (11). These efferent postganglionic sympa-

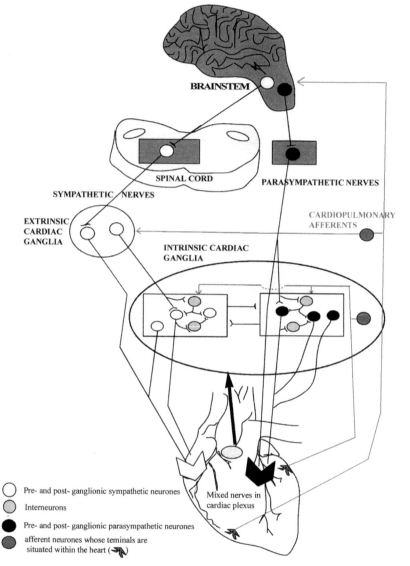

Fig. 1. Schematic diagram illustrating the possible neural interactions between extrinsic and intrinsic cardiac innervation. Within the intrinsic cardiac ganglia, note that some sympathetic and parasympathetic efferent projections are depicted as fibres of passage, whereas others terminate on cell bodies. The extrinsic ganglia consist of the stellate ganglion, the middle cervical ganglion, and the mediastinal ganglion. Two separate afferent populations are represented: one whose cell bodies are located extrinsically and a second population whose cell bodies are situated within the intrinsic ganglionated plexus.

thetic neurones, which may be located in any of the extracardiac ganglionic sites, project axons that extensively and concurrently innervate a number of different cardiac tissues *(13)*. Some even project axons in two or more cardiopulmonary nerves, thus permitting interactive integration between the cell bodies of adjacent efferent sympathetic neurones innervating different cardiac tissues *(14)*. Neurones displaying sympathetic activity have now been demonstrated also in intrinsic cardiac ganglia, structures thought previously to be exclusively parasympathetic in origin *(15–18)*. This finding is further supported by the localization of catecholaminergic intrinsic neurones in the mammalian heart (Fig. 2) *(2,19–21)*. Efferent parasympathetic nerve fibers (primarily cholinergic) reach the cardiac plexus through the large vagal nerves, which carry preganglionic fibers from their cell bodies in either the dorsal motor nucleus or the nucleus ambiguus of the medulla oblongata. Afferent sensory nerves also run to these nuclear regions from the heart *(22,23)*. Parasympathetic efferent neurons are located bilaterally in the medulla and, therefore, their axons innervate extensive regions of both the atrial and ventricular ganglionated plexuses in the majority of mammalian hearts *(17)*. The mixed nerves of the cardiac plexus, therefore, contain preganglionic and post-ganglionic parasympathetic and postganglionic sympathetic efferent fibers, as well as afferent fibers from cardiopulmonary receptors *(24,25)*.

2.2. Intrinsic (Intracardiac) Innervation

Efferent fibers of the cardiac plexus synapse with neuronal cell bodies of intracardiac ganglia. These collections of cell bodies are generally located on the epicardial surface, but can also be found within the myocardium and the nodal tissues of the conduction system. The number and distribution of intrinsic neurones varies among species *(2,26–29)*. Generally, their location is an indicator that their target is close by. For example, in the canine heart, neurones of the right atrial ganglionated plexus have been shown to control the sinus node *(30)*, whereas those adjacent to the inferior

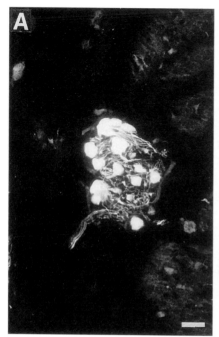
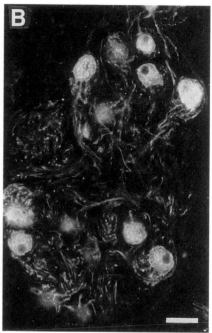

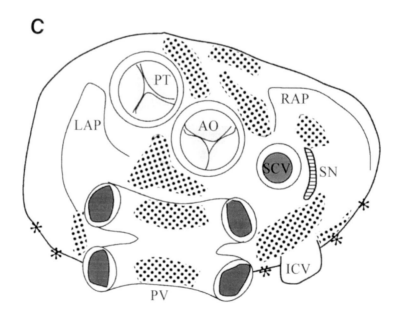

caval vein primarily modulate inferior atrial and atrioventricular nodal tissues *(31)*. Despite the fact that numerous investigators have studied the anatomy and electrophysiological properties of intracardiac neurones, little is known about the their overall contribution, in terms of the proportion of intrinsic nerve fibers, to the overall pattern of cardiac innervation. Temporal studies have been carried out on the extrinsically denervated bovine heart *(32,33)* and in human recipients of cardiac transplantation *(34,35)* that solely examined the occurrence of autonomic reinnervation. To date, there have been no investigations into the quantitative extent (or density) of the intrinsic nervous system within the intact heart. Nevertheless, intracardiac neurones have been cultured and their neurochemical and electrophysiological properties investigated *(36–38)*.

Exquisite microdissections of the intracardiac nervous system of humans have recently been reported *(28,29)*. These permitted the intracardiac ganglionated plexus of the human heart to be localized to approximately five atrial and five ventricular regions (*see* Fig. 2C). The atrial ganglionated plexus are located on the superior surface of the right atrium, the superior surface of the left atrium, the posterior surface of the right atrium, the posterior medial surface of the left atrium (which fuse medially and then extend anteriorly into the interatrial septum), and the inferior and lateral aspects of the posterior left atrium. The ventricular ganglionated plexuses can be found at the base of aorta, at the origins of

---

Fig. 2. Fluorescent photomicrographs showing immunoreactivity for the general neural marker protein gene product 9.5 **(A)** and tyrosine hydroxylase **(B)** in atrial epicardial intracardiac ganglia of humans **(A)** and pig **(B)**. Scale bar = 50 µm. The cell bodies in these ganglia are surrounded by many axodendritic processes. Schematic basal view of the mammalian heart **(C)** showing the locations of these intrinsic ganglia. Numerous populations of ganglion cell bodies are also found in the fatty tissues of the atrioventricular groove surrounding the posterior surface of the heart (*). AO, aorta; PT, pulmonary trunk; RAP, right atrial appendage; LAP, left atrial appendage; SCV, superior caval vein; ICV, inferior caval vein; PV, pulmonary veins.

the right and left coronary arteries (with the ganglia at the left coronary artery extending to the origins of the left anterior descending and circumflex arteries), at the origin of the posterior interventricular artery, adjacent to the origin of the right acute marginal artery, and at the origin of the left obtuse marginal artery. Ganglia have not been observed in either the left or right atrial free wall, in the ascending aorta or pulmonary trunk, nor in the ventricular myocardium of the heart (2,29). In effect, most intrinsic ganglionated plexuses are located on the posterior surfaces of the atria and the superior aspect of the ventricles. Subtle differences, however, exist between the number and location of intrinsic ganglia of the human heart compared to other mammalian hearts, such as that of the dog (27) and pig (2).

2.3. Afferent Innervation

Afferent fibers from mechanosensitive and/or chemosensitive endings respond to a variety of physical and/or chemical changes, respectively, via a number of different cardiac reflexes (39). These sensory endings play an important role in regulating blood pressure, blood volume, and heart rate during adjustments to circulatory demands by utilizing complex cardiac reflex pathways. Sensory nerve endings can be differentiated by their location, their natural stimulus (mechanical or chemical), the type of afferent fibers associated with them (myelinated or nonmyelinated), the morphology of the nerve endings (encapsulated or free), and the nerves that carry the afferent fibers (vagal or sympathetic). They are more commonly localized to the endocardial and epicardial tissues (40,41). Basically, cardiac sensory nerve endings can be functionally divided into two main groups; those with vagal (parasympathetic) projections and those with sympathetic afferents.

Afferent signals from cardiopulmonary "receptors" running with vagal fibers are known to be involved in the reflex control of sympathetic and parasympathetic efferent nerve traffic from the central nervous system. These vagal afferents have been shown to exert a continuous, tonic inhibition of central sympathetic outflow (42). Nevertheless, activation of the sensory endings of vagal afferent fibers results in a reflex stimulation of parasympathetic activity to the heart (43). Afferent input from cardiopulmonary "receptors" running with sympathetic fibers appear not to have any tonic inhibitory or excitatory influence over central sympathetic outflow (44). Nerve endings with vagal afferents are present in most mammals, in the myocardial, endocardial, and epicardial tissues of the majority of cardiac chambers, the lungs, and at the junctions of the great veins with the atria. These fibers ascend in the vagal nerves to the nodose ganglion, where impulses travel to the nucleus of the tractus solitarius. Interneurons then interface with the nucleus ambiguus and vasomotor centers to affect preganglionic efferent vagal and sympathetic nerve traffic descending in the bulbospinal tracts (39,45). Sympathetic afferents exit from most cardiac tissues, but are predominantly located in the myocardial tissues of the ventricles (39). Few morphological and neurochemical studies, however, have been carried out to support this observation. Furthermore, a recent study on the neurochemical localization of arborizations in the human heart found that catecholamine-containing endings are scattered extensively in the atrial chambers (41). Sympathetic afferents convey signals via cardiac nerves to the stellate ganglia of the sympathetic chain, from which impulses traverse the white rami communicans and dorsal root through spinothalamic and spinoreticular tracts in the spinal cord (39,45). Within the brainstem, interneurons interface with the nucleus ambiguus and vasomotor centers to affect efferent vagal and sympathetic nerve traffic (46). Some afferent fibers do not travel to the brainstem but, instead, traverse interneurons to alter efferent sympathetic nerves at the spinal level and even in the stellate ganglia as a cardiocardiac reflex (39). Additionally, there is evidence to suggest that some sensory nerve fibers are entirely intrinsic to the heart, with their neuronal cell bodies situated within intracardiac ganglia (47,48).

Vagal and sympathetic afferent nerve endings can be served by either myelinated or nonmyelinated fibers. This structural difference, however, does not appear to indicate any functional specialization. There is also no apparent correlation between specific morphological differences in nerve endings and their functional role. It has been suggested that different patterns of discharge represent different responses of a single type of nerve ending, which are determined by the stimulus profile as dictated by the anatomical location *(49)*. For example, the discharge patterns of receptors located in different regions of the heart can be "converted" to a different firing rate by a change of stimulus such as stretch, volume changes, or contractility changes *(50)*.

There have been numerous studies describing the morphology of the terminal nervous ramifications within the endocardium of several mammalian species *(51–57)*. Recent studies have also provided information with regard to the specific distribution, morphology, and neurochemistry of these nerve endings *(2,41)*. Two main types of terminal ramification have been observed. Plexus formations cover large areas and can be distinguished from so-called circumscribed end formations arising from single fibers *(56)*. Furthermore, plexus formations exhibit wide variation in morphology dependent on their location in the heart *(2,41)*. Circumscribed nerve endings (Fig. 3) usually arising from thick myelinated fibers *(2,56)*. The bewildering variety of afferent nerve endings in the human heart may be required to monitor the serious demands on the circulatory system caused by the upright stance of humans *(41,58)*. The four-legged stance of mammals, such as the pig *(2)*, does not impose such strong circulatory demands on the heart, and this is reflected in the differences in the distribution and morphology of nerve endings within their hearts compared to that of humans *(2)*.

2.4. Innervation of the Conduction System

Until recently, it was thought that autonomic neural inputs to the conduction system exhibited some degree of "imbalance" *(59)*. This notion is based on selective surgical ablation techniques and/or pharmacological interventions. These studies, thus far, have lacked morphological investi-

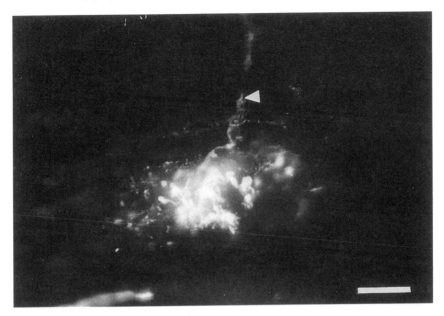

Fig. 3. Fluorescent photomicrographs showing a porcine endocardial circumscribed sensory nerve ending and its afferent nerve fibre (arrowhead) displaying immunoreactivity for tyrosine hydroxylase. Scale bar = 50 μm.

gations of neural distribution to support their findings. Nevertheless, it is known that in the canine heart, the right sympathetic and vagus nerves affect the sinus node more than the atrioventricular node, whereas the left sympathetic and vagus nerves affect the atrioventricular node more than the sinus node (24,59,60). On the right, the vagal input to the superior atrial and sinus nodal regions is by neural projections along the superior caval vein, right atrial junction, azygous vein, right pulmonary vein complex and dorsal surfaces of the common pulmonary venous complex (60). On the left, vagal input to the sinus nodal region is quantitatively less, but the pathways of innervation are similar to those on the right (60). These neural projections have yet to be clearly defined in the human heart. Nevertheless, the topography of cardiac ganglia and some of their neural projections have been described in humans (28,29). The conduction system of the mammalian heart is known to be extremely well inner-

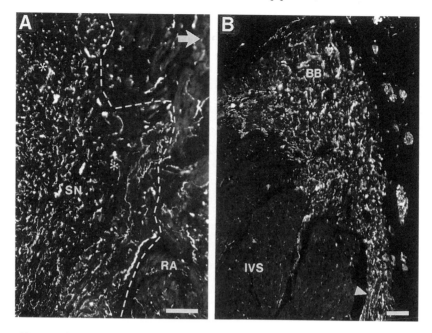

Fig. 4. Fluorescent photomicrographs showing nerve fibres immunoreactive for the general neural marker protein gene product 9.5 in the sinus node of the human heart **(A)** and in the ventricular conduction tissues of the guinea pig heart **(B)**. The border between the sinus node (SN) and the right atrial myocardium (RA) is shown by a dotted line. An arrow indicates the direction of the endocardial surface, and asterisks indicate branches of the sinus nodal artery. BB, branching bundle; IVS, interventricular septum; arrowhead, left bundle branch. Scale bar = 100 μm.

vated *(2,61–64)*. The total pattern of innervation and its component neural subpopulations have been described and quantitated in the human conduction system *(62)*. In humans, a significant regional variation of total innervation, as visualized by immunoreactivity for the general neural marker protein gene product 9.5, was observed throughout the different tissues of the conduction system *(62)*. The sinus node (Fig. 4) and the atrioventricular node were found to possess a much higher density of innervation compared to either the ventricular conduction system or their perinodal myocardium. This is in contrast to the conduction systems of other mammalian species, such as guinea pig (Fig. 4) *(63)*, cow *(64)*, and

Extrinsic sympathetic, parasympathetic and sensory-motor afferent nerve fibers terminate in these intrinsic ganglionated plexuses and influence the activity of intracardiac neurones via several different mechanisms *(80)*. The subsections which follow will describe, in brief, the localization and function of the multitude of neurotransmitters and neuromodulators found in the mammalian heart.

3.1. Classical Neurotransmitters

These are noradrenaline and acetylcholine and are the most abundant transmitters found in the cardiac autonomic nervous system. The predominant neurotransmitter released at cardiac sympathetic nerve terminals is noradrenaline, with important excitatory influences on the modulation of cardiac function, including heart rate and conduction *(81)*, coronary blood flow *(82)*, and the rate and force of contraction *(83)*. These excitatory influences come about through the binding of noradrenaline to a variety of adrenergic receptors that can be broadly classified into α- (α_1 and α_2) and β- (β_1 and β_2) adrenoceptor subtypes *(83–85)*. The normal signal transduction pathways for noradrenaline involve a cascade of events, including high-affinity β-adrenoceptor binding to multiple G-proteins, which then activates adenylyl cyclase to produce cAMP. This, in turn, improves the excitation–contraction coupling mechanisms in cardiac musculature *(83,86)*. Noradrenaline is synthesized from its precursor, L-tyrosine, within the cell body of the sympathetic neurone and is transported along the axon to nerve terminals, where it is stored *(85)*. It is primarily localized to postganglionic sympathetic fibers in the cardiac plexus, although catecholamine-containing intracardiac neuronal cell bodies and afferent nerve endings have been described in the mammalian heart *(2,41,64)*.

The predominant neurotransmitter released at the preganglionic and postganglionic vagal nerve terminals is acetylcholine. Two types of cholinergic receptor have been characterized: nicotinic and muscarinic. The main type of cholinergic receptor on the postganglionic neurone is nicotinic *(24)*. Nicotinic blocking agents such as hexamethonium can, therefore, interrupt transmission from the preganglionic to the postganglionic neurone. The main type of cholinergic receptor on the cardiac effector cell is muscarinic *(87)*. The gene families encoding the muscarinic and nicotinic receptor subtypes have now been cloned and manipulation of the endogenous gene products present in autonomic nerves will help to establish the range of cellular functions modulated by acetylcholine *(88)*. In contrast to noradrenaline, acetylcholine is synthesized mainly in the nerve endings, where it is stored in vesicles near the site of subsequent release *(89)*. The pathway for the synthesis of acetylcholine and its mechanism of release has been well described *(90)*. Following the arrival of an axonal action potential at a terminal varicosity, the subsequent influx of calcium through voltage-gated calcium channels causes the stored vesicular acetylcholine to be released. The released acetylcholine diffuses across the gap to either nicotinic or muscarinic receptors on the innervated target and induces a response. Junctions between autonomic cholinergic nerves and cardiac myocytes are wide and, therefore, lack postjunctional specialization *(91)*. In contrast, the cholinergic synapses of cardiac peripheral ganglia possess a much tighter apposition of presynaptic and postsynaptic elements *(90)*. This is also presumably true of sympathetic nerves. After release by the receptor, acetylcholine is rapidly hydrolyzed by acetylcholinesterase to choline and acetate, with a proportion of the choline generated reabsorbed by the presynaptic choline transporter and reused in acetylcholine synthesis.

3.2. Nonadrenergic Noncholinergic Transmitters

3.2.1. Purinergic Transmitters

Adenosine 5'-triphosphate (ATP) and other purines, such as adenosine, are known to play important roles in the autonomic neural control of cardiac function. ATP is known to be synthesized within many types of cells, including neurones, and it has been localized to nerves of sympathetic, parasympathetic, and sensory origin, where it is utilized as a transmitter *(76,92)*. Other purines, such as adenosine, adenosine 5'-monophosphate (AMP) and adenosine 5'-diphosphate are thought to have a neuromodulatory function in the peripheral autonomic nervous system *(92,93)*. ATP is known to be costored and coreleased with noradrenaline from sympathetic nerves in the heart *(94)*. It has also been localized to a subpopulation of intracardiac neurones *(95)* and colocalized to nerves containing acetylcholine or neuropeptides *(76,79)*. Enzymatic extracellular degradation of ATP results in the formation of ADP, AMP, and adenosine, the latter having potent local activity in the heart *(93,96)*. Both ATP and adenosine exert direct actions on the heart, which are mediated by the activation of different receptor subtypes *(93)*. Briefly, specific purinergic receptors have been divided into P_1- and P_2-purinoceptors, the former being more sensitive to adenosine and the latter to ATP. Two subtypes of the P_1-purinoceptor (A_1 and A_2) and P_2-purinoceptor (P_{2y} and P_{2x}) have been characterized *(92,96–98)*.

Adenosine 5'-triphosphate and adenosine exert a variety of actions on the heart that are beyond the scope of this review. Excellent accounts of these and other aspects of purinergic signal transduction mechanisms are given by Olsson and Pearson *(99)*, Rubino et al. *(96)*, and Pelleg et al. *(93)*. Adenosine is known to modulate release of transmitters from efferent nerve terminals of the heart, including noradrenaline *(100–102)* and nonadrenergic noncholinergic transmitters *(103,104)*, both via activation of the A_1 subtype of the P_1-purinoceptor. Interestingly, adenosine has also been shown to suppress release of acetylcholine in the guinea pig right atrium *(105)* and to attenuate the bradycardic response resulting from vagal stimulation in the rat heart *(106)*. Both ATP and adenosine cause negative inotropic and dromotropic effects on the sinus and atrioventricular nodes *(107)*. Despite this, ATP is known to trigger a cardio-cardiac depressor reflex by stimulating P_{2x}-purinoceptors on vagal afferent fibers, which, in turn, mediates its electrophysiological actions *(93)*. Only a small proportion of its effects are the result of its ectoenzyme hydrolysis to adenosine *(96)*. The relative abundance of the P_2-purinoceptor subtypes in cardiac effector tissues appears to be responsible for the actions of ATP. For example, in the atrial myocardium, ATP mimics the negative inotropic effect of adenosine via activation of P_1-purinoceptors *(108)*. Inactivation of G_i-proteins by pertussis, however, has revealed a positive inotropic effect of ATP, resulting from activation of P_2-purinoceptors *(109)*. It may follow, therefore, that the relative density or affinity of the P_2-purinoceptor subtypes seems to affect the inotropy of ATP in cardiac effector tissue *(96)*. The positive inotropic effect is synergistic with the stimulatory action of noradrenaline and contrasts with the apparent "vagal" action of adenosine. In addition, ATP can influence the activity of intracardiac neurones *(95,110)*, and when topically administered at certain epicardial sites, it can stimulate afferent sensory vagal C fibers *(111)*. Both adenosine and ATP play an important role in the extracardiac function of the autonomic nervous system. Adenosine is present in the central nervous system under physiological and pathological conditions. Here, it is considered to have a cytoprotective role because of its ability to suppress neurotransmission and enhance blood flow. The activation of adenosine receptors in specific brain regions results in the regulation of blood pressure and heart rate *(93)*, and microinjections of adenosine into the nucleus of the tractus solitarius of the rat produces dose-dependent reductions in these parameters *(112,113)*. Adenosine affects the activity of the carotid body, causing a stimulation of respiration concomitant with a decreased arterial blood pressure and heart rate *(114)*. Administration of adenosine into the human coronary arterial system evokes an increase in systemic blood pressure. This response is abolished in the denervated heart, indicating the involvement of an autonomic neural reflex mechanism *(115)*. ATP also plays an important role in the function of the autonomic nervous system, because it is a cotransmitter in sympathetic nerves, and extracellular ATP modulates the function of parasympathetic ganglia. There is also evidence in several species to indicate that P_{2x}-purinoceptors are capable of the mediation of the extracellular effects of ATP on the function of central and peripheral nerves in several species *(116–119).* Extracellular ATP is capable of activating sensory neurons and has been found to modulate the efferent function of capsaicin-sensitive neurones in isolated guinea pig preparations *(120).*

Large amounts of ATP are known to be released during hypoxic conditions, such as myocardial ischemia *(121).* It is tempting to speculate that ATP could be involved in the transmission of cardiac pain during episodes of myocardial ischemia. Furthermore, ATP can also trigger a cardio-cardiac depressor reflex by stimulating vagal afferent terminals and, therefore, could play a role in the onset of certain brady-arrhythmias. Central reflex mechanisms may also be involved here, as there is evidence that extracellular ATP can generate synaptic currents in specific regions of the brain associated with cardiac function *(116).* There is clinical evidence for this, because in patients predisposed for angina pectoris, neurostimulation therapy produces changes in myocardial blood flow *(122).* Nevertheless, the mechanism of action of neurostimulation therapy is unclear, and the safety of this treatment remains to be established. Further investigation is needed to establish its role in the transmission and perception of ischemic cardiac pain.

3.2.2. Cardiac Neuropeptides

Immunohistochemical techniques allow precise and accurate identification of the peptidergic neurotransmitters in cardiac nerves supplying the heart. Ultrastructural studies have provided strong evidence that, similar to the model put forward by Burnstock *(123),* terminal varicosities rather than synaptic contacts constitute the postganglionic nerve endings in the myocardium. These varicosities have been found to possess secretory vesicles of variable sizes. The smaller vesicles store the classical transmitters, whereas peptides were localized to the larger granular vesicles *(124).* Several peptides are colocalized and coreleased, together with noradrenaline and acetylcholine in sympathetic and parasympathetic nerve fibers, respectively. The following subsections describe and characterize the main peptides localized to the mammalian heart.

3.2.3. Neuropeptide Y

Neuropeptide Y (NPY) is found in abundance in the mammalian heart. Studies in animals and humans have described large numbers of NPY-immunoreactive nerves in the sinus and atrioventricular nodes, around coronary vessels, and in myocardial and endocardial tissues (Fig. 7) *(2,34,61–64,67,125–128)*. NPY is an amidated 36 amino acid peptide originally found and extracted from porcine brain *(129)*.

Neuropeptide Y-immunoreactive fibers are known to possess immunoreactivity for the catecholamine-synthesizing enzymes tyrosine and dopamine (β-) hydroxylase, indicating that they are largely derived from sympathetic nerves *(128)*. More conclusive evidence from studies involving ganglionectomy, or chemical sympathectomy, has demonstrated that the majority of NPY-containing nerves are of a postganglionic sympathetic origin *(130)*. Furthermore, a small number of NPY-containing nerves persist in the heart of some species after long-term destruction of sympathetic nerves. These constitute an intrinsic nerve subpopulation *(7,127,131)*. Even though NPY is costored with noradrenaline in sympathetic nerve terminals, its release is considered to be differential, because of contrasting subcellular storage sites *(128,132)*. The physiological role for the coexistence of NPY and noradrenaline remains to be solved, but NPY has been shown to inhibit catecholamine release and control the vasoconstrictor action of noradrenaline *(133)*. NPY produces vasoconstriction of small coronary arteries in most species, including humans *(134,135)*, but it has been reported to have variable effects on heart rate, which appear to be species dependent *(136)*. In the isolated, spontaneously beating guinea pig atrium NPY produces an increase in beating frequency *(135,137,138)*, whereas it decreases the heart rate in isolated rat hearts *(139)*. In contrast, NPY produces a direct negative ionotropic effect and reduces coronary blood flow in the isolated rabbit heart *(140)*. At present, the effect of NPY on the electrophysiology of cells in the conduction tissue of either normal or diseased human hearts remains to be elucidated. Although NPY appears to have little direct effect, it is

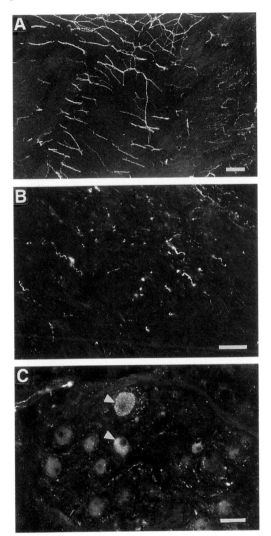

Fig. 7. Photomicrographs showing nerve fibres immunoreactive for neuropeptide Y in the right ventricular endocardium of the pig **(A)** and for vasoactive intestinal polypeptide in the sinus node of humans **(B)**. Immunoreactivity for somatostatin can be seen in a subpopulation of intrinsic neuronal cell bodies (arrowheads) from the right atrium of the pig **(C)**. Scale bar = 50 µm.

a powerful modulator of the actions of other neurotransmitters. Along with noradrenaline, it is released upon stimulation of sympathetic nerves and inhibits the cardiac responses to sympathetic field stimulation *(137)*. Some studies provide evidence to suggest that NPY produces a profound and persistent inhibition of the responses to vagal stimulation in the sinus and atrioventricular nodes *(136,141–143)*. It is important to note that NPY has no effect on the chronotropic responses to exogenously administered noradrenaline or acetylcholine. The effects of NPY, therefore, are the result of the inhibition of neurotransmitter release from sympathetic and vagal nerve endings *(137)*.

In the guinea pig, it has been demonstrated that NPY modulates atrial sensory-motor nerve activity by reducing the release of calcitonin gene-related peptide induced by electrical stimulation of these nerves *(144,145)*. It has also been suggested that NPY may affect the action of some neurotransmitters at the level of autonomic ganglia because it enhances inotropic and chronotropic responses to preganglionic sympathetic stimulation via a nicotinic mechanism *(146)*. The expression of NPY and NPY receptors by intrinsic neurones suggest that it is involved in the neural integration that occurs via nonadrenergic noncholinergic mechanisms in the local cardiac ganglia *(131,147)*. Therefore, NPY may play a vital role as a neuromodulator in the complex interactions between different branches of autonomic and sensory innervation of the heart.

3.2.4. Vasoactive Intestinal Polypeptide

Vasoactive intestinal polypeptide (VIP) is a 28 amino acid peptide thought to be a peptidergic cotransmitter in cholinergic parasympathetic neurones. It was originally isolated from porcine intestine and was later found to be localized mainly to central and peripheral neurons *(148)*. The origin of VIP-containing nerves in the cardiovascular system is unclear, with considerable species variation in the distribution of VIP-immunoreactive nerve fibers. Primarily, however, VIP-immunoreactive nerves are thought to represent postganglionic parasympathetic neurons and have been localized mainly to blood vessels in microvascular beds (Fig. 7) *(149)*. Apart from the presence of VIP-immunoreactive nerves in the perivascular plexus, other VIP-containing nerve fibers have been localized to the sinus and atrioventricular nodes, the atrial epicardium proximal to the sinus node, and to coronary vessels *(62,150,151)*. This species variation is most evident when comparisons are made with the dog. In this model, VIP-containing cardiac ganglion bodies have been demonstrated in the atria, around the large coronary arteries, and at the base of the great vessels *(151)*. The distribution of these cell bodies is similar to that reported for postganglionic cell bodies of the vagal nerve. It has been suggested that these nerves, as in other peripheral organs, are intrinsic in nature *(150,151)*. However, VIP-immunoreactive ganglion cells have been demonstrated in both the vagal nucleus after colchicine treatment *(152)* and in thoracic sympathetic ganglia *(153,154)*, whereas some primary sensory neurons have been shown to be VIP containing *(155,156)*.

In contrast to some of the other peptidergic neurotransmitters, VIP has potent, direct positive chronotropic and inotropic effects on the isolated human heart *(157)*. In the canine heart, it has been reported to be twice as potent as noradrenaline in increasing heart rate *(158)*. VIP may also play a role in the modulation of the activity of acetylcholine *(159,160)* and noradrenaline *(161)*. It is likely that the release of VIP from postganglionic parasympathetic neurons in the heart occurs over a different duration and frequency of stimulation to that of acetylcholine *(158)*. Acetylcholine and VIP appear also to have opposing actions on sinus node automaticity, atrioventricular nodal conduction time, and ventricular refractoriness, but a parallel action on atrial recovery *(160)*. Preliminary reports in isolated guinea pig atria have shown that the positive inotropic effect exhibited by VIP is affected by capsaicin treatment, which suggests that sensory-motor nerves are involved in the inotropic action of this peptide *(96)*.

3.2.5. Somatostatin

Somatostatin is a cyclic peptide of 14 amino acid residues, which was first isolated from ovine hypothalamus *(162)* and, later, it was also found to exist in a 28 amino acid form *(163)*. Somatostatinlike immunoreactivity has been extracted

from human, guinea pig, and rat hearts (164) and localized
to both nerve fibers in the myocardium (34,61), endocardium
(67), and, especially, the conduction system (62). Immunoreactivity for somatostatin has also been localized to atrial intracardiac neurones (Fig. 7) (165). Infusion of somatostatin, at
pharmacological doses, into human and guinea pig hearts
causes bradycardia, a fall in cardiac output (164,166,167), and
a restoration of sinus rhythm in cases of paroxysmal
supraventricular and junctional tachycardia (168,169).
Clinical studies have shown somatostatin to have a role in
depressing atrioventricular nodal conduction during sinus
rhythm and a prolonging of atrioventricular refractoriness
(169). These actions on the sinus and atrioventricular nodes
are in close resemblance to those caused by vagal stimulation, and cardiac nerves containing somatostatin may represent postganglionic parasympathetic neurones (165). This
"cholinergic-like" activity is further supported by its
inhibitory effect on electrical and noradrenaline-induced contractility in the isolated human atrium (157,165,170). It is
thought that somatostatin exerts its cardiopressant effects by
acting on calcium channels excited by β-adrenoceptor activation (167). Furthermore, somatostatin released from intracardiac neurones may have a neuromodulatory action on
cardiac sympathetic neurotransmission by acting at a
postjunctional site (96). There is also evidence that it can induce
the release of acetylcholine from intracardiac parasympathetic neurons in the dog heart (171), which corresponds
with the localization of somatostatin immunoreactivity both
in cell bodies of cardiac ganglia and to nerve fibers surrounding them (2,34,61).

Galanin is a 29-residue neuropeptide been found to be
colocalized with somatostatin in nerve fibers and to intracardiac neurones of the cat heart (172). Little is known about
the direct effects of galanin in the mammalian heart. Nevertheless, in isolated guinea pig atria, it reduces the cardiac
response to transmural electrical stimulation of sensory-motor
nerves without affecting the inotropic action of exogenous
calcitonin gene-related peptide (144). Galanin may, therefore,
act as a neuromodulator in the mammalian heart.

3.3. Substance P, Calcitonin Gene-Related Peptide, and Sensory-Motor Innervation

It is now well established that nonadrenergic noncholinergic neurotransmitters are capable of producing activation of the heart via sensory-motor pathways. Activation of cardiac capsaicin-sensitive sensory-motor fibers induces an increase in the discharge activity of both afferent nerve fibers and centrally mediated reflexes *(173)*. In conjunction with these effects, a peripheral release of the sensory peptides substance P (SP) and calcitonin gene-related peptide (CGRP) is also observed *(174–176)*. The coexistence of SP and CGRP in sensory nerve terminals has been well defined *(177–180)*. At the ultrastructural level, they are both contained in the same granular vesicles within nerve terminals and this provides the basis for their corelease *(181)*. Despite their coexistence, it is now thought that CGRP is the active transmitter of sensory-motor nerves, as SP does not appear to dramatically affect cardiac dynamics. Furthermore, SP and CGRP have no effect on sympathetic neurotransmission *(145)*, but they have been shown to interact with parasympathetic nerves *(147,182)*. The following two subsections will review the localization and actions of these sensory peptides within the heart.

3.3.1. Substance P (SP)

SP is a member of a group of bioactive peptides called tachykinins, which also includes neurokinin A and neurokinin B, and they are characterized by a common c-terminal amino acid sequence *(183–185)*. Studies using the sensory neurotoxin capsaicin demonstrated that SP predominantly occurs in primary sensory neurones and, therefore, it was deemed to be a major sensory neurotransmitter *(150,186–189)*. Nevertheless, it is also contained in sensory fibers resistant to capsaicin *(190,191)*. SP-immunoreactive nerve fibers are predominantly found surrounding large arteries and veins and around smaller vessels supplying many vascular beds both in the myocardium and in the sinus and atrioventricular nodes *(2,62,150,186,192)*. Immunocytochemical studies in

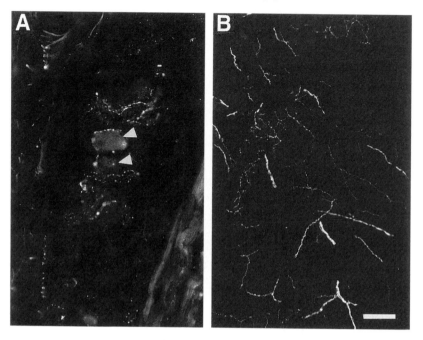

Fig. 8. Fluorescent photomicrographs demonstrating nerve fibres immunoreactive for substance P surrounding unreactive atrial ganglion cell bodies in humans **(A)** and for calcitonin gene-related peptide in the right atrial endocardial plexus of the pig **(B)**. Scale bar = 50 μm.

the guinea pig heart have revealed that, in addition to SP and other tachykinins, capsaicin-sensitive nerves also contain CGRP *(185)*. In the rat heart, however, CGRP and SP occur in a heterogeneous subpopulation of sensory neurones, and variations in capsaicin sensitivity have been demonstrated at different stages of neonatal development *(179,193,194)*. No immunoreactivity for SP has been demonstrated in cardiac ganglion cell bodies, which implies that these nerves are extrinsic in origin (Fig. 8). SP-binding sites, nonetheless, have been described in association with cardiac ganglia *(150,195)*. This, together with the fact that these nerves are partially depleted by bilateral stellatectomy and by capsaicin treatment of the vagus nerve, suggests that they are present in afferent sensory-motor nerves of both spinal and vagal origin *(196)*.

Substance P is a potent vasodilator but in vitro studies have revealed that it has no effect on heart rate *(197–200)*. It does produce a slow depolarizing synaptic action potential in cardiac parasympathetic ganglia in the guinea pig heart and a similar slow potential can be created by nerve stimulation and inhibited by SP antagonists *(182,196,201)*. It has, therefore, been suggested that SP may control parasympathetic activity in the heart, either in an afferent limb of a central reflex or when released from peripheral sensory nerves as part of a sensory-motor reflex *(59)*. SP is involved in the transmission of pain *(202)*; it is also involved in other bioactive properties such as the inducement of protein leakage from blood vessels *(203,204)*. In the rat cardiovascular system, SP and neurokinin A have been found to be associated with the modulation of cardiovascular homeostasis, where they were observed to increase blood pressure and heart rate, resulting in an increase in cardiac output by stimulating sympathetic activity *(205)*.

3.3.2. Calcitonin Gene-Related Peptide (CGRP)

CGRP is a 37-residue peptide produced from the expression of the calcitonin gene upon tissue-specific splicing of primary RNA transcripts *(206)*. Subsequently, two forms of the peptide, CGRPa and CGRPb, have been identified in both the rat *(207)* and in humans *(208)*. CGRP is present in high concentrations in both rat and guinea pig hearts and has been demonstrated in nerves supplying the sinus node, endocardium (Fig. 8), pericardium and coronary vasculature *(63,174,179,209)*. This is only partially representative of the findings in other species and, in contrast, the human heart possesses very few nerve fibers that display immunoreactivity to CGRP *(2,62,210)*.

CGRP is known to be a potent vasodilator, both in vivo and in vitro, of coronary and other peripheral blood vessels in the mammalian heart *(192,211–213)*. It may potentiate the effect of tachykinins, which induce plasma leakage from blood vessels during the inflammatory process, and this could be accentuated by inhibiting the breakdown of SP and attenuating its release (214,215). CGRP has direct inotropic and chronotropic actions on isolated rat and guinea pig hearts, and unlike SP, it is thought to be responsible for a long-lasting nonadrenergic, noncholinergic tachycardia in response to transmural nerve stimulation in the guinea pig heart (174). In the isolated human atrium, CGRP has been shown to elicit a positive inotropic effect (157), and in the isolated blood-perfused canine heart, the application of CGRP resulted in a negative chronotropic response in the atrial tissues (216). This apparent species variation may be a result of differing densities of CGRP-containing nerves (2,124). The injection of CGRP into epicardial regions containing parasympathetic ganglia is reported to attenuate the negative chronotropic action of vagal activity on the sinus node (217). Electrophysiological investigations have revealed that the inotropic and chronotropic effects of CGRP are based on its effects on the Ca^{2+} inward current via L-type calcium channels, the activation of a K^+ current, and its effects on guanidine triphosphate-binding proteins (218,219).

3.3.3. Other Peptides

These include neuropeptides such as opioids, peptide histidine isoleucine (which is colocalized with VIP), and neurotensin. They are all known to play a role, albeit minor, in nonadrenergic noncholinergic neurotransmission in the mammalian heart, however, their respective actions have yet to be clearly defined.

3.4. Other Nonadrenergic Noncholinergic Transmitters

3.4.1. Nitric Oxide and Carbon Monoxide

Nitric oxide is now thought to play a crucial role as a neurotransmitter and neuromodulator, both in the peripheral and central nervous systems. Immunoreactivity for the enzyme responsible for production of nitric oxide, nitric oxide synthase, has been described in a subpopulation of cultured intracardiac neurons isolated from newborn guinea pigs (220) and to intrinsic neuronal cell bodies as well as nerve fibers in guinea pig and rat hearts (221,222). Nitric oxide synthase has also been localized to nerve fibers innervating the wall of coronary arteries (221), and this raises the notion that nitric oxide could be involved in the control of coronary vascular tone (223). Bradycardia and a reduction in cardiac output have been observed when inhibitors to nitric oxide synthesis are administered systemically (224,225). Further investigation is required in order to define the origin of nitric oxide in mammalian cardiac innervation.

There is also increasing evidence to suggest that carbon monoxide, like nitric oxide, may be a neuronal transmitter or modulator. A population of newborn guinea pig intracardiac neurones have been shown to express carbon monoxide by displaying immunoreactivity for the enzyme responsible for its synthesis, namely heme oxygenase-2 (HO-2) (226). Double labeling also demonstrated that a subpopulation of these neurones also displayed nitric oxide synthase activity (226). The ubiquitous distribution of HO-2 in this population of intracardiac neurones, compared with nitric oxide synthase, suggests that carbon monoxide may be fundamental to their function, and this merits further investigation.

3.4.2. 5-Hydroxytryptamine and Histamine

The indoleamine 5-hydroxytryptamine (5-HT) has been detected in the heart of several species, including cat (227) and rat (228). Its actions are complex and species specific (*see* ref. 96 for a review). In general, it exerts positive inotropic and chronotropic effects that result from a direct action on cardiac tissue and/or are mediated by the release of transmitter from cardiac nerves. There is indirect evidence to suggest that 5-HT could activate sensory-motor nerves because the inotropy can be reduced by capsaicin treatment (229). More direct evidence is apparent by the release of CGRP via stimulation of 5-HT_3 receptors in the isolated guinea pig heart (230). Furthermore, the chronotropic response to 5-HT has been considered to be mediated by catecholamine release (231). These findings have lead to the suggestion that activation of both sympathetic and sensory-motor nerves could mediate the actions of 5-HT (96). Finally, 5-HT could be taken up and then released by intracardiac neurones in order to interact with autonomic and sensory nerves of the heart (232).

Histamine (HIST) is stored in mast cells and basophils. Nevertheless, high concentrations are present in sympathetic nerves, and immunoreactive fibers have been demonstrated in the developing rat heart (233,234). HIST produces a positive inotropic response and an increased action potential duration in guinea pig atria (235,236), which suggests that it may be involved in the mediation of sympathetic transmission. The mechanisms of HIST interaction with cardiac autonomic innervation are complex and remain to be elucidated.

4. The Denervated Cardiac Transplant and Prospects for Reinnervation

The question of whether cardiac reinnervation occurs after transplantation remains unresolved. It has been the focus of numerous investigations, most of which present convincing arguments either for or against the regrowth of extrinsic cardiac autonomic innervation. In general, most clinical investigations on this subject provide no morphological data to support their findings. Cardiac transplantation results in complete efferent and afferent denervation of the donor heart by the sectioning of neural axons. Afferent innervation may be considered as partial because a proportion of sensory afferent fibers are known to have their neuronal cell bodies within intrinsic cardiac ganglia (i.e., intracardiac reflexes). There is morphological evidence to suggest that the donor heart remains extrinsically denervated for at least a decade posttransplantation (34,237). Nevertheless, there is increasing functional evidence that reinnervation can occur in cardiac transplants (see ref. 238 for a review).

Evidence for sympathetic reinnervation has been derived from an increase in myocardial catecholamine content after transplantation (239), from an enhanced release of NA following intracoronary injections of tyramine in human patients (240), and from radioiodinated metaiodobenzylguanidine imaging, which demonstrated significant absorbance of this adrenergiclike neurotransmitter (241,242). Heart rate variability has also been used to assess the extent of sympathetic reinnervation to the sinus node in transplant recipients *(243)*. Interesting and somewhat convincing evidence has arisen from patients reporting classic anginal symptoms late after transplantation *(244)*. These symptoms have been attributed to sensory reinnervation, but evidence from induction of cardiac ischemic pain following intracoronary administration of adenosine, and this purine's coexistence with noradrenaline in sympathetic nerves, suggests that sympathetic afferent reinnervation may have occurred *(245)*. Furthermore, when employing metaiodobenzylguanidine imaging for the investigation of sympathetic reinnervation, it is important to be aware of the existence of NPY- and catecholamine-containing intrinsic nerve fibers within the heart. These would remain intact and functional after transplantation and they would be more than capable of metaiodobenzylguanidine uptake. Nevertheless, their does appear to be increasing evidence to suggest that extrinsic postganglionic sympathetic nerves could proceed from major arterial vessels across surgical suture lines and into the donor heart. Evidence for parasympathetic reinnervation has been much less forthcoming. Changes in heart rate variability *(246)*, the presence of a vasovagal response to head-up tilt *(247,248)*, and various cardiac dynamic responses to exercise *(249)*, albeit in a minor proportion of recipients, all support this notion. The problems that neural regrowth would encounter are, nonetheless, huge. The progress of axonal sprouting would be entirely dependent on the fact that it must grow through scar tissue and also accommodate the process of rejection *(238)*. This problem takes on a whole new meaning if reinnervation were to occur following the prospective transplantation of a cardiac xenograft from a transgenic pig donor *(250)*. This is extremely important because differences are known to exist between the innervation of the pig heart to that of the human heart *(2)*.

5. Conclusions and Clinical Implications

This review has provided an account of the neuroanatomy and neurochemistry of the mammalian heart. It has tried to emphasize the importance of the nonadrenergic noncholinergic neurotransmitters and of intrinsic neurones in the effective control of cardiac performance. Intrinsic cardiac ganglia possess a multitude of axodendritic processes and they are capable of exerting control over cardiac dynamics without influences from either preganglionic vagal or postganglionic sympathetic nerve fibers *(8,47,48).* Aberrant autonomic activity in the heart has been implicated in a variety of arrhythmogenic conditions *(251–254),* whereas myocardial ischemia is known to influence intrinsic neuronal function *(255).* It is, therefore, imperative that future work involves the further elucidation of the intracardiac nervous system and its interaction with efferent and/or afferent cardiac innervation.

References

1. Crick, S. J., Sheppard, M. N., Ho, S. Y., and Anderson, R. H. (1997) Anatomy and innervation of the conduction system, in *Recent Advances in Microscopy of Cells, Tissues and Organs* (Motta, P. M., ed.), Antonio Delfino Editore, Rome, pp. 301–309.
2. Crick, S. J. (1997) Innervation of the conduction system and other cardiac tissues in man and animal models, Ph.D. Thesis, University of London.
3. Loewy, A. D. and Spyer, K. M. (1990) *Central Regulations of Autonomic Functions,* Oxford University Press, New York.
4. Jänig, W. and Häbler, H.-J. (1995) Visceral-autonomic integration, in *Visceral Pain, Progress in Pain Research and Management,* vol. 5 (Gebhart, G. F., ed.), IASP, Seattle, WA, pp. 311–348.
5. Gutterman, D. D. (1996) Central integration of autonomic control of the heart including the coronary circulation, in *Nervous System of the Heart* (Shepherd, J. T. and Vatner, S. F., eds.), Harwood Academic, Amsterdam, 1996, pp. 253–294.
6. Ter Horst, G. J., Hautvast, R. W., De Jongste, M. J., and Korf, J. (1996) Neuroanatomy of cardiac activity-regulating circuitry: a transneuronal retrograde viral labelling study in the rat. *Eur. J. Neurosci.* **8(10),** 2029–2041.
7. Hassall, C. J. S., Penketh, R., Rodeck, C., and Burnstock, G. (1990) The intracardiac neurones of the fetal human heart in culture. *Anat. Embryol.* **182,** 329–337.
8. Ardell, J. L. (1994) Structure and function of mammalian cardiac neurons, in *Neurocardiology* (Armour, J. A. and Ardell, J. L., eds.), Oxford University Press, New York, pp. 95–114.

9. Horackova, M. J. and Armour, J. A. (1995) Role of peripheral autonomic neurones in maintaining adequate cardiac function. *Cardiovasc. Res.* **30,** 326–335.

10. Burnstock, G. (1986) Autonomic neuroeffector junctions: current developments and future directions. *J. Anat.* **146,** 1–30.

11. Armour, J. A. and Hopkins, D. A. (1984) Anatomy of the extrinsic efferent autonomic nerves and ganglia innervating the mammalian heart, in *Nervous Control of Cardiovascular Function* (Randall, W. C., ed.), Oxford University Press, New York, pp. 20–45.

12. Janes, R. D., Brandys, J. C., Hopkins, D. A., Johnstone, D. E., Murphy, D. A., and Armour, J. A. (1986) Anatomy of human extrinsic cardiac nerves and ganglia. *Am. J. Cardiol.* **57(4),** 299–309.

13. Randall, W. C. (1994) Changing perspectives concerning neural control of the heart, in *Neurocardiology* (Armour, J. A. and Ardell, J. L., eds.), Oxford University Press, New York, pp. 3–17.

14. Tomney, P. A., Hopkins, D. A., and Armour, J. A. (1985) Axonal branching of canine sympathetic postganglionic cardiopulmonary neurons: a retrograde fluorescent labelling study. *Brain Res. Bull.* **14(5),** 443–452.

15. Gagliardi, M., Randall, W. C., Beiger, D., Wurster, R. D., Hopkins, D. A., and Armour, J. A. (1988) Activity of in vivo canine cardiac plexus neurons. *Am. J. Physiol.* **255** (*Heart Circ. Physiol.* **24**) H789–H800.

16. Armour, J. A. and Hopkins, D. A. (1990) Activity of in vivo canine ventricular neurons. *Am. J. Physiol.* **258,** (*Heart Circ. Physiol.* **27**) H320–H336.

17. Armour, J. A. and Hopkins, D. A. (1990) Activity of in situ canine left atrial neurons. *Am. J. Physiol.* **259,** H1207–H1215.

18. Smith, F. M., Hopkins, D. A., and Armour, J. A. (1992) In vitro electrophysiological properties of intrinsic cardiac neurons in the pig (Sus scrofa). *Brain Res. Bull.* **28,** 715–725.

19. Moravec, M., Moravec, J., and Forsgren, S. (1990) Catecholaminergic and peptidergic nerve components of intramural ganglia in the rat heart. *Cell Tissue Res.* **262,** 315–327.

20. Horackova, M., Huang, M. H., Armour, J. A., Hopkins, D. A., and Mapplebeck, C. (1993) Co-cultures of ventricular myocytes with stellate ganglion and intrinsic cardiac neurons from adult guinea pig: spontaneous activity and pharmacological properties. *Cardiovasc. Res.* **27,** 1101–1108.

21. Crick, S. J., Sheppard, M. N., Anderson, R. H., Polak, J. M., Wharton, J. (1996) A qualitative assessment of innervation in the conduction system of the calf heart. *Anat. Rec.* **245,** 685–698.

22. Hopkins, D. A. and Armour, J. A. (1982) Medullary cells of origin of physiologically identified cardiac nerves in the dog. *Brain Res. Bull.* **8,** 359–365.

23. Hopkins, D. A. and Armour, J. A. (1984) Localisation of sympathetic postganglionic and parasympathetic preganglionic neu-

rons which innervate different regions of the dog heart. *J. Comp. Neurol.* **229,** 186–198.

24. Levy, M. N. and Martin, P. J. (1979) Neural control of the heart, in *Handbook of Physiology: The Cardiovascular System* (Berne, R. M., ed.), American Physiology Society, Bethesda, MD, pp. 581–620.

25. Owman, C. (1988) Autonomic innervation of the cardiovascular system, in *Handbook of Chemical Neuroanatomy: The Peripheral Nervous System,* vol. 6 (Bjorklund, A., Hokfelt, T., and Owman, C., eds.), Elsevier, Amsterdam, pp. 327–339.

26. King, T. S. and Coakley, J. B. (1958) The intrinsic nerve cells of the cardiac atria of mammals and man. *J. Anat.* **92,** 353–379.

27. Yuan, B. X., Ardell, J. L., Hopkins, D. A., Losier, A. M., and Armour, J. A. (1994) Gross and microscopic anatomy of the canine intrinsic cardiac nervous system. *Anat. Rec.* **239(1),** 75–87.

28. Armour, J. A., Murphy, D. A., Yuan, B. X., Macdonald, S., and Hopkins, D. A. (1997) Gross and microscopic anatomy of the human cardiac nervous system. *Anat. Rec.* **247,** 289–298.

29. Singh, S., Johnson, P. I., Lee, R. E., Orfei, E., Lonchyna, V. A., Sullivan, H. J., Montoya, A., Tran, H., Wehrmacher, W. H., and Wurster, R. D. (1996) Topography of cardiac ganglia in the adult human heart. *J. Thorac. Cardiovasc. Surg.* **112,** 943–953.

30. Randall, W. C., Ardell, J. L., Wurster, R. D., and Milosavljevic, M. (1987) Vagal postganglionic innervation of the canine sinoatrial node. *J. Auton. Nerv. Syst.* **20,** 13–23.

31. Randall, W. C., Ardell, J. L., Calderwood, D., Milosavljevic, M., and Goyal, S. C. (1986) Parasympathetic ganglia innervating the canine atrioventricular nodal region. *J. Auton. Nerv. Syst.* **16,** 311–323.

32. Gaer, J. A., Wharton, J., Gordon, L., Swift, R. I., Munsch, C., Inglis, G. C., Polak, J. M., and Taylor, K. M. (1992) Cardiac denervation in the calf using cryoablation: functional evidence and regional tissue catecholamine content. *Eur. J. Cardiothorac. Surg.* **6,** 201–208.

33. Gordon, L., Wharton, J., Gaer, J. A. R., Inglis, G. C., Taylor, K. M., and Polak, J. M. (1993) Quantitative immunohistochemical assessment of bovine myocardial innervation before and after cryosurgical cardiac denervation. *Cardiovasc. Res.* **27,** 318–326.

34. Wharton, J., Polak, J. M., Gordon, L., Banner, N. R., Springall, D. R., Rose, M., Khangani, A., Wallwork, J., and Yacoub, M. M. (1990) Immunohistochemical demonstration of human cardiac innervation before and after transplantation. *Circ. Res.* **66,** 900–912.

35. Arrowood, J. A., Goudreau, E., Minisi, A. J., Davis, A. B., and Mohanty, P. K. (1995) Evidence against reinnervation of cardiac vagal afferents after human orthotopic cardiac transplantation. *Circulation* **92,** 402–408.

36. Hassall, C. J. S. and Burnstock, G. (1986) Intrinsic neurons and associated cells of the guinea pig heart in culture. *Brain Res.* **364,** 102–113.

37. Allen, T. G. and Burnstock, G. (1987) Intracellular studies of the electrophysiological properties of cultured intracardiac neurones of the guinea pig. *J. Physiol.* **388**, 349–366.
38. Hassall, C. J. S., Penketh, R., Rodeck, C., and Burnstock, G. (1990) The intracardiac neurones of the fetal human heart in culture. *Anat. Embryol.* **182**, 329–337.
39. Smith, M. L. and Thames, M. D. (1994) Cardiac receptors: discharge characteristics and reflex effects, in *Neurocardiology* (Armour, J. A. and Ardell, J. L., eds.), Oxford University Press, New York, pp. 19–52.
40. Linden, R. J. (1979) Atrial receptors and heart rate, in *Cardiac Receptors* (Hainsworth, R., Kidd, C., and Linden, R. J., eds.), Cambridge University Press, Cambridge, pp. 165–192.
41. Marron, K., Wharton, J., Sheppard, M. N., Fagan, D., Royston, D., Kuhn, D. M., et al. (1995) Distribution, morphology and neurochemistry of endocardial and epicardial nerve terminal arborizations in the human heart. *Circulation* **92**, 2343–2351.
42. Mancia, G., Donald, D. E., and Shepherd, J. T. (1973) Inhibition od adrenergic outflow to peripheral blood vessels by vagal afferents from the cardiopulmonary region in the dog. *Circ. Res.* **33**, 713–721.
43. Cerati, D. and Schwartz, P. J. (1991) Single cardiac vagal fibre activity, acute myocardial ischaemia and risk for sudden death. *Circ. Res.* **69**, 1389–1401.
44. Thames, M. D., Smith, M. L., Dibner-Dunlap, M. E., and Minisi, A. J. (1996) Reflexes governing autonomic outflow to the heart, in *Nervous Control of the Heart* (Shepherd, J. T. and Vatner, S. F., eds.), Harwood, Amsterdam, pp. 295–327.
45. Kidd, C. (1979) Central neurons activated by cardiac receptors, in *Cardiac Receptors* (Hainsworth, R., Kidd, C., and Linden, R. J., eds.), Cambridge University Press, Cambridge, pp. 377–403.
46. Hopkins, D. A., Gootman, P. M., Gootman, N., Di Russo, S. M., and Zeballos, M. E. (1984) Brainstem cells of origin of the cervical vagus and cardiopulmonary nerves in the neonatal pig (Sus scrofa). *Brain Res. Bull.* **306**, 63–72.
47. Armour, J. A. (1996) Anatomy and function of peripheral autonomic neurons involved in cardiac regulation, in *Nervous Control of the Heart* (Shepherd, J. T. and Vatner, S. F., eds.), Harwood, Amsterdam, pp. 29–47.
48. Randall, W. C., Wurster, R. D., Randall, D. C., and Xi-Moy, S. X. (1996) From cardioaccelerator and inhibitory nerves to a "heart-brain," in *Nervous Control of the Heart* (Shepherd, J. T. and Vatner, S. F., eds.), Harwood, Amsterdam, pp. 173–199.
49. Hainsworth, R. (1991) Reflexes from the heart. *Physiol. Rev.* **71**, 617–658.
50. Kappagoda, C. T., Linden, R. J., and Sivananthan, N. (1977) Atrial receptors in dogs and rabbits. *J. Physiol.* **272**, 799–815.
51. Holmes, R. L. (1957) Structures in the atrial endocardium of the dog which stain with methylene blue, and the effects of unilateral vagotomy. *J. Anat.* **91**, 259–268.

52. Miller, M. R. and Kasahara, M. (1964) Studies on nerve endings in the heart. *Am. J. Anat.* **115,** 217–233.

53. Johnston, B. D. (1968) Nerve endings in the human endocardium. *Am. J. Anat.* **122,** 621–630.

54. Floyd, K., Linden, R. J., and Saunders, D. A. (1972) Presumed atrial receptors in the left atrial appendage of the dog. *J. Physiol.* **227,** 27–28.

55. Tranum-Jensen, J. (1975) The ultrastructure of the sensory end-organs (baroreceptors) in the atrial endocardium of young mini-pigs. *J. Anat.* **119,** 255–275.

56. Tranum-Jensen, J. (1979) Ultrastructural studies on atrial nerve-end formations in mini-pigs, in *Cardiac Receptors* (Hainsworth, R., Kidd, C., and Linden, R. J., eds.), Cambridge University Press, Cambridge, pp. 27–50.

57. Macdonald, A. A., Poot, P., and Wensing, J. G. (1983) Nerve endings in the pulmonary trunk, ductus arteriosus and aorta of intact and decapitated pig fetuses. *Anat. Embryol.* **168,** 395–404.

58. Folkow, B. (1979) Relevance of cardiovascular reflexes, in *Cardiac Receptors* (Hainsworth, R., Kidd, C., and Linden, R. J., eds.), Cambridge University Press, Cambridge, pp. 473–505.

59. Corr, L. (1992) Neuropeptides and the conduction system of the heart. *Int. J. Cardiol.* **35,** 1–12.

60. Zipes, D. P. and Miyazaki, T. (1990) The autonomic nervous system and the heart: basis for understanding interactions and effects on arrhythmia development, in *Cardiac Electrophysiology: From Cell to Bedside* (Zipes, D. P. and Jalife, J., eds.), W. B. Saunders, Philadelphia, pp. 312–329.

61. Gordon, L., Polak, J. M., Moscoso, C. J., Smith, A., Kuhn, D. M., and Wharton, J. (1993) Development of the peptidergic innervation of the human heart. *J. Anat.* **183,** 131–140.

62. Crick, S. J., Wharton, J., Sheppard, M. N., Royston, D., Yacoub, M. H., Anderson, R. H., and Polak, J. M. (1994) Innervation of the human cardiac conduction system: a quantitative immunohistochemical and histochemical study. *Circulation* **89,** 1697–1708.

63. Crick, S. J., Sheppard, M. N., Anderson, R. H., Polak, J. M., and Wharton, J. (1996) A quantitative study of nerve distribution in the conduction system of the guinea pig heart. *J. Anat.* **188,** 403–416.

64. Crick S. J., Sheppard M. N., Anderson R. H., Polak J. M., and Wharton J. (1996) A quantitative assessment of innervation in the conduction system of the calf heart, *Anat. Rec.* **245,** 685–698.

65. Mitrani, R. D. and Zipes, D. P. (1994) Clinical neurocardiology: arrhythmias, in *Neurocardiology* (Armour, J. A. and Ardell, J. L., eds.), Oxford University Press, New York, pp. 365–395.

66. Armour, J. A. (1994) Peripheral autonomic interactions in cardiac regulation, in *Neurocardiology* (Armour, J. A. and Ardell, J. L., eds.), Oxford University Press, New York, pp. 219–244.

67. Marron, K., Wharton, J., Sheppard, M. N., Gulbenkian, S., Royston, D., Yacoub, M. H., et al. (1994) Human endocardial innervation and its relationship to the endothelium: an immunohistochemical, histochemical and quantitative study. *Cardiovasc. Res.* **28,** 1490–1499.

68. Chow, L. T., Chow, S. S., Anderson, R. H., and Gosling, J. A. (1995) The innervation of the human myocardium at birth. *J. Anat.* **187,** 107–114.

69. Dae, M. W., O'Connell, J. W., Botvinick, E. H., Ahearn, T., Yee, E., Huberty, J. P., et al. (1989) Scintigraphic assessment of regional cardiac adrenergic innervation. *Circulation* **79,** 634–644.

70. Dae, M. W., DeMarco, T., Botvinick, E. H., O'Connell, J. W., Heltner, R. S., Huberty, J. P., et al. (1992) Scintigraphic assessment of MIBG uptake in globally denevated human and canine hearts—implications for clinical studies. *J. Nucl. Med.* **33,** 1444–1450.

71. Chilson, D. A., Peigh, P., Mahomed, Y., and Zipes, D. P. (1985) Encircling endocardial incision interrupts efferent vagal-induced prolongation of endocardial and epicardial refractoriness in the dog. *J. Am. Coll. Cardiol.* **5,** 290–296.

72. Takahishi, N., Barber, M. J., and Zipes, D. P. (1985) Efferent vagal innervation of canine ventricle. *Am. J. Physiol.* **248** (*Heart Circ. Physiol.* **17**), H89–H97.

73. Lundberg, J. M. and Hökfelt, T. (1986) Multiple co-existence of peptides and classical transmitters in peripheral autonomic neurones. Functional and pharmacological implications, in *Progress in Brain Research*, vol. 68 (Hökfelt, T., Fuxe, K., and Pernow, B., eds.), Elsevier Science Publishers, New York, pp. 241–262.

74. Burnstock, G. (1986) The changing face of autonomic neurotransmission. *Acad. Physiol. Scand.* **126,** 67–91.

75. Burnstock, G. (1976) Do some nerve cells release more than one transmitter? *Neuroscience* **1,** 239–248.

76. Burnstock, G. (1990) Co-transmission. *Arch. Int. Pharmacodyn. Ther.* **304,** 7–33.

77. Burnstock, G. (1985) Nervous control of smooth muscle by transmitters, cotransmitters and modulators. *Experientia* **41,** 869–874.

78. Wetzel, G. T., Goldstein, D., and Heller Brown, J. (1985) Acetylcholine release from rat atria can be regulated through an alpha$_1$-adrenergic receptor. *Circ. Res.* **56,** 763–766.

79. Morris, J. L. and Gibbins, I. L. (1992) Co-transmission and neuromodulation, in *Autonomic Neuroeffector Mechanisms* (Burnstock, G. and Hoyle, C. H. V., eds.), Harwood, Chur, Switzerland, pp. 33–119.

80. Allen, T. G. J., Hassall, C. J. S., and Burnstock G. (1994) Mammalian intrinsic cardiac neurons in cell culture, in *Neurocardiology* (Armour, J. A. and Ardell, J. L., eds.), Oxford University Press, New York, pp. 115–138.

81. Levy, M. N. and Martin, P. J. (1996) Autonomic control of cardiac conduction and automaticity, in *Nervous Control of the Heart*

(Shepherd, J. T. and Vatner, S. F., eds.), Harwood, Amsterdam, pp. 201–225.

82. Feigl, E. O. (1996) Autonomic control of coronary blood flow, in *Nervous Control of the Heart* (Shepherd, J. T. and Vatner, S. F., eds.), Harwood, Amsterdam, pp. 227–252.

83. Vatner, S. F. (1996) Autonomic control of the myocardium: β-adrenoceptor mechanisms, in *Nervous Control of the Heart* (Shepherd, J. T. and Vatner, S. F., eds.), Harwood, Amsterdam, pp. 79–110.

84. Hwa, J., De Young, M. B., Perez, D. M., and Graham, R. M. (1996) Autonomic control of the myocardium: α-adrenoceptor mechanisms, in *Nervous Control of the Heart* (Shepherd, J. T. and Vatner, S. F., eds.), Harwood, Amsterdam, pp. 49–77.

85. Fillenz, M. (1992) Transmission: noradrenaline, in *Autonomic Neuroeffector Mechanisms* (Burnstock, G. and Hoyle, C. H. V., eds.), Harwood, Chur, Switzerland, pp. 323–365.

86. Lindemann, J. P. and Watanabe, A. M. (1990) Sympathetic control of cardiac electrical acitvity, in *Cardiac Electrophysiology: From Cell to Bedside* (Zipes, D. P. and Jalife, J., eds.), W. B. Saunders, Philadelphia, pp. 277–283.

87. Hartzell, H. C. (1988) Regulation of cardiac ion channels by catecholamines, acetylchjoline and second messenger systems. *Prog. Biophys. Mol. Biol.* **52,** 165–247.

88. Roeske, W. R. and Yamamura, H. I. (1996) Autonomic control of the myocardium: muscarinic cholinergic receptor mechanisms, in *Nervous Control of the Heart* (Shepherd, J. T. and Vatner, S. F., eds.), Harwood, Amsterdam, pp. 111–137.

89. Loffelholz, K. and Papano, A. J. (1985) The parasympathetic neuroeffector junction of the heart, *Pharmacol. Rev.* **37,** 1–24.

90. Buckley, N. J. and Caulfield, M. (1992) Transmission: acetylcholine, in *Autonomic Neuroeffector Mechanisms* (Burnstock, G. and Hoyle, C. H. V., eds.), Harwood Academic Publishers, Chur, Switzerland, pp. 257–322.

91. Kilbinger, H. (1988) The autonomic cholinergic neuroeffector junction, in *Handbook of Experimental Pharmacology*, vol. 86 (Whittaker, V. P., ed.), Springer-Verlag, Berlin, pp. 581–595.

92. Hoyle, C. H. V. (1992) Transmission: purines, in *Autonomic Neuroeffector Mechanisms* (Burnstock, G. and Hoyle, C. H. V., eds.), Harwood, Chur, Switzerland, pp. 367–407.

93. Pelleg, A., Katchanov, G., and Xu, J. (1997) Autonomic neural control of cardiac function: modulation by adenosine and adenosine 5'-triphosphate. *Am. J. Cardiol.* **79(12A),** 11–14.

94. Burnstock, G. (19900 Noradrenaline and ATP as cotransmitters in sympathetic nerves. *Neurochem. Int.* **17,** 357–368.

95. Allen, T. G. J. and Burnstock, G. (1990) The actions of adenosine 5'-triphosphate on guinea pig intracardiac neurons in culture. *Br. J. Pharmacol.* **100,** 269–276.

96. Rubino, A., Hassall, C. J. S., and Burnstock, G. (1996) Autonomic control of the myocardium: non-adrenergic non-cholinergic (NANC) mechanisms, in *Nervous Control of the Heart* (Shepherd, J. T. and Vatner, S. F., eds.), Harwood2, Amsterdam, pp. 139–171.

97. Burnstock, G. and Buckley, N. J. (1985) The classification of receptors for adenine nucleotides, in *Methods Used in Adenosine Research* (Paton, D. M., ed.), Plenum, New York, pp. 193–212.

98. Burnstock, G. and Kennedy, C. (1985) Is there a basis for distinguishing more than one type of P_2-purinoceptor. *Gen. Pharmacol.* **16,** 433–440.

99. Olsson, R. A. and Pearson, J. D. (1990) Cardiovascular purinoceptors. *Physiol. Rev.* **70,** 761–845.

100. Hedquist, B. P. and Fredholm, B. B. (1979) Inhibitory effect of adenosine on adrenergic neuroeffector transmission in the rabbit heart. *Acta Physiol. Scand.* **105,** 120–122.

101. Wennmalm, M., Fredholmn, B. B., and Hedquist, P. (1988) Adenosine as a modulator of sympathetic nerve-stimulation-induced release of noradrenaline from the isolated rabbit heart. *Acta Physiol. Scand.* **132,** 487–494.

102. Richardt, G., Waas, W., Kranzhofer, R., Cheng, B., Lohse, M. J., and Schomig, A. (1989) Interaction between the release of adenosine and noradrenaline during sympathetic stimulation: a feedback mechanism in the rat heart. *J. Mol. Cell. Cardiol.* **21,** 269–277.

103. Robino, A., Mantelli, L., Amerini, S., and Ledda, F. (1990) Adenosine modulation of non-adrenergic non-cholinergic neurotransmission in isolated guinea pig atria. *Naunyn Schmiedebergs Arch. Pharmacol.* **342,** 520–522.

104. Robino, A., Mantelli, L., Amerini, S., and Ledda, F. (1991) Adenosine receptors involved in the inhibitory control of non-adrenergic non-cholinergic neurotransmission in guinea pig atria belong to the A_1 subtype. *Naunyn Schmiedebergs Arch. Pharmacol.* **344,** 464–470.

105. Nakatsuka, H., Nagano, O., Foldes, F. F., Nagashima, H., and Vizi, E. S. (1995) Effects of adenosine on norepinephrine and acetylcholine release from guinea pig right atrium: role of A_1-receptors. *Neurochem. Int.* **27,** 345–353.

106. Monteiro, E. C. and Ribeiro, J. A. (1991) Adenosine and the bradycardiac response to vagus nerve stimulation in rats. *Eur. J. Pharmacol.* **204,** 193–202.

107. Pelleg, A. (1987) Cardiac electrophysiology and pharmacology of adenosine and ATP: modulation by the autonomic nervous system. *J. Clin. Pharmacol.* **27,** 366–372.

108. Collis, M. G. and Pettinger, S. J. (1982) Can ATP stimulate P1-receptors in guinea pig atrium without conversion to adenosine? *Eur. J. Pharmacol.* **81,** 521–529.

109. Mantelli, L., Amerini, S., Filippi, S., and Ledda, F. (1993) Blockade of adenosine receptors unmasks a stimulating effect of ATP on cardiac contractility. *Br. J. Pharmacol.* **109,** 1268–1271.

110. Fieber, L. A. and Adams, D. J. (1991) Adenosine triphosphate-evoked currents in cultured neurons dissociated from rat parasympathetic cardiac ganglia. *J. Physiol.* **434,** 239–256.

111. Armour, J. A., Huang, M. H., Pelleg, A., and Sylven C. (1994) Responsiveness of in situ canine nodose ganglion afferent neurons to epicardial mechanical or chemical stimuli. *Cardiovasc. Res.* **28,** 1218–1225.

112. Barraco, R. A., Januz, C. J., Polasck, P. M., Parizon, M., and Roberts, P. A. (1988) Cardiovascular effects of microinjection of adenosine into the nucleus tractus solitarius. *Brain Res. Bull.* **20,** 129–132.

113. Tao, S. and Abdel-Rahman, A. A. (1993) Neuronal and cardiovascular responses to adenosine microinjection into the nucleus tractus solitarius. *Brain Res. Bull.* **32,** 407–417.

114. Monteiro, E. C. and Ribeiro, J. A. (1987) Ventilatory effects of adenosine mediated by carotid body chemoreceptors in the rat. *Naunyn Schmiedebergs Arch. Pharmacol.* **335,** 143–148.

115. Cox, D. A., Vita, J. A., Treasure, C. B., Fish, R. D., Selwyn, A. P., and Ganz, P. (1989) Reflex increase in blood pressure during intracoronary administration of adenosine in man. *J. Clin. Invest.* **84,** 592–596.

116. Edwards, F. A., Gibb, A. J., and Colquhoun, D. (1992) ATP receptor-mediated synaptic currents in the central nervous system. *Nature* **359,** 144–147.

117. Tresize, D. J., Kennedy, I, and Humphrey, P. P. A. (1993) Characterisation of purinoceptors mediating depolarization of rat isolated vagus nerve. *Br. J. Pharmacol.* **110,** 1055–1060.

118. Khakh, B., Humphrey, P. A. A., and Surprenant, A. (1995) Electrophysiological properties of P2x-purinoceptors in rat superior cervical, nodose and guinea pig coeliac neurones. *J. Physiol.* **484,** 385–395.

119. Pelleg, A. and Hurt, C. M. (1996) Mechanism of ATP's action on canine pulmonary vagal fibre nerve terminals. *J. Physiol.* **490,** 265–275.

120. Rubino, A., Amerinin, S., Ledda, F., and Mantelli, L. (1992) ATP modulates the efferent function of capsaicin-sensitive neurons in guinea pig isolated atria. *Br. J. Pharmacol.* **105,** 516–520.

121. Forrester, T. and Williams, C. A. (1976) Release of adenosine triphosphate from isolated adult heart cells in response to hypoxia. *J. Physiol.* **268,** 371–390.

122. Hautvast, R. W., De Jongste, M. J., Ter Horst, G. J., Blanksma, P. K., and Lie, K. I. (1996) Angina pectoris refractory for conventional therapy—is neurostimulation a possible alternative treatment? *Clin. Cardiol.* **19(7),** 531–535.

123. Burnstock G., Purinergic nerves, *Pharmacol Rev,* **24** (1972) 509–581.

124. Wharton, J., Polak, J. M., McGregor, G. P., Bishop, A. E., and Bloom, S. R. (1981) The distribution of substance P-like immunoreactive nerves in the guinea pig heart. *Neuroscience* **6,** 2193–2204.

125. Gu, J., Polak, J. M., Allen, J. M., Huang, W. M., Sheppard, M. N., Tatemoto, K., et al. (1984) High concentrations of a novel peptide, neuropeptide Y, in the innervation of the mouse and rat heart. *J. Histochem. Cytochem.* **32,** 467–472.
126. Sternini, C. and Brecha, N. (1985) Distribution and co-localisation of neuropeptide Y- and tyrosine hydroxylase-like immunoreactive nerves in the guinea pig heart. *Cell Tissue Res.* **241,** 93–102.
127. Corr, L. A., Aberdeen, J. A., Milner, P., Lincoln J., and Burnstock, G. (1990) Sympathetic and non-sympathetic neuropeptide Y (NPY)-containing nerves in the rat myocardium and coronary arteries. *Circ. Res.* **66,** 1602–1609.
128. Forsgren, S. (1989) Neuropeptide Y-like immunoreactivity in relation to the distribution of sympathetic nerve fibres in the heart conduction system. *J. Mol. Cell. Cardiol.* **21,** 279–290.
129. Tatemoto, K., Carlquist, M., and Mutt, V. (1982) Neuropeptide Y—a novel brain peptide with structural similarities to peptide YY and pancreatic polypeptide. *Nature* **296,** 659–660.
130. Wharton, J. and Gulbenkian, S. (1987) Peptides in the mammalian cardiovascular system. *Experientia* **43,** 821–832.
131. Hassall, C. J. S. and Burnstock, G. (1984) Neuroeptide Y-like immunoreactivity in cultured intrinsic neurones of the heart. *Neurosci. Lett.* **52,** 111–115.
132. Lundberg, J. M., Rudehill, A., Solleau, A., Theodorsson-Norheim, A., and Hamberger, B. (1986) Frequency- and reserpine-dependent chemical coding of sympathetic transmission: differential release of noradrenaline and neuropeptide Y from pig spleen. *Neurosci. Lett.* **63,** 96–100.
133. Millar, B. C., Piper, H. M., and McDermott, B. J. (1988) The antiadrenergic effect of NPY on the ventricular cardiomyocyte. *Naunyn Schmiedebergs Arch. Pharmacol.* **338,** 426–429.
134. Michel, M. C., Wirth, S. C., Zerkowski, H. R., Maisel, A. S., and Motulsky, H. J. (1989) Lack of inotropic effects of neuropeptide Y in human myocardium. *J. Cardiovasc. Pharmacol.* **14,** 919–922.
135. Franco-Cereceda, A. and Lundberg, J. M. (1987) Potent effects of neuropeptide Y and calcitonin gene-related peptide on human coronary vascular tone in vitro. *Acta Physiol. Scand.* **137,** 159–160.
136. Warner, M. R. and Levy, M. N. (1989) Inhibition of cardiac vagal effects by neurally released and exogenous neuropeptide Y. *Circ. Res.* **65,** 1536–1546.
137. Lundberg, J. M., Hua, X. Y., and Franco-Cereceda, A. (1984) Effects of neuropeptide Y (NPY) on mechanical activity and neurotransmission in the heart, vas deferens and urinary bladder of the guinea pig. *Acta Physiol. Scand.* **121,** 325–332.
138. Franco-Cereceda, A., Lundberg, J. M., and Dahlof, C. (1985) Neuropeptide Y and sympathetic control of heart contractility and coronary vascular tone. *Acta Physiol. Scand.* **124,** 361–369.

139. Balasubramanian, A., Grupp, I., and Matlib, M. A. (1988) Comparison of the effects of neuropeptide Y (NPY) and 4-norleucine-NPY on isolated perfused rat hearts: effects of NPY on atrial and ventricular strips of rat heart and on rabbit heart mitochondria. *Reg. Pept.* **21,** 289–299.

140. Allen, J., Birchman, P. M. N., Edwards, A. V., Tatemoto, K., and Bloom, S. R. (1983) Neuropeptide Y (NPY) reduces myocardial perfusion and inhibits the force of contraction of the isolated perfused rabbit heart. *Regul. Pept.* **6,** 247–253.

141. Warner, M. R. and Levy, M. N. (1990) Sinus and atrioventricular nodal distribution of sympathetic fibres that contain NPY. *Circ. Res.* **67(3),** 713–721.

142. Potter, E. K. (1985) Prolonged non-adrenergic inhibition of cardiac vagal action following sympathetic stimulation: neuromodulation by neuropeptide Y? *Neurosci. Lett.* **54,** 117–121.

143. Potter, E. K. (1987) Presynaptic inhibition of cardiac vagal postganglionic nerves by neuropeptide Y. *Neurosci. Lett.* **83,** 101–106.

144. Giuliani, S., Maggi, C. A., and Meli, A. (1989) Prejunctional modulatory action of neuropeptide Y on peripheral terminals of capsaicin-sensitive sensory nerves. *Br. J. Pharmacol.* **98,** 407–412.

145. Amerini, S., Rubino, A., Filippi, S., Ledda, F., and Mantelli, L. (1991) Modulation by adrenergic transmitters of the efferent function of capsaicin-sensitive nerves in cardiac tissue. *Neuropeptides* **20,** 225–232.

146. Armour, J. A. (1989) Peptidergic modulation of efferent sympathetic neurones in intrathoracic ganglia regulating the canine heart. *Proc. Soc. Exp. Biol. Sci.* **191,** 60–68.

147. Armour, J. A., Huang, M. H., and Smith, F. M. (1993) Peptidergic modulation of in situ canine intrinsic cardiac neurons. *Peptides* **14,** 191–202.

148. Larsson, L. I., Fahrenkrug, J., Schaffalitzky de Muckadell, O., Sundler, F., Hakanson, R., and Rechfeld, J. F. (1976) Localisation of vasoactive intestinal polypeptide (VIP) to central and peripheral neurons. *Proc. Natl. Acad. Sci.* **73,** 3197–3200.

149. Della, N. G., Papka, R. E., Furness, J. B., and Costa M. (1983) Vasoactive intestinal polypeptide-like immunoreactivity in nerves associated with the cardiovascular system of guinea pigs. *Neuroscience* **9(3),** 605–619.

150. Weihe, E. and Reinecke, M. (1981) Peptidergic innervation of the mammalian sinus nodes: vasoactive intestinal polypeptide, neurotensin, substance P. *Neurosci. Lett.* **26,** 283–288.

151. Weihe, E., Reinecke, M., and Forssmann, W. G. (1984) Distribution of vasoactive intestinal polypeptide-like immunoreactivity in the mammalian heart: interrelation with neurotensin- and substance P-like immunoreactive nerves. *Cell Tissue Res.* **236,** 527–540.

152. Triepel, J. (1982) Vasoactive intestinal polypeptide in the medulla oblongata of the guinea pig. *Neurosci. Lett.* **29,** 73–78.

153. Hökfelt, T., Johansson, O., Ljungdahl, A., Lundberg, J. M., and Schultzberg, M. (1980) Peptidergic neurones. *Nature* **284,** 515–521.
154. Heym, C. H., Reinecke, M., Weihe, E., and Forssmann, W. G. (1984) Dopamine β-hydroxylase, neurotensin-, substance P-, vasoactive intestinal polypeptide-, and enkephalin- immunohistochemistry of cat paravertebral and prevertebral ganglia. *Cell Tissue Res.* **235,** 411–418.
155. Yaksh, T. L., Abay, E. O., and Go, V. L. W. (1982) Studies on the location and release of cholecystokinin and vasoactive intestinal polypeptide in rat and cat spinal cord. *Brain Res.* **242,** 279–290.
156. Anderson, F. L., Wynn, J. R., Kimball, J., Hanson, G. R., Hammond, E., Hershberger R., et al. (1992) Vasoactive intestinal polypeptide in canine hearts: effect of total cardiac denervation. *Am. J. Physiol.* **262,** H598–H602.
157. Franco-Cereceda, A., Bengtsson, L., and Lundberg, J. M. (1987) Inotropic effects of calcitonin gene-related peptide, vasoactive intestinal polypeptide and somatostatin on the human right atrium in vitro. *Eur. J. Pharmacol.* **134,** 69–76.
158. Rigel, D. (1988) Effects of neuropeptides on heart rate in dogs: comparison of VIP, PHI, NPY, CGRP and NT. *Am. J. Physiol.* **255,** H311–H317.
159. Lundberg, J. M., Hedlund, B., and Bartfai, T. (1982) Vasoactive intestinal polypeptide enhances muscarinic ligand binding in cat submandibular salivary gland. *Nature* **295,** 417–149.
160. Rigel, D. and Lathrop, D. A. (1990) Vasoactive intestinal polypeptide facilitates atrioventricular nodal conduction and shortens atrial and ventricular refractory periods in conscious and anaesthetised dogs. *Circ. Rec.* **67,** 1323–1333.
161. Ferron, A., Siggins, G. R., and Bloom, S. R. (1985) Vasoactive intestinal polypeptide acts synergistically with norepinephrine to depress spontaneous discharge rate in cerebral cortical neurons. *Proc. Natl. Acad. Sci.* **82,** 8810–8812.
162. Brazeau, S. G., Vale, W., Burgus, R., Ling, W., Butcher, M., Riner, J., et al. (1973) Hypothalamic peptide that inhibits the secretion of immunoreactive pituitary growth hormone. *Science* **179,** 77–79.
163. Pradayrol, L., Jornvall, H., Mutt V., and Ribet, A. (1980) N-terminally extended somatostatin: the primary structure of somatostatin-28. *FEBS Lett.* **109,** 55–58.
164. Day, S. M., Gu, J., Polak, J. M., and Bloom, S. R. (1985) Somatostatin in the human and comparison with guinea pig and rat heart. *Br. Heart J.* **53,** 153–157.
165. Franco-Cereceda, A., Lundberg, J. M., and Hökfelt, T. (1986) Somatostatin: an inhibitory parasympathetic transmitter in the human heart? *Eur. J. Pharmacol.* **132,** 101–102.
166. Rioux, F., Kerouac, R., and St-Pierre, S. (1981) Somatostatin: interaction with sympathetic nervous system in guinea pigs. *Neuropeptides* **1,** 319–327.

167. Diez, J., Tamargo, J., and Valenzuela, C. (1985) Negative inotropic effect of somatostatin in guinea pig atrial fibres. *Br. J. Pharmacol.* **86,** 547–558.
168. Greco, A. V., Ghirlanda, G., Barone, C., Bertoli, A., Caputo, S., Uccioli, L., et al. (1984) Somatostatin in paroxysmal supraventricular and junctional tachycardia. *Br. Med. J.* **188,** 28–29.
169. Webb, S. C., Krikler, D. M., Hendry, W. G., Adrian, T. E., and Bloom, S. R. (1986) Electrophysiological actions of somatostatin on the atrioventricular junction in sinus rhythm and reentry tachycardia. *Br. Heart J.* **56,** 236–241.
170. Hou, Z. Y., Lin, C. I., Chiu, T. H., Chiang, B. N., Cheng, K. K., and Ho, L. T. (1987) Somatostatin effects in isolated human atrial fibres. *J. Mol. Cell. Cardiol.* **19,** 177–185.
171. Wiley, J. W., Uccioli, L., Owyang, C., and Yamada, T. (1989) Somatostatin stimulates acetylcholine release in the canine heart. *Am. J. Physiol.* **257,** H483–H487.
172. Zhu, W. and Dey, R. D. (1992) Distribution of the neuropeptide galanin in the cat heart and coexistence with vasoactive intestinal polypeptide, substance P and neuropeptide Y. *J. Mol. Cell. Cardiol.* **24,** 35–41.
173. Malliani, A., Lombardi, F., and Pagani, M. (1986) Sensory innervation of the heart. *Prog. Brain Res.* **67,** 39–48.
174. Saito, A., Kimura, S., and Goto, K. (1986) Calcitonin gene-related peptide as potential neurotransmitter in guinea pig right atrium. *Am. J. Physiol.* **250,** H693–H698.
175. Saito, A., Ishikawa, T., Kimura, S., and Goto, K. (1987) Role of calcitonin gene-related peptide as cardiotonic neurotransmitter in guinea pig left atria. *J. Pharmacol. Exp. Ther.* **243,** 731–736.
176. Franco-Cereceda, A., Saria, A., and Lundberg, J. M. (1989) Differential release of calcitonin-gene-related peptide and neuropeptide Y from the isolated heart by capsaicin, ischaemia, nicotine, bradykinin and ouabain. *Acta Physiol. Scand.* **135,** 173–187.
177. Lundberg, J. M., Franco-Cereceda, A., Hua, X., Hökfelt, T., and Fischer, J. A. (1985) Co-existence of substance P and calcitonin gene-related peptide-like immunoreactivities in sensory nerves in relation to cardiovascular and bronchoconstrictor effects of capsaicin. *Eur. J. Pharmacol.* **108,** 315–319.
178. Gibbins, I. L., Furness, J. B., Costa, M., MacIntyre, I., Hillyard, C. J., and Girgis, S. (1985) Co-localisation of calcitonin gene-related peptide-like immunoreactivity with substance P in cutaneous, vascular and visceral sensory neurons of guinea pigs. *Neurosci. Lett.* **57,** 125–130.
179. Wharton, J., Gulbenkian, S., Mulderry, P. K., Ghatei, M. A., McGregor, G. P., Bloom, S. R., et al. (1986) Capsaicin induces depletion of calcitonin gene-related peptide (CGRP)-like immunoreactive nerves in the cardiovascular system of the guinea pig and rat. *J. Auton. Nerv. Syst.* **16,** 289–309.

180. Franco-Cereceda, A., Henke, H., Lundberg, J. M., Petermann, J. B., Hökfelt, T., and Fischer, J. A. (1987) Calcitonin gene-related peptide (CGRP) in capsaicin-sensitive substance P-immunoreactive sensory neurons in animals and man: distribution and release by capsaicin. *Peptides* **8,** 399–410.

181. Gulbenkian, S., Merighi, A., Wharton, J., Varndell, I. M., and Polak, J. M. (1986) Ultrastructural evidence for the existence of calcitonin gene-related peptide and substance P in secretory vesicles of peripheral nerves in the guinea pig. *J. Neurocytol.* **15,** 535–542.

182. Armour, J. A., Yuan, B., and Butler, C. K. (1990) Cardiac responses elicited by peptides administered to canine intrinsic cardiac neurones. *Peptides* **11,** 753–761.

183. Kangawa, K., Minamino, N., Fukuda, A., and Matsuo, H., Neuromedin, K. (1983) a novel mammalian tachykinin identified in porcine spinal cord. *Biochem. Biophys. Res. Commun.* **114,** 533–540.

184. Kimura, S., Okada, M., Sugita, Y., Kanazawa, I., and Munekatat, E. (1983) Novel neuropeptides, neurokinin α and β isolated from porcine spinal cord. *Proc. Jpn. Acad.* **59B,** 101–104.

185. Hua, X.-Y., Theodorsson-Norheim, E., Brodin, E., Lundberg, J. M., and Hökfelt, T. (1985) Multiple tachykinins (neurokinin A, neuropeptide K, and substance P) in capsaicin sensitive neurons in the guinea pig. *Regul. Pept.* **13,** 1–19.

186. Reinecke, M., Weihe, E., and Forssmann, W. G. (1980) Substance P-immunoreactive nerve fibres in ther heart. *Neurosci. Lett.* **20,** 265–269.

187. Wharton, J., Polak, J. M., McGregor, G. P., Bishop, A. E., and Bloom, S. R. (1981) The distribution of substance P-like immunoreactive nerves in the guinea pig heart. *Neuroscience* **6,** 2193–2204.

188. Furness, J. B., Elliot, J. M., Murphy, R., Costa, M., and Chambers, J. P. (1982) Baroreceptor reflexes in conscious guinea pigs are unaffected by depletion of cardiovascular substance P nerves. *Neurosci. Lett.* **32,** 285–290.

189. Papka, R. E., Furness, J. B., Della, N. G., and Costa, M. (1984) Time course of effect of capsaicin on ultrastructure and histochemistry of substance P-immunoreactive nerves associated with the cardiovascular system of the guinea pig. *Neurosacience* **12,** 1277–1292.

190. Forsberg, K., Karlson, J. A., Theodorsson, E., Lundberg, J. M., and Persson, C. G. (1988) Cough and brochoconstriction mediated by capsaicin-sensitive sensory neurons in the guinea pig. *Pulm. Pharmacol.* **1(1),** 33–39.

191. Brauer, M. M., Lincoln, J., Sarner, S., Blundell, D., Milner, P., Passaro, M., et al. (1994) Maturational changes in sympathetic and sensory innervation of the rat uterus: effects of neonatal capsaicin treatment. *Int. J. Dev. Neurosci.* **12(2),** 157–171.

192. Uddmann, R., Edvinsson, L., Owman, C., and Sundler, F. (1981) Perivascular substance P: occurrence and distribution in mammalian pial vessels. *J. Cerebr. Blood Flow Metab.* **1,** 221–232.

193. Lee, Y., Takami, K., Kawai, Y., Girgis, S., Hillyard, C. J., MacIntyre, I.,
     et al. (1985) Distribution of calcitonin gene-related peptide in the
     rat peripheral nervous system with reference to its coexistence with
     substance P. *Neuroscience* **15,** 1227–1237.
194. Matsuyama, T., Wanaka, A., Yoneda, S., Kimura, K., Kamada, T.,
     Girgis, S., et al. (1986) Two distinct calcitonin gene-related pep-
     tide-containing peripheral nervous systems: distribution and quan-
     titative differences between the iris and cerebral artery with special
     reference to substance P. *Brain Res.* **373,** 205–212.
195. Hoover, D. B. and Hancock, J. C. (1988) Distribution of substance P
     binding sites in guinea pig heart and pharmacological effects of
     substance P. *J. Auton. Nerv. Syst.* **23,** 189–197.
196. Dalsgaard, C.-J., Franco-Cereceda, A., Saria, A., Lundberg, J. M.,
     Theodorsson-Norheim, E., and Hökfelt, T. (1986) Distribution and
     origin of substance P- and neuropeptide Y- immunoreactive nerves
     in the guinea pig heart. *Cell Tissue Res.* **243,** 477–485.
197. Burcher, E., Alterhog, J. H., Pernow, B., and Rosell, S. (1977) Car-
     diovascular effects of substance P: effects on the heart and regional
     blood flow in the dog, in *Substance P* (Von Euler, U. S. and
     Pernow, B., eds.), Raven, New York, pp. 261–268.
198. Bury, R. W. and Mashford, M. L. (1977) Cardiovascular effects of
     synthetic substance P in several species. *Eur. J. Pharmacol.* **45,**
     335–340.
199. Quirion, R., Regoli, D., Rioux, F., and St-Pierre, S. (1980) The stimu-
     latory effects of neurotensin and related peptides in rat stomach
     strips and guinea pig atria. *Br. J. Pharmacol.* **68,** 83–91.
200. Iven, H., Pursche, R., and Zelter, G. (1980) Field stimulus response
     of guinea pig atria as influenced by the peptides angiotensin, bradyki-
     nin and substance P. *Naunyn Schmiedebergs Arch. Pharmacol.* **312,** 63–68.
201. Konishi, S., Okamoto, T., and Otsuka, M. (1985) Substance P as
     a neurotransmitter released from peripheral branches of pri-
     mary afferent neurones producing slow synaptic excitation in
     autonomic ganglion cells, in *Substance P—Metabolism and Bio-
     logical Actions* (Jordon, C. C. and Oehme, P., eds.), Taylor
     Francis, London, pp. 121–136.
202. Hökfelt, T., Ljungdahl, A., Terenius, L., Elde, R., and Nilsson, G.
     (1977) Immunohistochemical analysis of peptide pathways possi-
     bly related to pain and analgesia: enkephalin and substance P. *Proc.
     Natl. Acad. Sci.* **74,** 3081–3085.
203. Gamse, R., Holzer, P., and Lembeck, F. (1980) Decrease of substance
     P in primary afferent neurones and impairment of neurogenic
     plasma extravasation by capsaicin. *Br. J. Pharmacol.* **68(2),** 207–213.
204. Saria, A., Lundberg, J. M., Skofitsch, G., and Lembeck, F. (1983)
     Vascular protein leakage in various tissues induced by substance
     P, capsaicin, tachykinin, serotonin, histamine and by antigen chal-
     lenge. *Naunyn Schmiedebergs Arch. Pharmacol.* **324,** 212–218.

205. Takano, Y., Nagashima, A., Hagio, T., Tateishi, K., and Kamiya, H. (1990) Role of central tachykinin peptides in cardiovascular regulation in rats. *Brain Res.* **528,** 231–237.
206. Rosenfeld, M. G., Mermod, J. J., Amara, S. G., Swanson, L. W., Sawchenko, P. E., Rivier, J., et al. (1983) Production of a novel neuropeptide encoded by the calcitonin gene via tissue-specific RNA processing. *Nature* **304,** 129–135.
207. Amara, S. G., Arriza, J. L., Leff, S. E., Swanson, L. W., Evans, R. M., and Rosenfeld, M. G. (1985) Expression in brain of the messenger RNA encoding a novel neuropeptide homologous to calcitonin gene-related peptide. *Science* **229,** 1094–1097.
208. Steenbergh, P. H., Hoppener, J. W. M., Zandberg, J., Lips, C. J. M., and Jansz, H. S. (1985) A second human calcitonin/CGRP gene. *FEBS Lett.* **184,** 403–407.
209. Mulderry, P. K., Ghatei, M. A., Rodrigo, J., Allen, J. M., Rosenfeld, M. G., Polak, J. M., et al. (1985) Calcitonin gene-related peptide in cardiovascular tissues of the rat. *Neuroscience* **14,** 947–954.
210. Wharton, J., Gulbenkian, S., Merighi, S., Kuhn, D. M., Jahn, R., Taylor, K. H., et al. (1988) Immunohistochemical ultrastructural localisation of peptide-containing nerves and myocardial cells in the human atrial appendage. *Cell Tissue Res.* **254,** 155–166.
211. McEwan, J., Larkin, S., Davies, G., Chierchia, S., Brown, M., Stevenson, J., et al. (1986) Calcitonin gene-related peptide: a potent dilator of human epicardial coronary arteries. *Circ.* **74,** 1243–1247.
212. Franco-Cereceda, A. and Rudehill, A. (1989) Capsaicin-induced vasodilatation of human coronary arteries in vitro is mediated by calcitonin gene-related peptide rather than substance P or neurokinin A. *Acta Physiol. Scand.* **136,** 575–580.
213. Franco-Cereceda, A. (1991) Calcitonin gene-related peptide and human epicardial coronary arteries: presence, release and vasodilator effects. *Br. J. Pharmacol.* **102,** 506–510.
214. Brain, S. D., Williams, T., Tippins, J. R., Morris, H. R., and MacIntyre, I. (1985) Calcitonin gene-related peptide is a potent vasodilator. *Nature* **313,** 54–56.
215. Gamse, R. and Saria, A. (1985) Potentiation of tachykinin-induced plasma protein extravasation by calcitonin gene-related peptide. *Eur. J. Pharmacol.* **114,** 61–66.
216. Sugiyama, A., Kobayashi, M., Tsujimoto, G., Motomura, S., and Hashimoto, K. (1989) The first demonstration of CGRP-immunoreactive fibres in canine hearts: coronary vasodilator, inotropic and chronotropic effects of CGRP in canine isolated, blood-perfused heart preparations. *Jpn. J. Pharmacol.* **50,** 421–427.
217. Xi, X., Duff, M. J., Weber, M., Fiscus, B. I., Thomas, J. X., O'Toole, M. F., et al. (1989) In vivo effects of calcitonin gene-related peptide (CGRP) on intracardiac vagal ganglia. *FASEB J.* **3,** A413 (abstract).

218. Ono, K., Delay, M., Nakajima, T., Irisawa, H., and Giles, W. R. (1989) Calcitonin gene-related peptide regulates calcium current in heart muscle. *Nature* **340,** 721–724.
219. Ono, K. and Giles, W. R. (1991) Electrophysiological effects of calcitonin gene-related peptide in bull frog and guinea pig atrial myocytes. *J. Physiol.* **436,** 195–217.
220. Hassall, C. J. S., Saffrey, M. J., Belai, A., Hoyle, C. H. V., Moules, E. W., Moss, J., et al. (1992) Nitric oxide synthase immunoreactivity and NADPH-diaphorase activity in a subpopulation of intrinsic neurones of the guinea pig heart. *Neurosci. Lett.* **143,** 65–68.
221. Klimaschewski, L., Kummer, W., Mayer, B., Courand, J. Y., Preissler, U., Philippin B., et al. (1992) Nitric oxide synthase in cardiac nerve fibres and neurones of rat and guinea pig heart. *Circ. Rec.* **71.** 1533–1537.
222. Tanaka, K., Hassall, C. J. S., and Burnstock, G. (1993) Distribution of intracardiac neurones and nerve terminals that contain a marker for nitric oxide, NADPH-diaphorase, in the guinea pig heart. *Cell Tissue Res.* **273,** 293–300.
223. Smith, R. E. A., Palmer, R. M. J., and Moncada, S. (1991) Coronary-vasodilatation induced by endotoxin is nitric oxide dependent and inhibited by dexamethasone in the isolated perfused rabbit heart. *Br. J. Pharmacol.* **104,** 5,6.
224. Gardiner, S. M., Compton, A. M., Kemp, P. A., and Bennett, T. (1990) Regional and cardiac haemodynamic effects of N^G-nitro-L-arginine methyl ester in conscious, Long Evans rats. *Br. J. Pharmacol.* **101,** 625–631.
225. Klabunde, R. E., Kimber, N. D., Kuk, J. E., Helgren, M. C., and Forstermann, U. (1992) N^G-Methyl-L-arginine decreases contractility, cGMP and cAMP in isoproterenol-stimulated rat hearts in vitro. *Eur. J. Pharmacol.* **223,** 1–7.
226. Hassall, C. J. S. and Hoyle, C. H. V. (1997) Heme oxygenase-2 and nitric oxide synthase in guinea pig intracardiac neurones. *Neuroreport* **8,** 1043–1046.
227. Votavova, M., Boullin, D. J., and Costa, E. (1971) Specificity of action of 6-hydroxydopamine in peripheral cat tissues: depletion of noradrenaline without depletion of 5-hydroxytryptamine. *Life Sci.* **10,** 87–91.
228. Berkowitz, B., Lee C.-H., and Spector, S. (1974) Disposition of serotonin in the rat blood vessels and heart. *Clin. Exp. Pharmacol. Physiol.* **1,** 397–400.
229. Bernoussi, A. and Rioux, F. (1989) Effects of capsaicin desensitisation on the stimulatory effect of kinins, prostaglandins, biogenic amines and various drugs in guinea pig isolated atria. *Br. J. Pharmacol.* **96,** 563–572.
230. Tramontana, M., Giuliani, S., Del Bianco, E., Lecci, A., Maggi, C. A., Evangelista, S., et al. (1993) Effects of capsaicin and 5-HT$_3$ antagonists

on 5-hydroxytryptamine-evoked release of calcitonin gene-related peptide in the guinea pig heart. *Br. J. Pharmacol.* **108**, 431–435.

231. de Boer, H. J., Dhasmana, K. M., and Saxema, P. R. (1986) The tachycardic response to 5-hydroxytryptamine in the spinal guinea pig. *Br. J. Pharmacol.* **89**, 545P.

232. Hassall, C. J. S. and Burnstock, G. (1987) Evidence for uptake and synthesis of 5-hydroxytryptamine by a subpopulation of intrinsic neurones in the guinea pig heart. *Neuroscience* **22**, 413–423.

233. Ryan, M. J. and Brody, M. J. (1972) Neurogenic and vascular stores of histamine in the dog. *J. Pharmacol. Exp. Ther.* **181**, 83–91.

234. Häppölä, O., Ahonen, M., and Panula, P. (1991) Distribution of histamine in the developing peripheral nervous system. *Agents Actions* **33**, 112–115.

235. Hattori, Y. and Kanno, M. (1985) Effect of Ni^{2+} on the multiphasic positive inotropic response to histamine mediated by H_1-receptors in left atria of guinea pigs. *Naunyn Schmiedebergs Arch. Pharmacol.* **329**, 188–194.

236. Hattori, Y., Nakaya, H., Tohse, N., and Kanno, M. (1988) Effects of Ca^{2+} channel antagonists and ryanodine on H_1-receptor mediated electromechanical response to histamine in guinea pig left atria. *Naunyn Schmiedebergs Arch. Pharmacol.* **337**, 323–330.

237. Rowan, R. R. and Billingham, M. E. (1988) Myocardial innervation in long-term heart transplant survivors: a quantitative ultrastructural survey. *J. Heart Transplant.* **7**, 448–452.

238. Mancini, D. (1997) Surgically denervated cardiac transplant: rewired or permanently unplugged? *Circulation* **96**, 6–8.

239. Mohanty, P. K., Sowers, J. R., Thames, M. D., Beck, F. W. J., Kawaguchi, A., and Lower, R. R. (1986) Myocardial norepinephrine, epinephrine and dopamine concentrations after cardiac autotransplantation in dogs. *J. Am. Coll. Cardiol.* **7**, 419–424.

240. Wilson, R. F., Christensen, B. V., Olivari, M. T., Simon, A., White, C. W., and Laxson, D. D. (1991) Evidence for structural sympathetic reinnervation after orthotopic cardiac transplantation in humans. *Circulation* **83**, 1210–1220.

241. Gill, J. S., Hunter, G. J., Gane, G., and Camm, A. J. (1993) Heterogeneity of the human myocardial sympathetic innervation: in vivo demonstration of iodine 123-labeled metaiodobezylguanidine scintigraphy. *Am. Heart J.* **126**, 390–398.

242. DeMarco, T., Dae, M., Yuen-Green, M. S., Kumar, S., Sudhir, K., Keith, F., et al. (1995) Iodine-123 metaiodobezylguanidine scintigraphic assessment of the transplanted human heart: evidence for late reinnervation. *J. Am. Coll. Cardiol.* **25**, 927–931.

243. Lord, S. W., Clayton, R. H., Mitchell, L., Dark, J. H., Murray, A., and McComb, J. M. (1997) Sympathetic reinnervation and heart rate variability after cardiac transplantation. *Heart* **77**, 532–538.

244. Stark, R. P., McGinn, A. L., and Wilson, R. F. (1991) Chest pain in cardiac transplant recipients: evidence of sensory reinnervation after cardiac transplantation. *N. Engl. J. Med.* **324,** 1791–1794.
245. Crea, F., Pupita, G., Galassi, A. R., El-Tamimi, H., Kaski, J. C., Davies, G., et al. (1990) Role of adenosine in pathogenesis of anginal pain. *Circulation* **81,** 164–172.
246. Fallen, E., Damath, M., Ghista, D., and Fitchett, D. (1988) Spectral analysis of heart rate variability following human heart transplantation. *J. Auton. Nerv. Syst.* **23,** 199–206.
247. Rudas, L., Pflugfelder, P. W., and Kostuk, W. J. (1992) Vasodepressor syncope in a cardiac transplant recipient: a case of vagal reinnervation? *Can. J. Cardiol.* **8,** 403–405.
248. Fitzpatrick, A. P., Banner, N., Cheng, A., Yacoub, M., and Sutton, R. (1993) Vasovagal reactions may occur after orthotopic heart transplantation. *J. Am. Coll. Cardiol.* **21,** 1132–1137.
249. Paulus, W. J., Bronzwaer, J. G. F., Felice, H., Dishan, N., and Wellens, F. (1992) Deficient acceleration of left ventricular relaxation during exercise after heart transplantation. *Circulation* **86,** 1175–1185.
250. Cozzi, E. and White, D. J. G. (1995) The generation of transgenic pigs as potential organ donors for humans. *Nat. Med.* **1,** 964–966.
251. Brandys, J. C., Hopkins, D. A., and Armour, J. A. (1984) Cardiac responses to stimulation of discrete loci within canine sympathetic ganglia following hexamethonium. *J. Auton. Nerv. Syst.* **11,** 243–255.
252. Butler, C. K., Smith, F. M., Nicholson, J., and Armour, J. A. (1990) Cardiac effects induced by chemically activated neurons in canine intrathoracic ganglia. *Am. J. Physiol.* **259,** H1108–H1117.
253. Cardinal, R., Scherlag, B. J., Vermeulen, M., and Armour, J. A. (1992) Distinct epicardial activation patterns of iodoventricular rhythms and sympathetically-induced ventricular tachycardias in dogs with atrioventricular block. *Pace* **15,** 1300–1316.
254. Yuan, B.-X., Hopkins, D. A., Ardell, J. L., and Armour, J. A. (1993) Differential cardiac responses induced by nicotinic sensitive canine intrinsic atrial and ventricular neurons. *Cardiovasc. Res.* **27,** 760–769.
255. Huang, M. H., Ardell, J. L., Hanna, B., Wolf, S., and Armour, J. A. (1993) Effects of transient coronary artery occlusion on canine intrinsic cardiac neuronal activity. *Integr. Physiol. Behav. Sci.* **28,** 5–21.

CHAPTER 2

Emotions and Heart-Activity Control

Neurocircuitries and Pathway Interactions

Gert J. Ter Horst

1. Introduction

Happiness, sadness, anger, anxiety, fear, love, hate, panic, and many other conditions that affect the emotional state of human beings are accompanied by alterations of heart rate and blood pressure, as everyone may know from own experience. Anger and chronic stress have been associated with the occurrence of cardiac diseases like sudden death, arrhythmias, and myocardial infarctions. Regional damage to the central nervous system also may affect emotions and the functioning of the cardiovascular system.

Emotions are associated with nervous activity in forebrain circuitry. Many, if not all, of the structures that compose this circuitry belong to the so-called "limbic system."

Heart rate, blood pressure, and plasma parameters such as glucose levels, pH, and osmolarity, are monitored by the central nervous system in its capacity as guardian of metabolic homeostasis. It has been established that through activity of the autonomic nervous system, the brain can modulate these parameters. To achieve maintenance of metabolic homeostasis, nervous circuitry has developed that controls gain setting and the balance of parasympathetic and

From: *The Nervous System and the Heart*
Ed: G. J. Ter Horst © Humana Press Inc.

sympathetic activities. This complex steering circuitry involves nuclei located at various levels of the neuraxis, but the hypothalamus is considered the command center for the regulation of such autonomic activity. The hypothalamus belongs to the limbic system as defined by Papez. Thus, in the limbic system overlapping or parallel circuitry may generate alterations of cardiovascular activity during emotional states.

Limbic system circuitry related to emotions and heart-activity regulation will be described in this chapter, as well as the input and output pathways of the limbic system, and the modulating effects of various neurotransmitters and peptides.

2. Neural Substrate of Emotions

In *The Expression of Emotion in Man and Animals*, Charles Darwin (1872) defined the concept of basic or primary emotions that serve to protect the survival needs of the individual and the species. Since the beginning of 20th century, emotions have been the subject of intensive research and neurobiological studies of brain circuitry of emotion have progressed considerably, although much remains unknown. In our current concepts, we distinguish emotional experience, expression, and memory, each involving the participation of selective neuronal circuitry. Emotional experience refers to the conscious aspects of emotions and emotional expression to the behavioral, autonomic, and other physiological responses. Emotional memory has been recognized as an important aspect of emotions much later and fulfills a role in evaluating the emotional load of sensory stimuli. This system safeguards that not all sensory stimuli received by the brain evoke an emotional expression or conscious emotional experience. A distorted emotional memory system, generated somehow by genetic factors, life events, or other conditions, may be a possible cause of neuropsychiatric diseases, such as depression and anxiety disorders that are associated with inappropriate or exaggerated emotional responses.

2.1. History

Four major developments at the beginning of this century have contributed significantly to our current understanding of the neurobiological basis of emotion. These include Canon and Bard's work on sham rage, Papez' anatomical model of emotion, the "psychic blindness" studies of Kluver and Bucy, and the limbic system or visceral brain concept of MacLean. In the last decades, the fear-conditioning studies of LeDoux have increased our knowledge of neuronal substrates of emotions (1,2). In the nineties, Nieuwenhuys et al. (3,4) and Holstege (5) introduced new definitions for the limbic system that are based on modern tract tracing and immunocytochemical and biochemical studies.

2.1.1. Sham-Rage Studies of Canon and Bard

Sham rage is the hyperexpression of anger in decorticated animals. From studies in such decorticated animals, Cannon concluded that the expression of emotional behavior does not depend on the cerebral cortex. Decorticated animals exhibited signs such as diffuse autonomic activation, including hypertension, sweating, piloerection, and secretion of adrenal medullary catecholamines, that were associated with emotional arousal. Cannon (6) argued that this diffuse autonomic activation was part of processes needed for increased physiological efficiency as part of the struggle to live. This theory is still widely discussed, but the fundamental aspect of a diffuse sympathetic autonomic activation as part of fight-or-flight responses has been accepted. Cannon's pupil, Bard, has contributed to the understanding of nervous circuitry of sham rage. He elaborated on previous findings that transection at the midbrain level could eliminate emotional responses (7). Accordingly, Bard later illustrated that structures lying below the cortex and above the midbrain were responsible for mediating emotional responses in sham rage (8). He identified the caudal hypothalamus and the ventral thalamus as the areas responsible for the diffuse autonomic activation in sham rage.

2.1.2. Circuitry of Papez

The anatomist Papez was the first to construct a neuronal circuitry for emotions (9) that was instigated by the physiological findings of Cannon and Bard. He accepted their conclusion that the hypothalamus and the cerebral cortex respectively mediate emotional expression and experience. Using anatomical data, Papez constructed his neuronal circuitry model of emotions, in which he included the hypothalamus, the anterior thalamic nuclei, the hippocampus, and the cingulate gyrus (9). Fundamental to his neuronal circuitry was the inclusion of the cingulate gyrus, which he saw as the cortical area for emotional experience. In Papez circuitry, the thalamus is activated by sensory information from the external and internal environments and serves to distribute this information to the hypothalamus and the neocortex via the ventral and dorsal thalamic nuclei, respectively. Both the hypothalamus and neocortex can funnel the sensory information to the cingulate gyrus. The neocortical route to the cingulate gyrus involves, according to Papez' theory, the hippocampus and its projections to the hypothalamus. The projections of the mammillary body, a part of the posterior hypothalamus, mediate the hypothalamic activity to the cingulate gyrus through the anterior thalamic area. Central to Papez' theory was that the emotional load of sensory information was acquired in the hypothalamus and only after such information was processed by the hypothalamus was it tagged with emotional meaning. Papez attempted to validate his model with clinical data. Tumors located in the cingulate gyrus were associated with apathy. Lesions of the mammillary body were thought to result in emotional inactivity, whereas anterior thalamic and hippocampal lesions caused respectively spontaneous laughing and crying, and intense emotions. Much of the connections described by Papez have been identified later with modern neuroanatomical techniques, although the interrelations between the components were more complex, very often also reciprocal, and they involved additional relay areas, like the amygdala and septum. Nonetheless, even with these inconsistencies, the neu-

"core of the neuraxis" and lateral and medial *"paracores" (3,4)*. He based this definition on immunocytochemical and biochemical studies, which showed that certain parts of the brain exhibit a rich neurotransmitter, peptide, and receptor diversity. In particular, the limbic system can be characterized this way. These neuromediator-rich areas seem to participate somehow in visceral effector mechanisms, agonistic behavior, locomotion or forward progression related to fight-or-flight responses, nociception, and reproductive and feeding behaviors. Like Darwin before him, Nieuwenhuys concluded that these neuromediator-rich areas are involved in mechanisms that support the survival of the individual animal or the species. The core of the neuraxis according to Nieuwenhuys' definition is divided in caudal and rostral parts. The caudal core is composed of the preoptic region, the hypothalamus, the periaqueductal gray matter, the parabrachial nuclei, the dorsal motor nucleus of the vagus nerve including the nucleus of the solitary tract, and the spinal substantia intermedia centralis. The septum, the amygdala, the bed nucleus of the stria terminalis, and the hippocampus comprise the rostral core. The hippocampus and/or the amygdala are intermediate structures for information from the neocortex, the unimodal sensory association areas, and the polymodal entorhinal and perirhinal cortices. The medial and (bi)lateral paracores are comprised respectively of the serotonergic raphe nuclei, and the noradrenergic and adrenergic cell groups in the brainstem. All ascending and descending fiber connections of the paracore cell groups are covered by the definition. The medial paracore is situated near or adjacent to the core of the neuraxis, and its descending projections supposedly fulfill a role in level setting in the sensory and motor systems. The lateral paracores are located near the large ascending and descending fiber systems of the brain in the lateral parts of the brainstem and are continuous with the medial forebrain bundle in the lateral hypothalamus. This lateral paracore system may mediate output of the core of the neuraxis for specific physiological and behavioral activities because it projects to visceromotor and skeletomotor areas. The core–

paracore definition of Nieuwenhuys has some resemblance with the endocrine–autonomic-integration and regulation system previously described by Stumpf and Jennes (25) and conforms to the earlier broad definition of the limbic system, which included all regions connected to the hypothalamus.

In the nineties Holstege (5) introduced the Emotional Motor System (EMS), which basically may be viewed at as output system of the limbic forebrain to the visceromotor and skeletomotor systems in the brainstem and spinal cord. Largely, the EMS is homologous to the lateral paracore system of Nieuwenhuys and co-workers (3,4). Like the lateral paracore, the emotional motor system mediates information from the limbic forebrain to the various autonomic and somatic premotor areas of the brainstem. Here, the EMS guides/regulates/modulates the coordination of visceral autonomic and locomotor responses associated with activities such as agonistic behavior and feeding and reproductive behaviors that are aimed at the survival of the organism.

In conclusion, although, recently, some new concepts regarding the definition of the limbic system as neuronal substrate of emotions have been put forward, these new definitions have not found much support in the scientific literature yet. Most papers involving anatomical and pharmacological aspects of emotional behavior employ the term *limbic system* or *limbic forebrain*.

2.2. Lesions and Electrical Stimulation in Humans

Regarding neurobiological substrates of emotions, much was learned from behavior analysis in patients who suffer from local neuropathology or from studies that used electrical stimulation of selected brain regions during neurosurgery. In particular, lesions of the frontal lobes have been associated with distinctive syndromes, including mood disturbances, obsessive–compulsive disorders, mania, personality changes, and disorders of executive functions. Cummings (26), however, has reviewed abnormal human behavior states after localized frontal lobe and subcortical lesions and concludes that damage within three distinct pathways, all arising from the frontal lobe, may be responsible for the various disorders shown by the patients. He recognized frontal–subcortical circuits originating in the dorsolateral prefrontal cortex, the lateral orbital cortex, and the anterior cingulate cortex as the substrate for human behavioral disorders and illustrated this with different clinical observations. The dorsal prefrontal circuit originates in Brodman's areas 9 and 10 and includes the head of the caudate nucleus, the dorsomedial globus pallidus, and the rostral substantia nigra. Feedback is supplied through the ventral anterior and medial dorsal thalamic nuclei. Localized lesions in any part of this circuitry are characterized primarily by deficits of executive function and motor programming, although, in some patients, depression has been observed with left-hemisphere lesions located in the dorsolateral prefrontal and caudate nucleus *(27,28)*. The lateral orbitoprefrontal circuitry according to Cummings *(26)* arises from Brodman's area 10 and includes the ventromedial caudate nucleus, the dorsomedial pallidum, and the rostromedial substantia nigra. Both the pallidum and the substantia nigra supply feedback to the orbitofrontal gyrus through the ventral anterior and medial dorsal thalamic nuclei. Lesions located somewhere in the orbitofrontal circuitry are characterized by marked personality changes, such as irritability, less worrying, euphoria, and lability. Mania for example, has been reported after lesions in the medial orbitofrontal cortex, the caudate nucleus, and the right thalamus *(29,30)*. The anterior cingulate circuitry originates in Brodman's area 24 and includes the ventral striatum—the nucleus accumbens, olfactory tubercle and the ventromedial caudate nucleus—the putamen, the ventral, and rostral globus pallidus, and the rostrodorsal substantia nigra. The nigra and globus pallidus both innervate the paramedian parts of the medial dorsal thalamic nucleus, the habenula, the ventral tegmental area, the hypothalamus, and the amygdala. Feedback to the anterior cingulate gyrus is supplied by the medial dorsal thalamic nucleus. Damage in the anterior cingulate circuitry according to Cummings *(26)* is associated with akinetic mutism, apathy,

incontinence, and lack of emotional responses to painful stimuli
(31). Other studies have associated lesions in the anterior cingulate area with depression and deficits of attention (32).

Electrical stimulation of the anterior cingulate gyrus
induced feelings of fear and pleasure, agitation (33), and
euphoria (34). Seizures attributed to anterior cingulate dysfunction were associated with sudden bursts of laughing and
crying, irritability, sexual deviancy, and emotional lability
(32). Patients with anterior cingulate tumors (32) showed a
variety of emotional responses from apathy, sexual disinhibition, depression, aggression, anxiety, obsessive–compulsive disorders (OCD), to bulimia. On the other hand,
cingulatomy has been used for treatment of obsessive–compulsive disorders, tics, anxiety, aggression, and depression.
Ablation of area 24 of the anterior cingulate gyrus, in particular, was associated with long-lasting positive effects on
OCD and anxiety symptoms (26,31). Lesions of the medial
thalamic nucleus, a region included in the anterior cingulate
circuitry of Cummings (26), also caused reduction of tics and
symptoms of OCD (35). Stimulation applied to the temporal
lobe (36) and insular cortex (37) were not associated with
emotional responses. However, injuries of the insular cortex
generated multimodal neglect syndromes, in which the
patients did not show appropriate motor and emotional
responses to offensive visual and auditory stimuli. Augustine
(37) has attributed this syndrome to interruption of the
somatosensory–insular–amygdala pathway.

A selective bilateral damage to the human amygdala is
rare, but when found, it impaired recognition of facial
expressions of emotion, and fear and anger responses (38–40).
Studies employing electrical stimulation of the human
amygdala substantiated the role of the amygdaloid complex
in fear and anger responses, as it could evoke strong fearful
emotional responses (41). Aversive emotional responses were
associated to the right amygdala (42).

Small lesions of the posteromedial hypothalamus effec-
tively reduced occurrence of violence, aggression, restlessness, and rage in human patients (43). On the other hand,

naturally occurring human hypothalamic damage mainly induced appetitive disorders without significant impairments of emotional function *(44)*.

2.3. In Vivo Neuroimaging

The identification of neuronal substrates of emotions entered a new era with the introduction of neuroimaging techniques. Today, we have possibilities to investigate in vivo human brain activity during well-defined emotional states and in psychiatric diseases that consist of a pathologic disturbance of mood and affect, like unipolar and bipolar depression, anxiety disorders, phobia, and obsessive–compulsive disorders. In the past, neuroanatomical, behavioral, and pharmacological studies in animals have dictated the definition of a neuronal substrate for emotions—in particular, studies involving fear conditioning. Substrates defined with such animal studies are informative, but they remain questionable because it is hard for the investigators to characterize the emotional load for the animals of the various experimental conditions. To unravel the full neuronal substrate of emotions and not only circuitry for emotional expression but also that for emotional experience and memory, human subjects are needed. The challenge of present-day research is to verify and substantiate neuronal substrates of emotions with in vivo neuroimaging techniques like positron emission tomography (PET) and functional magnetic resonance imaging (fMRI). However, these imaging methods have limitations too, because alterations of regional cerebral blood flow (rCBF) are employed as an indirect measure for increased or decreased regional brain activity. The relationships between alterations of rCBF and brain activity are debated.

2.3.1. Normal Human Emotion

To delineate neuroanatomical substrates of internally and externally generated human emotion, PET imaging of regional brain activity has been employed during various experimental conditions. The earlier studies used anticipatory anxiety of a painful electrical shock and found increased rCBF in regions of the limbic system—in particular, in the anterior insular, anterior temporal, temporoparietal, and lateral prefrontal cortical regions, the thalamus, the midbrain, and the anterior cingulate and medial prefrontal cortex. The nonlimbic caudate nucleus and cerebellar vermis also were affected by this condition *(45)*. Using film- and recall-generated emotions, brain activity associated with happiness, sadness, and disgust has been studied, both independent of and dependent on the emotional type or valence. Film-generated emotional states were associated with symmetrical increases in brain activity in the medial prefrontal cortex, the thalamus, the occipitotemporoparietal cortex, the lateral cerebellum, the hypothalamus, the hippocampal formation, the midbrain, and the region that includes the anterior temporal cortex and the amygdala *(45)*. Recall of the emotional states triggered increased rCBF in the thalamus, the medial prefrontal cortex, the vicinity of the anterior insular cortex, and in the orbitofrontal and the anterior temporal cortex *(45)*. The activity in the vicinity of the anterior insular area may be localized in the lateral putamen, the claustrum, and the anterior insular cortex. The medial prefrontal cortex and thalamus activity could not be related to a selective emotional state, valence, or method of induction, in contrast to the anterior insular cortex activity, which appeared to be associated with recall of negative emotions *(46)*. Lane et al. *(46)* therefore concludes that the anterior insular region may be involved in assigning negative emotional significance to information about the self. This conclusion is supported by findings showing increased rCBF in the insular cortex during lactate-induced panic *(47)*, anticipatory anxiety *(48)*, phobia *(49)*, and perception of temperature and pain *(50–53)*.

George et al. (54) studied alterations of rCBF in subjects who recalled from own personal experience happy or sad situations while viewing a picture that displayed a corresponding facial expression. In contrast to the studies using recall from film-generated emotions *(45,46)*, lateralization of rCBF activity changes was found. Moreover, some regions exhibited decreased instead of increased flow. Again, in this experimental design, sad situations were associated with increased rCBF in limbic regions, including the anterior cingulate, medial prefrontal and temporal cortices, the brainstem, the thalamus, and the caudate/putamen. Happiness, however, did not induce increases of rCBF but generated decreased flows only in the right prefrontal and temporal–parietal cortical regions. These observations suggest that in healthy volunteers, different neuronal networks mediate specific emotions, an hypothesis that was later substantiated by Paradiso et al. *(55)* in film-generated emotions.

2.3.2. Depression

The major depressive syndrome consists of a pathologic disturbance of mood and affect in which a persistent negative emotional state is accompanied by changes in energy, sleep, appetite, activity, and cognition. Sometimes, major depression is considered as a state of "emotional pain." The neuronal substrate underlying occurrence of depressive syndromes is not clear and investigators have used PET or MRI to visualize neurobiological substrates of both unipolar and bipolar depression. This has led to the definition of neuroanatomical circuits. Some imaging studies point to localized lesions within this circuitry; others argue in favor of generalized structural alterations as an underlying cause of these mood disorders.

Some fluorine-18 fluorodeoxyglucose (FDG) or H_2 ^{15}O PET or single photon emission computed tomography (SPECT) imaging studies showed decreased global brain metabolism or blood flow in untreated unipolar depressive patients *(56,57)*. More often, however, regional decreases of blood flow or metabolism have been reported. In unipolar depressive patients, such decreases were localized to the dorsolateral prefrontal cortex, bilateral or on the left side, the caudate nucleus, the thalamus, the temporal, cingulate and parietal cortices, and the left putamen *(58–61)*. Various antidepressive treatments, either pharmacological, sleep-deprivation, or electroconvulsive therapy, generated alterations of baseline activity in the left prefrontal cortex, the anterior cingulate cortex, the amygdala, the orbitofrontal cortex, the hippocampus, the infratemporal cortex, the right putamen, or the right thalamus *(62–64)*. Drevets et al. *(59)* have reported increased regional blood flow in the left prefrontal cortex and the left amygdala in a unipolar familiar-type depression. Left prefrontal activity was elevated in the depressed but not in the remitted phase, whereas the activity of the left amygdala was unrelated to the phase of the depression. This finding suggests that the activity of the left amygdala and prefrontal cortex are respectively trait and state abnormalities of unipolar depression. The prefrontal region in the Drevets et al. *(59)* study contained a portion of the lateral orbital cortex and extended beyond the orbital gyrus into the inferior frontal gyrus and the anterior cingulate gyrus. Interestingly, a recent FDG PET study has provided evidence for a role of the rostral anterior cingulate cortex in treatment responses. Nonresponders were characterized by hypometabolism in the rostral anterior cingulate cortex compared to controls, in contrast to the responders who showed hypermetabolism in this part of the cerebral cortex *(60)*.

Using MRI on depressive patients, structural abnormalities have been identified in the frontal lobe of unipolar, but not of bipolar, depressives. Other studies showed temporal lobe asymmetries in bipolar depressive patients that could not be reproduced. Also, evidence of thalamic abnormalities and reduced amygdala–hippocampus complex volumes await further replication. Smaller putamen and caudate volumes, reported in unipolar depression, highlight a potential role of the basal ganglia in mood disorders. Interestingly, both in the unipolar and bipolar patients, the cerebellar volume was reduced also. For a review on structural abnormalities in depression ref. *65*.

2.3.3. Phobia, Anxiety, and Obsessive–Compulsive Disorder

The central nervous system correlates of simple phobic fear were sparsely investigated using rCBF PET. Visual phobogenic (pictures of spiders) and neutral stimuli triggered increased rCBF in the secondary visual cortex and reduced flow in the hippocampus, the prefrontal, the orbitofrontal, the temporopolar, and the posterior cingulate cortex in patients suffering from symptomatic spider phobia *(66).* However, Rauch et al. *(67),* using a similar approach, observed elevated rCBF in the right inferior frontal cortex, right posterior orbitofrontal cortex, bilateral in the insular cortex, the putamen, and the brainstem during symptom-provocation tests in a patient group composed of simple phobic, obsessive–compulsive (OCD), and posttraumatic stress disorder patients. rCBF changes in the brainstem were significantly correlated to subjective anxiety ratings and, most likely, localized in a region composed of the locus coeruleus, the parabrachial nucleus, the ventral tegmental area, and the periaqueductal gray *(67).*

The most common differences between OCD and control subjects observed with FDG PET or metabolic scanning was hypermetabolism of the orbitofrontal and the anterior cingulate cortex, the caudate nucleus, and the thalamus *(68).* Treatment responses were associated to decreased hypermetabolism in the right caudate and orbitofrontal cortex *(69,70).* However, the value of such observations can be questioned when other studies report hypometabolism in these same structures.

McGuire et al. *(71),* not using the common region of interest method but a statistical parametric pixel-by-pixel approach to analyze rCBF data from 12 successive scans to correlate symptom intensity to both positive and negative flow changes, found positive correlation's with blood-flow changes in the right orbitofrontal cortex, the ventral putamen and tail of the caudate nucleus, the right thalamus, the left posterior cingulate gyrus, the left hippocampus, and the left cuneus nucleus. The flow in the right temporoparietal region, the left middle temporal gyrus, and the right middle frontal gyrus were negatively correlated to symptom intensities.

A number of neuroimaging studies have characterized rCBF during lactate- *(47)* or cholecystokinin 4 (CCK4)-induced *(72)* anxiety attacks in healthy volunteers and patients suffering of panic disorder. Both studies showed provocation-induced increases of rCBF bilateral in the temporal poles. There is some discussion about activation of this temporal region in anxiety because Benkelfat et al. *(72)* noted that the locus of activation was situated outside of the cortical rim, most likely in the domain of the temporal artery. Lactate-induced anxiety produced increased rCBF in a number of other regions, including bilateral the insular cortex, the claustrum, the lateral putamen, and the superior colliculus and the left cerebellar vermis. More or less the same regions showed increased rCBF during CCK4-induced anxiety, albeit that the left-hemisphere activation dominated and the claustrum–insular–amygdala region was attributed a significant role in anxiety. Moreover, CCK4-induced anxiety triggered a rCBF increase within the left anterior cingulate cortex. Anticipatory anxiety to CCK4 treatment caused rCBF increases in the orbitofrontal cortex and the cerebellar vermis.

2.3.4. Summary

Neuroimaging studies aimed at characterization of nervous circuitry of mood and affect have implicated a large number of brain structures in regulation of emotional states. Although this has not yet led to a clear image of nervous circuitry of emotions, all imaging studies share altered metabolism and/or regional brain activity in a limited number of tightly interconnected forebrain regions (Fig. 1). In both patients and volunteers, emotional stimuli triggered alterations of regional brain activity in the following cortical areas: the prefrontal (dorsolateral, lateral, and medial), anterior insular, anterior cingulate, orbitofrontal, and temporal fields. Subcortical regions showing altered metabolism or flow in the various designs were the hippocampus and amygdala, the caudate nucleus, the putamen, the thalamus and hypothalamus, and parts of the midbrain, including the locus coeruleus, ventral tegmental area, periaqueductal gray, and the parabrachial region. A number of recent studies implicated the cerebellum in regulation of mood and affect.

In general, healthy subjects showed mainly hypermetabolism or increased rCBF during various emotional stimuli.

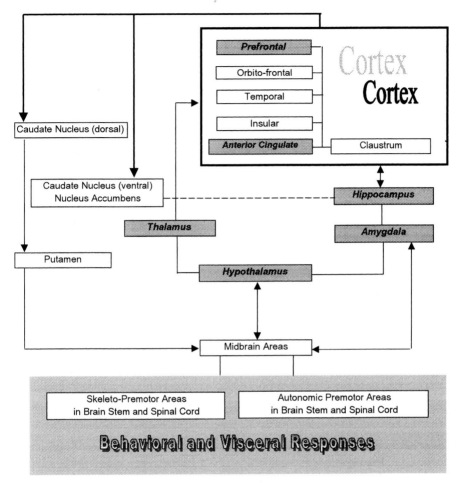

Fig. 1. Hypothetical model of limbic forebrain circuitry for emotions emerging from neuroimaging studies in mood disorders. Connections between highlighted structures illustrate the limbic system as originally defined by Papez *(9)*.

Only incidentally, a decreased metabolism or rCBF was reported in volunteers during film-generated recall of happy situations. Patients suffering of disorders of mood and affect showed mainly hypometabolism and/or decreased rCBF after exposure to symptom-inducing stimuli. Various treatments of mood disorders were reflected in alterations of rCBF in the aforementioned areas, which implies that, indeed, a dysfunction of these regions may be part of the pathophysiological mechanism underlying the disease.

3. Neuronal Substrates of Cardiovascular Regulation

For a longtime, scientists have shown interest in the neuronal substrate for cardiovascular regulation to understand, among others the autonomic changes associated with emotions. Various methods have been and are utilized to characterize this circuitry in experimental animals. First, selective electrolytic brain lesions were employed and, later, tract tracing and neurophysiological and neuropharmacological examinations were introduced. Recently, human in vivo neuroimaging has been added to these research tools (see Chapter 10). In this section, results of fundamental research in this field will be reviewed.

3.1. Autonomic Innervation of the Heart

The heart is innervated both by sympathetic and parasympathetic autonomic nerves, like all other visceral organs. The autonomic heart innervation is comprised of afferent sensory and efferent motor fibers, which are associated to ganglia that contain either the primary sensory and/or the postganglionic autonomic cells. Two ganglion types have been recognized at the efferent level: the intrinsic and extrinsic cardiac ganglia that contain respectively, apart from the local circuit neurons, sympathetic and parasympathetic, and sympathetic postganglionic cells *(73)*. The neurotransmitters of the postganglionic parasympathetic and sympathetic neurons, acetylcholine and norepinephrine, are colocalized with various neuropeptides. The cardiac postganglionic sympathetic cells are located predominantly in the cranial poles of the stellate ganglia bilaterally. A small number of such postganglionic cells have been identified in the middle cervical and the mediastinal ganglia and in the superior cervical ganglia of dogs and primates. Isolated sympathetic postganglionic cells have been found in the intrinsic cardiac ganglia as well. These latter cells can modulate cardiac activity to a considerable degree, as neurophysiological studies have demonstrated *(73,74)*. The parasympathetic postganglionic cells are situated in the intrinsic cardiac ganglia, which are located in the fatty connective tissue lying on the epicardium, in intimate association with one or more nerve trunks *(73)*. Seven such intrinsic ganglia have been identified in the dog: four associated to the atrial and three to the ventricular tissue. Intrinsic cardiac ganglia located on the atria modify primarily, but not exclusively, atrial activities, whereas those located on the ventricles modify primarily, but not exclusively, ventricular activity *(73,74)*. The intrinsic cardiac ganglia have been referred to as the "brain of the heart" because, apparently, they can fulfill an important role in regulation of cardiac activity. To fulfill such a role, it is important that the intrinsic ganglia also contain local circuit neurons and, as indicated earlier, sympathetic postganglionic cells.

Classically, the nodose and dorsal root ganglia have been recognized as locations of primary sensory neurons associated with the central cardiovascular reflexes. Recently, however, it has become clear from neurophysiological studies that some primary afferent neurons also are located in the intrinsic cardiac ganglia *(73,74)*. The nerve supply of the heart is reviewed in detail in Chapter 1 and discussed here briefly only to show the relation with the preganglionic cells in the brainstem and thoracic spinal cord, which serve as the common final path in central nervous system cardiovascular control.

3.2. Preganglionic Autonomic Neurons

Preganglionic sympathetic cells of the heart have been localized in the intermediolateral cell group (IML) of the thoracic spinal cord. The levels from which such cardiac sympathetic efferent nerves originate are a matter of discussion and may be species dependent. Retrograde-labeled cells were found in the IML from the cervical 8 (C8) to the thoracic 9 (Th9) levels after tracer injections into the stellate ganglion of the rat *(75,76)*. Transneuronal retrograde viral tracing showed virus-infected cells in the IML of Th1–Th8 both after inoculation of the stellate ganglion *(77,78)* and the ventricular myocardium *(79,80)* of the rat. Some additional viral labeling of IML cells occurred at the Th8–Th11 level in the latter study. However, this Th8–Th11 IML labeling was attributed to transneuronal infection in the spinal cord, as it was present only after long postinoculation survival times and not after 3 d, when Th1–Th8 infections were shown. Pyner and Coote *(75,76)* and Jansen et al. *(77)* have demonstrated that double labeling of preganglionic sympathetic cells is limited to less than 1% of the population after tracer injections into the stellate ganglion and the adrenal gland. These observations support the suggestion from viral tracing that the preganglionic sympathetic cells for the left and right ventricular myocardium and sinus node regions occupy slightly different positions in the upper thoracic IML *(80)*. Morphological studies, however, have not shown any spatial representation and no left/right localization of efferent nerves innervating different cardiac regions in the dog *(74)*.

Preganglionic parasympathetic cells of the heart have been identified in the brainstem bilaterally, in the periambiguus area (AMB), the dorsal motor vagus nucleus (DMnX) and dispersed in the parvocellular reticular formation (PCRt) between these two nuclei *(74,79–84)*. The majority of the preganglionic parasympathetic cells are situated in the posterior periambiguus area (80%) and only a small proportion is located in the lateral part of the dorsal motor vagus nucleus (15%) and the lateral PCRt (5%) *(80)*. Lateralization of viral-labeling patterns was reported in the DMnX and the AMB after myocardial pseudorabies infection in the rat *(80)*. DMnX and AMB left- and right-side dominance occurred after inoculation of the right and left ventricular myocardium, respectively. Evidence of lateralization at the preganglionic parasympathetic level, however, is not supported by other studies using different tracing techniques and/or injection size, virus strains, or species *(74,82–85)*. Physiological investigations in the dog do support a lateralization, and have shown distinct effects of right and left vagus nerve stimulation on the sinoatrial and atrioventricular node activity, and on regional contractile functions of the heart *(86,87)*.

3.3. Higher-Order Cardiovascular Circuitry

Higher-order circuitry for cardiovascular regulation has been characterized with different anatomical tract-tracing techniques. Much information was obtained with the current classical retrograde and anterograde tracing methods such as horseradish peroxidase (HRP), tritiated aminoacid autoradiography, and lectin immunocytochemistry that gave us overwhelming information about connections of selected regions in the brain. By combining the results from these studies with neurophysiological and neuropharmacological data, a hypothetical model of cardiovascular control circuitry has been constructed. An important drawback has been the lack of a direct anatomical verification method that could show labeling of higher-order structures after injections of tracers in the heart. Recently, this has become possible after the introduction of a retrograde transneuronal viral-labeling technique *(88–90)*. Using pseudo-rabies virus and inoculation of various parts of the heart or the stellate ganglion, others and we have characterized cardiovascular control circuitry in the rat *(77–83,91)*. Data from these studies will be used here to illustrate the cytoarchitecture of the cardiac control circuitry (Fig. 2).

3.3.1. Medulla Oblongata

In addition to the parasympathetic preganglionic cells in the DMnX and the AMB, higher-order viral infections have been identified in a limited number of areas in the medulla oblongata (Fig. 3) after myocardial inoculations. Infected cells were located in the rostral (RVL) and caudal ventrolateral reticular formation (CVL), the raphe pallidus, raphe obscures and raphe magnus nuclei, the nucleus of the solitary tract (NTS), the parvocellular and gigantocellular reticular formation, the caudal spinal trigeminal nucleus, and the prepositus hypoglossal nucleus *(79,80,82,83)*. Using spinal cord transection at Th1, we have corroborated earlier studies showing a role for the raphe pallidus *(88,92–94)* and the ventral reticular formation *(88,89)* in control of sympathetic heart innervation. The raphe magnus, as a final pathway of limbic descending modulating systems, controls the transfer of sen-

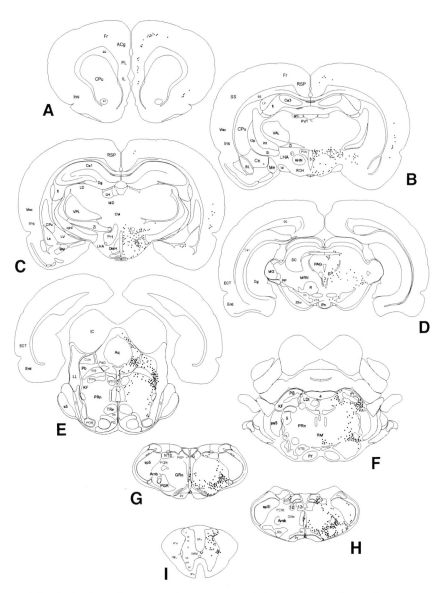

Fig. 2. Series of transverse sections of the rat brain from the rostral forebrain (A) to the thoracic spinal level (I), illustrating the locations of retrograde transneuronally labeled cells after Pseudorabies virus infection of the left ventricular myocardium *(79,80)*. The infection pattern was bilateral but for topographical clarification shown on the right side only. Legend: 10, dorsal motor vagus nucleus; 5, trigeminal motor nucleus; ac, anterior commissure; ACg, anterior cingulate gyrus; AHN, anterior hypothalamic area; Amb, nucleus ambiguus; BL, basolateral amygdala; BM, basomedial amygdala; cc, corpus callosum; Ce, central amygdala; CM, central–medial thalamic nucleus; CPu, caudate putamen;

brainstem. The amygdaloid complex comprises a heterogeneous group of cytoarchitectonically, histochemically, and connectionally distinct nuclei. With respect to the regulation of cardiovascular functions, the central amygdala (CEA) has been identified as the most important structure in the amygdaloid complex. Viral-tracing studies have shown retrograde transneuronal infections in the central amygdala after inoculation of the myocardium *(79,80)* and the stellate ganglion *(78,81)*. Much of the infection pattern in the central amygdala remained after spinal cord transection at Th1 *(81)*, suggesting a close relation of the CEA to the parasympathetic nervous system. Accordingly, bilateral lesions of the central amygdala have caused disruption of characteristic parasympathetic responses both to conditioned and unconditioned aversive foot shock *(167,168)*. Electrical stimulations of the central amygdala have produced a complex pattern of cardiovascular changes. Bradycardic responses were elicited during electrical stimulation of the medial–anterior CEA in conscious rabbits *(169)*. However, electrical stimulation of the CEA yielded pressor and tachycardic responses in conscious rats *(170)* and depressor and bradycardic effects in anesthetized rats *(170)*. This latter response in anesthetized animals was attributed to depressant effects of anesthetics on the vasoconstriction in renal and mesenteric system that causes the rise in arterial pressure in awake animals *(171)*. More recent literature *(172)* attributes the central amygdala an important role in neuronal circuitry that controls effects mediated by the parasympathetic nervous system. Infusion of CRH in the central amygdala, for example, diminished the cardiac parasympathetic drive in awake rats *(173)*. These effects are most likely mediated by peptidergic [CRH, neurotensin, somatostatin, substance P, and galanin *(174)*] efferent projections from the CEA to the caudal medulla oblongata and, in particular, to the NTS and the preganglionic parasympathetic DMnX and AMB *(100,107,175,176)*. Projections from the CEA have been traced also to higher-order cardioresponsive sites, including the PVN, the LHA, and the DMH, and to the parabrachial complex, the locus coeruleus, and the PAG

(177–179). This connectivity pattern illustrates the important role of the central amygdala in cardiovascular control. As a key component of the limbic system, the CEA can affect cardiovascular responsiveness by modulation of neuronal activity at various levels of the cardiovascular control circuitry, including the autonomic preganglionic parasympathetic level and the baroreceptor reflex arc.

3.3.3.4. CEREBRAL CORTEX

Dampney *(102)*, Loewy *(132)*, and Verberne and Owens *(133)* have reviewed the role of various parts of the cerebral cortex in cardiovascular regulation. For information about connections and functions of the various cortical areas in cardiovascular regulation, the previous reviews are recommended.

Clinical, physiological, and anatomical observations have yielded evidence for a role of the medial prefrontal and insular cortex in cardiovascular regulation. Recently, we have added further anatomical evidence by identifying virus-infected cells in these cortical fields after myocardial inoculation *(80,81)*. Other virus-infected cells were located in the anterior cingulate, frontal, and retrosplenial cortical fields.

3.3.3.4.1. Prefrontal Cortex. The medial prefrontal cortex has been subdivided in the dorsal prelimbic and ventral infralimbic cortices on bases of different afferent and efferent connectivities. The mediodorsal thalamic nucleus innervates the prelimbic, but not the infralimbic cortex *(180)*. The infralimbic, but not the prelimbic, cortex projects to the NTS *(133)*. Descending projections to the preganglionic sympathetic cell groups of the thoracic cord originate from the infralimbic area *(181)*. Bacon and Smith *(182)* provided anatomical and neurophysiological evidence for a direct projection from the prelimbic cortex to the central autonomic area of the thoracic cord. Both the pre-limbic and the infralimbic cortices innervate various other areas that have been implicated in cardiovascular regulation, including the ventrolateral reticular formation, the PAG, the amygdala, and the hypothalamus *(133)*. Medial prefrontal afferent innervation originates from the ventrolateral reticular formation, the mediodorsal thalamus, the insular cortex, and the hippocampus *(133)*, but not from the baroreceptive part of the NTS *(23)*.

Electrical stimulation of the medial prefrontal cortex has generated depressor responses in anesthetized rats *(182,183)* and pressor and depressor responses in awake rats *(184)* and rabbits *(185)*, respectively. Chemical stimulations repeatedly have elicited hypotension and bradycardic responses and this has led to the conclusion that the medial prefrontal cortex exerts an inhibitory influence on sympathoexcitatory systems *(133)*. Recent investigations of the medial prefrontal cortex provided evidence for a role in the occurrence of differential hemodynamic effects in various vascular beds, but this mechanism awaits further characterization *(183)*.

Polysynaptic descending pathways most likely mediate medial prefrontal sympathoinhibitory effects, because ablation of the LHA could reduce renal sympathetic responses elicited by stimulation of the infralimbic cortex *(186)*. Moreover, blood pressure and heart rate responses triggered from the infralimbic cortex were decreased after glutamate microinjections into the LHA *(187)*. The PAG and the ventrolateral reticular formation are other terminal fields of the medial prefrontal cortex that exert a strong sympathoexcitatory influence. It is tempting to speculate that inhibitory medial prefrontal effects in the PAG and/or the ventrolateral brainstem yield the depressor responses. Indeed, Verberne *(183)* has provided evidence for inhibition of ventrolateral reticular sympathoexcitatory neurons by the medial prefrontal cortex. Alternatively, medial prefrontal–NTS pathways could mediate depressor responses. This mechanism has found support in a study that showed the induction of Fos expression in the baroreceptive part of the NTS and in the sympathoinhibitory CVL after electrical stimulation of the infralimbic cortex *(133)*.

Anatomical and neurophysiological studies have demonstrated a projection from the CA1 field of the hippocampus to the pre-limbic and infralimbic cortex *(188–190)*. This, most likely, glutamatergic pathway has been shown to mediate the cardiorespiratory responses elicited by electrical stimulation of the hippocampus *(191,192)*. Terminal fields of hippocampal efferents in the infralimbic cortex have been identified near cells that project to the NTS *(192)*. This pathway may relate the hippocampus to alteration of baroreceptor reflex arc sensitivity in emotional situations.

        3.3.3.4.2. Insular Cortex. The insular cortex (IC) is a long structure situated dorsally from the rhinal sulcus, which extends rostrally to the level of the olfactory bulb and caudally to the amygdala. The rostral insular cortex may also be referred to as lateral prefrontal cortex.

        In both the rostral and caudal insular cortices, virus-infected neurons were identified after inoculation of the myocardium *(80,81)* and substantiated evidence of insular cortex participation in cardiovascular control circuitry *(193,194)*. Spinal cord transection at Th1 prohibited virus infection of the rostral IC and reduced the number of virus-positive cells in the posterior IC *(81)*. Afferent innervation of the insular cortex originates from the parabrachial nucleus, the ventral posterior and mediodorsal thalamic nuclei, and the lateral hypothalamic area *(96,133,195)*. Inputs from the visceral/baroreceptive caudal NTS have not been demonstrated *(23)* and a sparse innervation arising from the ventrolateral reticular formation is debated *(133)*.

        Electrical stimulation of the rostral insular cortex elicited depressor responses *(133)*. Direct projections from the rostral IC to the preganglionic parasympathetic and sympathetic heart innervation have not been described; therefore, this response must be mediate by polysynaptic pathways. Inhibition of sympathoexcitatory neurons in the RVL by a GABAergic mechanism has been demonstrated during rostral IC stimulation *(196)*. GABAergic cells recruited by the rostral IC most likely are located in the CVL, the region that can inhibit the baroreceptor reflex. Alternatively, projections from the rostral IC to the NTS *(197,198)* could mediate the depressor response, which, however, is highly unlikely because the response is inhibited by neurochemical lesions of the lateral hypothalamic area *(133)*, implicating a key role for the LHA in rostral IC-induced cardiovascular events.

Stimulation of the caudal IC has triggered both depressor and pressor responses that were associated respectively with tachycardia and bradycardia depending on the location *(133)*, pressor responses deriving from the rostral and depressor responses from the caudal part. Viral-tracing studies nicely corroborated this viscerotopy of the caudal IC *(81,199)*, infection of the posterior caudal IC. Projections from the posterior insular cortex to the NTS have been described in several species *(133)* but this pathway does not mediate cardiovascular events elicited by IC stimulation. Interruption of synaptic transmission in the NTS with cobalt could not prevent posterior IC-induced pressor responses in the rat *(186)*. Intermediate structures in polysynaptic descending pathways from the posterior IC are the ventrolateral reticular formation, the parabrachial complex *(96)*, the central amygdala *(169)*, and the hypothalamus *(96,186,195)*. Projections from the posterior IC to the sympathoexcitatory RVL have not been demonstrated, and inhibition of the synaptic transmission in the parabrachial complex with cobalt could not block IC-induced cardiovascular responses *(186)*. Firing patterns of central amygdaloid cells were affected by IC stimulation in conscious rabbits *(200)*, but other studies have shown that IC-central amygdala projections do not participate in the generation of conditioned bradycardic responses *(201,202)*. Microinjections of cobalt into the posterior LHA blocked pressor responses elicited by stimulation of the posterior IC *(186)*, implicating participation of the lateral hypothalamic–rostral ventrolateral reticular pathway *(100)* in cardiovascular control from the posterior IC *(96,133,186,187)*.

3.3.3.4.3. Anterior Cingulate Cortex. Participation of the anterior cingulate cortex (ACg) in regulation of autonomic functions has been demonstrated in various species, including humans *(32,203)*. Anatomical evidence for a role of the ACg in cardiovascular control circuitry has been obtained with retrograde transneuronal viral tract tracing. Virus-posi-

tive cells were identified in the ACg after myocardial inoculation both in spinal cord transected *(81)* and intact rats
(79,80). Monosynaptic tract-tracing studies have shown ACg
projections to the sympathetic thoracic intermediolateral cell
group *(181)*, the parasympathetic preganglionic DMnX *(181)*,
the NTS *(197)*, the PAG and the amygdala *(32,107)*. This set
of connections gives the ACg access to both the preganglionic parasympathetic and sympathetic heart innervating systems and to autonomic balance and baroreceptor sensitivity
modulating areas at higher-order levels of the neuraxis. As
may be predicted from this connectivity pattern, both
increases and decreases of heart rate and blood pressure have
been elicited during ACg electrical stimulation in cats, dogs,
and monkeys *(32)*. In particular, areas 24c and 25 of the
human cingulate gyrus have been associated to regulation
of cardiovascular, respiratory, digestive, and thermoregulatory systems and to release of the gonadal and adrenal hormones *(32,203,204)*.

Apart from projections from ACg areas 24 and 25 to
autonomic nervous system controlling regions, the rostral
ACg innervates all major components of the basal ganglia,
including the nucleus accumbens, the ventral striatum, and
the dorsolateral caudate nucleus *(205)*. These connections
illustrate a role for the rostral ACg in modulation of
skeletomotor system activity too. Devinsky et al. *(32)* postu-
late, on the basis of this set of connections, that the rostral
ACg, including areas 24 and 25 are engaged in executive functions associated with affect. Functional neuroimaging
(51–53,206) and neurophysiological *(207)* studies have
implicated the ACg in (cardiac) pain perception and in the
affective components of pain and motor-response selection
in particular.

Various cortical and subcortical areas supply input to
areas 24 and 25 of the ACg, including the retrosplenial,
orbitofrontal, insular, temporopolar, perirhinal, entorhinal,
parasubicular, and parahippocampal areas *(203)*. Subcortical afferents originate from the nucleus accumbens *(205)*, the
midline and anterior thalamic nuclei *(208)*, the amygdala

like body temperature, body weight, and diurnal rhythms. Most likely, this is achieved via genetically programmed or "learned" autonomic and neuroendocrine responses. Typical behavioral responses related to a fight-or-flight response have been elicited from the hypothalamus (217), which may be an additional argument for a hierarchical strucure of emotion and heart controlling sytems.

5. Conclusions

Possible interactions at different levels of the neuraxis of emotion and cardiovascular regulation circuitry were described to define an anatomical substrate for emotion-related cardiovascular responses. Clinical and preclinical anatomical data related to substrates for emotions and cardiovascular regulation and neurophysiological studies yield an image of a hierarchically organized system for occurrence of such emotion-related responses. Forebrain limbic circuitry, basically structured around the limbic system model of Papez, is held responsible for emotional responses and dysfunction in various psychiatric diseases, such as mood and anxiety disorders. Cardiovascular activity is regulated by a system comprised of various tightly connected diencephalic, midbrain, brainstem, and spinal structures, in which the hypothalamus is functioning as the highest level of command. The hypothalamus controls metabolic homeostasis, including cardiovascular functions, around setpoints of body weight, temperature, blood glucose levels, and so forth by using genetically programmed or learned response patterns, involving a fine-tuned behavior, neuroendocrine and autonomic interaction. Spontaneously or in response to selective stimuli, emotions can be generated in the forebrain limbic circuitry. The emotional response involves initiation of appropriate behavior from the hypothalamus, the output structure of the limbic forebrain circuitry. The behavioral response, initiated by the limbic forebrain circuitry, emerges from the programmed or learned patterns of behavior, neuroendocrine and autonomic interaction that are "stored" at the hypothalamic level as part of its role in the maintenance of metabolic homeostasis. The limbic forebrain monitors the emotional load of incoming sensory information that is supplied by feedback systems after initiation of the emotional response. This monitoring is important for fine-tuning or the termination of the response and may involve interventions from the limbic forebrain through selective output pathways at hypothalamic and/or midbrain, brainstem, or spinal level.

References

1. LeDoux, J. E. (1987) Emotion, in *Handbook of Physiology, The Nervous System, V: Higher Cortical Functions in the Brain* (Plum, F. and Mountcastle, V. B., eds.), American Physiological Society, Bethesda, MD, pp. 419–459.
2. LeDoux, J. E. (1996) *The Emotional Brain.* Simon and Schuster, New York.
3. Nieuwenhuys, R., Voogd, J., and Van Huijzen, C. (1988) *The Human Central Nervous System: A Synopsis and Atlas*, 3rd ed., Springer-Verlag, Berlin.
4. Nieuwenhuys, R. (1996) The greater limbic system, the emotional motor system and the brain. *Prog. Brain Res.* **107**, 551–580.
5. Holstege, G. (1992) The emotional motor System. *Eur. J. Morph.* **30**, 67–81.
6. Cannon, W. B. (1927) The James–Lange theory of emotions: a critical examination and an alternative theory. *Am. J. Physiol.* **39**, 106–124.
7. Bard, P. (1928) A diencephalic mechanism for the expression of rag with special reference to the sympathetic nervous system. *Am. J. Physiol.* **84**, 490–515.
8. Bard, P. (1929) The central representation of the sympathetic nervous system. *Arch. Neurol. Psychiatry* **22**, 230–246.
9. Papez, J. W. (1937) A proposed mechanism of emotion. *Arch. Neurol. Psychiatry* **79**, 217–224.
10. Kluver, H. and Bucy, P. C. (1937) "Psychic blindness" and other symptoms following bilateral temporal lobectomy in rhesus monkeys. *Am. J. Physiol.* **119**, 352–353.
11. Kluver, H. and Bucy, P. C. (1939) Preliminary analysis of functions of the temporal lobe in monkeys. *Arch. Neurol. Psychiatry* **42**, 979–1000.
12. McLean, P. D. (1949) Psychosomatic disease and the visceral brain. Recent developments bearing on Papez theory of emotion. *Psychosom. Med.* **11**, 338–353.
13. McLean, P. D. (1952) Some psychiatric implications of physiological studies on frontotemporal portion of limbic system (visceral brain). *Electroencephalogr. Clin. Neurophysiol.* **4**, 407–418.

14. Nauta, W. J. H. (1958) Hippocampal projections and related neural pathway to the mid-brain in the cat. *Brain* **81**, 319–341.
15. Domesick, V. (1986) Cross-roads of limbic and basal ganglia circuitry: neuroanatomical substrates of mood and movement. 4th World Congress of Biological Psychiatry. *Int. J. Neurosci.* **39**, 18.
16. Brodal, A. (1982) *Neurological Anatomy*, Oxford University Press, New York.
17. Swanson, L. W. (1983) The hippocampus and the concept of the limbic system, in *Neurobiology of the Hippocampus* (Seifert, W., ed.), Academic, London, pp. 3–19.
18. Livingston, K. E. and Escobar, A. (1971) Anatomical bias of the limbic system concept. *Arch. Neurol.* **24**, 17–21.
19. Quirk, G. J., Armony, J. L., and LeDoux, J. E. (1997) Fear conditioning enhances different temporal components of tone-evoked spike trains in auditory cortex and lateral amygdala. *Neuron* **19**, 613–624.
20. LeDoux, J. E., Ruggiero, D. A., and Reis, D. J. (1985) Projections from anatomically defined regions of the medial geniculate body in the rat. *J. Comp. Neurol.* **242**, 182–213.
21. LeDoux, J. E., Farb, C. F., and Ruggiero, D. A. (1990) Topographic organization of neurons in the acoustic thalamus that project to the amygdala. *J. Neurosci.* **10**, 1043–1054.
22. Romanski, L. M., and LeDoux, J. E. (1993) Information cascade from primary auditory cortex to the amygdala: corticocortical and corticoamygdaloid projections of the temporal cortex in the rat. *Cereb. Cortex* **3**, 515–532.
23. Ter Horst, G. J. and Streefland, C. (1994) Ascending projections of the solitary tract nucleus, in *Nucleus of the solitary tract.* (Barraco, I. R. A., ed.), CRC, Boca Raton, FL, pp. 93–103.
24. Charney, D. S. and Deutch, A. (1996) A functional neuroanatomy of anxiety and fear: implications for the pathophysiology and treatment of anxiety disorders. *Crit. Rev. Neurobiol.* **10**, 419–446.
25. Stumpf, W. E. and Jennes, L. (1984) The A-B-C (allocortex–brainstem–core) circuitry of endocrine–autonomic integration and regulation: a proposed hypothesis on the anatomical functional relationships between estradiol sites of action and peptidergic–aminergic neuronal systems. *Peptides* **5**, 221–226.
26. Cummings, J. L. (1993) Frontal-Subcortical circuits and human behavior. *Arch. Neurol.* **50**, 873–880.
27. Robinson, R. G., Kubos, K. L., Starr, L. B., Rao, K., and Price, T. R. (1984) Mood disorders in stroke patients: importance of location of lesion. *Brain* **107**, 81–93.
28. Starkstein, S. E., Robinson, R. G., and Price, T. R. (1987) Comparison of cortical and subcortical lesions in the production of post-stroke mood disorders. *Brain* **110**, 1045–1059.

29. Cummings, J. L. and Mendez, M. F. (1984) Secondary mania with focal cerebrovascular lesions. *Am. J. Psychiatry* **141,** 1084–1087.

30. Starkstein, S. E., Boston, J. D., and Robinson, R. G. (1988) Mechanisms of mania after brain injury: 12 case reports and review of the literature. *J. Nerv. Ment. Dis.* **176,** 87–100.

31. Foltz, E. L., and White, L. E. (1962) Pain 'relief' by frontal cingulumotomy. *J. Neurosurg.* **19,** 89–100.

32. Devinsky, O., Morrell, M. J., and Vogt, B. A. (1995) Contributions of the anterior cingulate cortex to behaviour. *Brain* **118,** 279–306.

33. Meyer, G., McElhaney, M., Martin, W., and McGraw, C. P. (1973) Stereotactic cingulotomy with results of acute stimulation and serial psychological testing, in *Surgical Approaches in Psychiatry* (Laitinen, L. V. and Livingston, K. E., eds.), University Park Press, Baltimore, MD, pp. 39–58.

34. Laitinen, L. V. and Vilkki, J. (1973) Observations on the transcallosal emotional connections, in *Surgical Approaches in Psychiatry* (Laitinen, L. V. and Livingston, K. E., eds.), University Park Press, Baltimore, MD, pp. 74–80.

35. Hassler, R. and Dieckmann, G. (1970) Stereotatic treatment of tics and inarticulate cries or corporalia consideed as motor obsessional phenomena in Gilles de la Tourette's disease. *Rev. Neurol. (Paris)* **123,** 89–100.

36. Halgren, E., Walter, R. D., Cherlow, D. G., and Crandall, P. H. (1978) Mental phenomena evoked by electrical stimulation of the human hippocampal formation and amygdala. *Brain* **101,** 83–117.

37. Augustine, J. R. (1996) Circuitry and functional aspects of the insular lobe in primates including humans. *Brain Res. Rev.* **22,** 229–244.

38. Breiter, H. C., Etcoff, N. L., Whalen, P. J., Kennedy, W. A., Rauch, S. L., Buckner, R. L., et al. (1996) Responses and habituation of the human amygdala during visual processing of facial expression. *Neuron* **17,** 875–887.

39. LeBar, K. S., LeDoux, J. E., Spencer, D. D., and Phelps, E. A. (1995) Impaired fear conditioning following unilateral temporal lobectomy in humans. *J. Neurosci.* **15,** 6846–6855.

40. Scott, S. K., Young, A. W., Calder, A. J., Hellawell, D. J., Aggleton, J. P. and Johnson, M. (1997) Impaired auditory recognition of fear and anger following bilateral amygdala lesions. *Nature* **385,** 254–257.

41. Morris, J. S., Frith, C. D., Perrett, D. I., Rowland, D., Young, A. W., Calder, A. J., et al. (1996) A differential neural response in the human amygdala to fearful and happy facial expressions. *Nature* **383,** 812–815.

42. Angrilli, A., Mauri, A., Palomba, D., Flor, H., Birbaumer, N., Sartori, G., et al. (1996) Startle reflex and emotion modulation impairment after a right amygdala lesion. *Brain* **119,** 1991–2000.

43. Sano, K. and Mayanagi, Y. (1988) Posteromedial hypothalamotomy in the treatment of violent, aggressive behaviour. *Acta Neurochir. Suppl. Wien* **44**, 145–151.
44. Weddell, R. A. (1994) Effects of subcortical lesion site on human emotional behavior. *Brain Cogn.* **25**, 161–193.
45. Reiman, E. M., Lane, R. D., Ahern, G. L., Schwartz, G. E., Davidson, R. J., Friston, K. J., et al. (1997) Neuroanatomical correlates of externally and internally generated human emotion. *Am. J. Psychiatry* **154**, 918–925.
46. Lane, R. D., Reiman, E. M., Ahern, G. L., Schwartz, G. E., and Davidson, R. J. (1997) Neuroanatomical correlates of happiness, sadness, and disgust. *Am. J. Psychiatry* **154**, 926–933.
47. Reiman, E. M., Raichle, M. E., Robins, E., Mintun, M. A., Fusselman, M. J., Fox, P. T., et al. (1989) Neuroanatomical correlates of a lactate-induced anxiety attack. *Arch. Gen. Psychiatry* **46**, 493–500.
48. Reiman, E. M., Fusselman, M. J., Fox, P. T., and Raichle, M. E. (1989) Neuroanatomical correlates of anticipatory anxiety. *Science* **243**, 1071–1074.
49. Rauch, S. L., Savage, C. R., Alpert, N. M., Miguel, E. C., Baer, L., Breiter, H. C., et al. (1995) A positron emission tomography study of simple phobic symptom provocation. *Arch. Gen. Psychiatry* **52**, 20–28.
50. Craig, A. D., Reiman, E. M., Evans, A., and Bushnell, M. C. (1996) Functional imaging of an illusion of pain. *Nature* **384**, 258–260.
51. Rosen, S. D., Paulesu, E., Frith, C. D., Frackowiak, R. S. J., Davies, G. J. D., Jones, T., et al. (1994) Central nervous pathways mediating angina pectoris. *Lancet* **344**, 147–150.
52. Rosen, S. D., Paulesu, E., Nihoyannopoulos, P., Tousoulis, D., Frackowiak, R. S. J., Frith, C. D., et al. (1996) Silent ischemia as a central problem: regional brain activation compared in silent and painful myocardial ischemia. *Ann. Intern. Med.* **124**, 939–949.
53. Hautvast, R. W. M., Ter Horst, G. J., DeJong, B. M., DeJongste, M. J. L., Blanksma, P. K., Paans, A. M. J., et al., (1997) Relative changes in regional cerebral blood flow during spinal cord stimulation in patients with refractory angina pectoris. *Eur. J. Neurosci.* **9**, 1178–1183.
54. George, M. S., Ketter, T. A., Parekh, P. I., Horwitz, B., Herscovitch, P., and Post, R. M. (1995) Brain activity during transient sadness and happiness in healthy women. *Am. J. Psychiatry* **152**, 341–351.
55. Paradiso, S., Robinson, R. G., Andreasen, N. C., Downhill, J. E., Davidson, R. J., Kirchner, P. T., et al. (1997) Emotional activation of limbic circuitry in elderly normal subjects in a PET study. *Am. J. Psychiatry* **154**, 384–389.
56. Martinot, J. L., Hardy, P., Feline, A., Huret, J. D., Mazoyer, B., Attar-Levey, D., et al. (1990) Left prefrontal glucose hypome-

tabolism in the depressed state: a confirmation. *Am. J. Psychiatry* **147,** 1313–1317.

57. Baxter, L. R., Schwartz, J. M., Phelps, M. E., Mazziota, J. C., Guze, B. H., Selin, C. E., et al. (1989) Reduction of prefrontal cortex glucose metabolism common to three types of depression. *Arch. Gen. Psychiatry* **46,** 243.

58. Bremner, J. D., Innis, R. B., Salomon, R. M., Staib, L. H., Ng, C. K., Miller, H. L., et al. (1997) Positron Emission Tomography measurement of cerebral metabolic correlates of tryptophan depletion-induced depressive relapse. *Arch. Gen. Psychiatry* **54,** 364–374.

59. Drevets, W. C., Videen, T. O., Price, J. L., Preskom, S. H., Carmichael, S. T., and Raichle, M. E. (1992) A functional anatomical study of unipolar depression. *J. Neurosci.* **12,** 3628–3641.

60. Mayberg, H. S., Brannan, S. K., Mahurin, R. K., Jerabek, P. A., Brickman, J. S., Tekell, J. L., et al. (1997) Cingulate function in depression: a potential predictor of treatment response. *Neuroreport* **8,** 1057–1061.

61. Cummings, J. L. (1993) The neuroanatomy of depression. *J. Clin. Psychiat.* **54(Suppl.),** 14–20.

62. Ebert, D., Feistel, H., and Barocka, A. (1991) Effects of sleep deprivation on the limbic system and the frontal lobes in affective disorders: a study with Tc-99m-HMPAO SPECT. *Psychiatry Res.* **40,** 247–251.

63. Goodwin, G. M., Austin, M. P., Dougall, N., Ross, M., Murray, C., O'Carroll, R. E., et al. (1993) State changes in brain activity shown by the uptake of 99mTc-exametazine with single photon emission tomography in major depression before and after treatment. *J. Affect. Disord.* **29,** 245–255.

64. Wu, J. C., Gillin, J. C., Buchsbaum, M. S., Hershey, T., Johnson, J. C., and Bunney, W. E. (1992) Effect of sleep deprivation on brain metabolism of depressed patients. *Am. J. Psychiatry* **149,** 538–543.

65. Soares, J. C. and Mann, J. J. (1997) The anatomy of mood disorders—review of the structural neuroimaging studies. *Biol. Psychiatry* **41,** 86–106.

66. Fredrikson, M., Wik, G., Annas, P., Ericson, K., and Stone-Elander, S. (1995) Functional neuroanatomy of visually elicited simple phobic fear: additional data and theoretical analysis. *Psychophysiology* **32,** 43–48.

67. Rauch, S. L., Savage, C. R., Alpert, N. M., Fischman, A. J., and Jenike, M. A. (1997) The functional neuroanatomy of anxiety: a study of three disorders using positron emission tomography and symptom provocation. *Biol. Psychiatry* **42,** 446–452.

68. Maliza, A. L. and Nutt, D. J. (1997) Obsessive–compulsive disorder and the brain: what do brain-imaging techniques tell us? in *Obsessive-Compulsive Spectrum Disorders* (den Boer, J. A. and Westenberg, H. G. M., eds.), Synthesis, Amsterdam, pp. 107–122.

69. Baxter, L. R., Schwartz, J. M., Bergman, K., Szuba, M. P., Guze, B. H., Mazziota, J. C., et al. (1992) Caudate glucose metabolic rate changes with both drug and behavior therapy for obsessive compulsive disorder. *Arch. Gen. Psychiatry* **49**, 681–689.

70. Perani, D., Colombo, C., Bressi, S., Bonfanti, A., Grassi, F., Scarone, S., et al. (1995) [18F] FDG PET study in obsessive compulsive disorder. A clinical/metabolic correlation study after treatment. *Br. J. Psychiatry* **166**, 224–250.

71. McGuire, P. K., Bench, C. J., Frith, C. D., Marks, I. M., Frackowick, R. S. J., and Dolan, R. J. (1994) Functional anatomy of obsessive compulsive phenomena. *Br. J. Psychiatry* **164**, 459–468.

72. Benkelfat, C., Bradwejn, J., Meyer, E., Ellenbogen, M., Milot, S., Gjedde, A., et al. (1995) Functional neuroanatomy of CCK4-induced anxiety in normal healthy volunteers. *Am. J. Psychiatry* **152**, 1180–1184.

73. Ardell, J. L. (1994) Structure and function of mammalian intrinsic cardiac neurons, in *Neurocardiology* (Armour, J. A. and Ardell, J. L., eds.), Oxford University Press, New York, pp. 95–114.

74. Armour, J. A. (1994) Peripheral autonomic neuronal interactions in cardiac regulation, in *Neurocardiology* (Armour, J. A. and Ardell, J. L., eds.), Oxford University Press, New York, pp. 219–244.

75. Pyner, S. and Coote, J. H. (1994) A comparison between the adult rat and neonate rat of the architecture of sympathetic preganglionic neurons projecting to the superior cervical ganglion, stellate ganglion and adrenal medulla. *J. Auton. Nerv. Syst.* **48**, 153–166.

76. Pyner, S. and Coote, J. H. (1994) Evidence that sympathetic preganglionic neurons are arranged in target specific columns in the thoracic spinal cord of the rat. *J. Comp. Neurol.* **342**, 15–22.

77. Jansen, A. S. P., Farwell, D. G., and Loewy, A. D. (1993) Specificity of pseudorabies virus as a retrograde marker of sympathetic preganglionic neurons: implications for transneuronal labeling studies. *Brain Res.* **617**, 103–112.

78. Jansen, A. S. P. (1996) CNS cell groups that regulate the cardiosympathetic system, Thesis, University of Groningen, Groningen, The Netherlands.

79. Ter Horst, G. J., Van den Brink, A., Homminga, S. A., Hautvast, R. W. M., Rakhorst, G., Mettenleiter, T. C., et al. (1993) Transneuronal viral labelling of rat heart left ventricle controlling pathways. *Neuroreport* **4**, 1307–1310.

80. Ter Horst, G. J., Hautvast, R. W. M., De Jongste, M. J. L., and Korf, J. (1996) Neuroanatomy of cardiac activity-regulating circuitry: a transneuronal retrograde viral labeling study in the rat. *Eur. J. Neurosci.* **8**, 2029–2041.

81. Ter Horst, G. J. and Postema, F. (1997) Forebrain parasympathetic control of heart activity: retrograde transneuronal viral labeling in rats. *Am. J. Physiol.* **273**, H2926–H2930.

82. Standish, A., Enquist, L. W., and Schwaber, J. S. (1994) Innervation of the heart and its central medullary origin defined by viral tracing. *Science* **263,** 232–234.

83. Standish, A., Enquist, L. W., Escardo, J. A., and Schwaber, J. S. (1995) Central neural circuit innervating the rat heart defined by transneuronal transport of pseudorabies virus. *J. Neurosci.* **15,** 1998–2012.

84. Armour, J. A. and Hopkins, D. A. (1984) Anatomy of extrinsic efferent autonomic nerves and ganglia innervating the mammalian heart, in *Nervous Control of Cardiovascular Function* (Randall, W. C., ed.), Oxford University Press, New York, pp. 20–45.

85. Kalia, M. and Mesulam, M.-M. (1980) Brainstem projections of sensory and motor components of the vagus complex in the cat. II. Laryngeal, tracheobronchial, pulmonary, cardiac, and gastrointestinal branches. *J. Comp. Neurol.* **193,** 467–508.

86. Ardell, J. L. and Randall, W. C. (1986) Selective vagal innervation of sinoatrial and atrioventricular nodes in canine heart. *Am. J. Physiol.* **251,** H764–H773.

87. Ardell, J. L., Randall, W. C., Cannon, W. J., Schmacht, D. C., and Tasdemiroglu, E. (1988) Differential sympathetic regulation of autonomic, conductile and contractile tissue in dog heart. *Am. J. Physiol.* **255,** H1050–H1059.

88. Strack, A. M., Sawyer, W. B., Platt, K. B., and Loewy, A. D. (1989) CNS cell groups regulating the sympathetic outflow to the adrenal gland as revealed by transneuronal cell body labeling with pseudorabies virus. *Brain Res.* **491,** 274–296.

89. Strack, A. M. and Loewy, A. D. (1990) Pseudorabies virus: a highly specific transneuronal cell body marker in the sympathetic nervous system. *J. Neurosci.* **10,** 2139–2147.

90. Card, J. P., Rinaman, L., Lynn, R. B., Lee, B.-H., Meade, R. P., Miselis, R. R., and Enquist, L. W. (1993) Pseudorabies virus infection of the rat central nervous system: ultrastructural characterization of viral replication, transport and pathogenesis. *J. Neurosci.* **13,** 2515–2539.

91. Jansen, A. S. P., Van Nguyen, X., Karpitsky, V., Mettenleiter, T. C., and Loewy, A. D. (1995) Central command neurons of the sympathetic nervous system: basis of the flight-or-fight response. *Science* **270,** 644–646.

92. Loewy, A. D. (1981) Raphe pallidus and raphe obscurus projections to the intermediolateral cell column in the rat. *Brain Res.* **222,** 129–133.

93. Bacon, S. J., Zagon, A., and Smith, A. D. (1990) Electron microscopic evidence of a monosynaptic pathway between cells in the caudal raphe nuclei and the sympathetic preganglionic neurons in the rat spinal cord. *Exp. Brain Res.* **79,** 589–602.

94. Morrison, S. F. (1993) Raphe pallidus excites a unique class of sympathetic preganglionic neurons. *Am. J. Physiol.* **265,** R82–R89.

95. Ross, C. A., Ruggiero, D. A., and Reis, D. J. (1985) Projections from the nucleus tractus solitarii to the rostral ventrolateral medulla. *J. Comp. Neurol.* **242,** 511–531.

96. Saper, C. B. (1995) Central autonomic nervous system, in *The Rat Nervous System*, 2nd ed. (Paxinos, G., ed.), Academic, San Diego, CA, pp. 107–135.

97. Ciriello, J., Hochstenbach, S. L., and Roder, S. (1994) Central projections of baroreceptor and chemoreceptor afferent fibers in the rat, in *Nucleus of the Solitary Tract* (Barraco, I. R. A., ed.), CRC, Boca Raton, FL, pp. 35–51.

98. Ricardo, J. A. and Koh, E. T. (1978) Anatomical evidence of direct projections from the nucleus of the solitary tract to the hypothalamus, amygdala and other forebrain structures in the rat. *Brain Res.* **153,** 1–26.

99. Ter Horst, G. J., De Boer, P., Luiten, P. G. M., and Van Willigen, J. D. (1989) Ascending projections from the solitary tract nucleus to the hypothalamus. A phaseolus vulgaris lectin tracing study in the rat. *Neuroscience* **31,** 785–797.

100. Luiten, P. G. M., Ter Horst, G. J., and Steffens, A. B. (1987) The hypothalamus, intrinsic connections and output pathways to the endocrine system in relation to the control of feeding and metabolism. *Prog. Neurobiol.* **28,** 1–54.

101. Ruggiero, D. A., Cravo, S. L., Arango, V., and Reis, D. J. (1989) Central control of the circulation by the rostral ventrolateral reticular nucleus: Anatomical substrates, in *Progress in Brain Research*, vol. 81 (Ciriello, J., Caverson, M. M., and Polosa, C., eds.), Elsevier Science, Amsterdam, pp. 49–79.

102. Dampney, R. A. L. (1994) Functional organization of central pathways regulating the cardiovascular system. *Physiol. Rev.* **74,** 321–363.

103. Pyner, S. and Coote, J. H. (1998) Rostroventrolateral medulla neurons preferentially project to target-specified sympathetic preganglionic neurons. *Neuroscience* **83,** 617–631.

104. Brown, D. L. and Guyenet, P. G. (1985) Electrophysiological study of cardiovascular neurons in the rostral ventrolateral medulla in the rat. *Circ. Res.* **56,** 359–369.

105. Herbert, H., Moga, M. M., and Saper, C. B. (1990) Connections of the parabrachial nucleus with the nucleus of the solitary tract and the medullary reticular formation in the rat. *J. Comp. Neurol.* **293,** 540–580.

106. Herbert, H. and Saper, C. B. (1992) Organization of medullary adrenergic and noradrenergic projections to the periaqueductal gray matter in the rat. *J. Comp. Neurol.* **315,** 34–52.

107. Ter Horst, G. J., Luiten, P. G. M., and Kuipers, F. (1984) Descending pathways from hypothalamus to dorsal motor vagus and ambiguus nuclei in the rat. *J. Auton. Nerv. Syst.* **11,** 59–75.

108. Ter Horst, G. J. and Luiten, P. G. M. (1986) Projections of the dorsomedial hypothalamic nucleus in the rat. *Brain Res. Bull.* **16,** 231–248.

109. Beitz, A. J. (1995) Periaqueductal gray, in *The Rat Nervous System*, 2nd ed. (Paxinos, G., ed.), Academic, New York, pp. 173–182.
110. Alheid, G. F., De Olmos, J. S., and Beltramino, C. A. (1995) Amygdala and extended amygdala, in *The Rat Nervous System*, 2nd ed. (Paxinos, G., ed.), Academic, New York, pp. 495–578.
111. Chamberlin, N. L. and Saper, C. B. (1992) Topographic organization of cardiovascular responses to electrical and glutamate microstimulation of the parabrachial nucleus in the rat. *J. Comp. Neurol.* **326**, 245–262.
112. Bandler, R. P. and Shipley, M. (1994) Columnar organization in midbrain periaqueductal gray: modules for emotional expression? *Trends Neurosci.* **17**, 379–389.
113. Clement, C. I., Keay, K. A., Owler, B. K., and Bandler, R. P. (1996) Common patterns of increased and decreased Fos expression in midbrain and pons evoked by noxious deep somatic and noxious visceral manipulations in the rat. *J. Comp. Neurol.* **366**, 495–515.
114. Lovick, T. A. (1992) Inhibitory modulation of the cardiovascular defence response by the ventrolateral periaqueductal gray matter in rats. *Exp. Brain Res.* **89**, 133–139.
115. Veening, J., Buma, P., Ter Horst, G. J., Roeling, T. A. P., Luiten, P. G. M., and Nieuwenhuys, R. (1991) Hypothalamic projections to the PAG in the rat: topographical, immunoelectronmicroscopical and functional aspects, in *The Midbrain Periaqueductal Gray Matter: Functional, Anatomical and Neurochemical Organization* (Depaulis, A. and Bandler, R. P., eds.), Plenum, New York, pp. 387–415.
116. Jansen, A. S. P., Farkas, E., MacSams, J., and Loewy, A. D. (1998) Local connections between the columns of the periaqueductal gray matter: a case for intrinsic neuromodulation. *Brain Res.* **784**, 329–336.
117. Holstege, G. (1995) The basic, somatic, and emotional components of the motor system in mammals, in *The Rat Nervous System*, 2nd ed. (Paxinos, G., ed.), Academic, New York, pp. 139–154.
118. Farkas, E., Jansen, A. S. P., and Loewy, A. D. (1997) Periaqueductal gray matter projection to vagal preganglionic neurons and the nucleus tractus solitarius. *Brain Res.* **764**, 257–261.
119. Carrive, P. and Bandler, R. P. (1991) Viscerotopic organization of neurons subserving hypotensive reactions within the midbrain periaqueductal grey—a correlative functional and anatomical study. *Brain Res.* **460**, 339–345.
120. Carrive, P. and Bandler, R. P. (1991) Control of extracranial and hindlimb blood flow by the midbrain periaqueductal grey of the cat. *Exp. Brain Res.* **84**, 599–606.
121. Halliday, G., Harding, A., and Paxinos, G. (1995) Serotonin and tachykinin systems, in *The Rat Nervous System*, 2nd ed. (Paxinos, G., ed.), Academic, New York, pp. 929–974.
122. Aston-Jones, G., Shipley, M. T., and Grzanna, R. (1995) The locus coeruleus, A5 and A7 noradrenergic cell groups, in *The Rat Ner-*

vous System, 2nd ed. (Paxinos, G., ed.), Academic, New York, pp. 183–213.

123. Ter Horst, G. J., Toes, G. J., and Van Willigen, J. D. (1991) Locus coeruleus projections to the dorsal motor vagus nucleus in the rat. *Neuroscience* **45**, 153–160.

124. Haselton, J. R., Winters, R. W., Liskowsky, D. R., Haselton, C. L., McCabe, P. M., and Schneiderman, N. (1988) Cardiovascular responses elicited by electrical and chemical stimulation of the rostral medullary raphe of the rabbit. *Brain Res.* **453**, 167–175.

125. Robinson, S. E., Rice, M. A., and Davidson, W. (1986) A GABA cardiovascular mechanism in the dorsal raphe of the rat. *Neuropharmacology* **25**, 611–615.

126. Sved, A. F., and Felsten, G. (1987) Stimulation of the locus coeruleus decreases arterial pressure. *Brain Res.* **414**, 119–132.

127. Murase, S., Takayama, M., and Nosaka, S. (1993) Chemical stimulation of the nucleus locus coeruleus: cardiovascular responses and baroreflex modification. *Neurosci. Lett.* **153**, 1–4.

128. Banks, D. and Harris, M. C. (1984) Lesions of the locus coeruleus abolish baroreceptor-induced depression of supraoptic neurons in the rat, *J. Physiol. London* **355**, 383–389.

129. Gurtu, S., Pant, K. K., Sinha, J. N., and Bhargava, K. P. (1984) An investigation into the mechanism of cardiovascular responses elicited by electrical stimulation of locus coeruleus and subcoeruleus in the cat. *Brain Res.* **301**, 59–64.

130. Oppenheimer, S. M. and Cechetto, D. F. (1990) The cardiac chronotropic organization of the rat insular cortex. *Brain Res.* **533**, 66–72.

131. Cechetto, D. F. and Chen, S. J. (1992) Hypothalamic and cortical sympathetic responses relay in the medulla of the rat. *Am. J. Physiol.* **263**, R245–R262.

132. Loewy, A. D. (1991) Forebrain nuclei involved in autonomic control. *Prog. Brain Res.* **87**, 253–268.

133. Verberne, A. J. M. and Owens, N. C. (1998) Cortical modulation of the cardiovascular system. *Prog. Neurobiol.* **54**, 149–168.

134. Soltis, R. P. and DiMicco, J. A. (1991) GABAA and excitatory amino acid receptors in the dorsomedial hypothalamus and heart rate in rats. *Am. J. Physiol.* **260**, R13–R20.

135. Soltis, R. P. and DiMicco, J. A. (1992) Hypothalamic excitatory amino acid receptors mediate stress-induced tachycardia in rats. *Am. J. Physiol.* **262**, R689–R697.

136. Foreman, R. D., Blair, R. W., and Weber, R. N. (1984) Viscerosomatic convergence onto T2–T4 spinoreticular, spinoreticular-spinothalamic, and spinothalamic tract neurons in the cat. *Exp. Neurol.* **85**, 597–619.

137. Bolser, D. C., Hobbs, S. F., Chandler, M. J., Ammons, W. S., Brennan, T. J., and Foreman, R. D. (1991) Convergence of phrenic and cardiopulmonary spinal afferent information on cervical and thoracic

spinothalamic tract neurons in the monkey. Implications for referred pain from the diaphragm and the heart. *J. Neurophysiol.* **65**, 1042–1054.
138. Sawchenko, P. E. and Swanson, L. W. (1983) The organization of forebrain afferents to the paraventricular and supraoptic nuclei in the rat. *J. Comp. Neurol.* **218**, 121–144.
139. Kannan, H., Hayshida, Y., and Yamashita, H. (1989) Increase of sympathetic outflow by paraventricular nucleus stimulation in awake rats. *Am. J. Physiol.* **256**, R1325–R1330.
140. Martin, D. S. and Haywood, J. R. (1992) Sympathetic nervous system activation by glutamate injections into the paraventricular nucleus. *Brain Res.* **577**, 261–267.
141. Blair, M. L., Piekut, D., Want, A., and Olschowka, J. A. (1996) Role of the hypothalamic paraventricular nucleus in cardiovascular regulation. *Clin. Exp. Pharmacol. Physiol.* **23**, 161–165.
142. Martin, D. S., Rodrigo, M. C., Egland, M. C., and Barnes, L. U. (1997) Disinhibition of the hypothalamic paraventricular nucleus increases mean circulatory filling pressure in conscious rats. *Brain Res.* **756**, 106–113.
143. Diz, D. I. and Jacobowitz, D. M. (1984) Cardiovascular effects of discrete hypothalamic and preoptic injections of bradykinin. *Brain Res. Bull.* **12**, 409–417.
144. Martin, D. S., Segura, T., and Haywood, J. R. (1991) Cardiovascular responses to bicuculline in the paraventricular nucleus of the rat. *Hypertension* **18**, 48–55.
145. Armstrong, W. E. (1995) Hypothalamic supraoptic and paraventricular nuclei, in *The Rat Nervous System*, 2nd ed. (Paxinos, G., ed.), Academic, New York, pp. 377–390.
146. Sawchenko, P. E. and Swanson, L. W. (1990) Organization of CRF immunoreactive cells, and fibers in the rat brain: immunohistochemical studies, in *Corticotropin-Releasing Factor: Basic and Clinical Studies of a Neuropeptide* (De Souza, E. B. and Nemeroff, C. B., eds.), CRC, Boca Raton, FL, pp. 29–52.
147. Curtis, G. C., Abelson, J. L., and Gold, P. W. (1997) Adrenocorticotropic hormone and cortisol responses to corticotropin releasing hormone: changes in panic disorder and effects of alprazolam treatment. *Biol. Psychiatry* **41**, 76–85.
148. Linthorst, A. C., Flachskamm, C., Hopkins, S. J., Hoadley, M. E., Labeur, M. S., Holsboer, F., et al. (1997) Long-term intracerebroventricular infusion of corticotropin-releasing hormone alters neuroendocrine, neurochemical, autonomic, behavioral, and cytokine responses to a systemic inflammatory challenge. *J. Neurosci.* **17**, 4448–4460.
149. Korte, S. M., Bouws, G. A. H., and Bohus, B. G. (1993) Central actions of corticotropin-releasing hormone (CRH) on behavioral, neuroendocrine and cardiovascular regulation. *Horm. Behav.* **27**, 167–183.

Progress in Brain Research, vol. 85 (Uylings, H. B. M., van Eden, C. G., De Bruin, J. P. C., Corner, M. A., and Feenstra, M. G. P., eds.), Elsevier Science, Amsterdam, pp. 147–165.

205. Kunishio, K. and Haber, S. N. (1994) Primate cingulostriatal projection: Limbic striatal versus sensorimotor striatal input. *J. Comp. Neurol.* **350,** 337–356.

206. Vogt, B. A., Derbyshire, S., and Jones, A. K. (1996) Pain processing in four regions of human cingulate cortex localized with co-registered PET and MR imaging. *Eur. J. Neurosci.* **8,** 1461–1473.

207. Sikes, R. W. and Vogt, B. A. (1992) Nociceptive neurons in area 24 of rabbit cingulate cortex. *J. Neurophysiol.* **68,** 1720–1732.

208. Bentivoglio, M., Kultas-Ilinsky, K., and Ilinsky, I. (1993) Limbic thalamus: structure, intrinsic organization and connections, in *Neurobiology of Cingulate Cortex and Limbic Thalamus: A Comprehensive Handbook* (Vogt, B. A. and Gabriel, M., eds.), Birkhauser, Boston, pp. 71–122.

209. Van Hoesen, G. W., Morecraft, R. J., and Vogt, B. A. (1993) Connections of the monkey cingulate cortex, in *Neurobiology of Cingulate Cortex and Limbic Thalamus: A Comprehensive Handbook* (Vogt, B. A. and Gabriel, M., eds.), Birkhauser, Boston, pp. 249–284.

210. Neafsey, E. J., Bold, E. L., Haas, G., Hurley-Gius, K. M., Quirk, G., Sievert, C. F., et al. (1986) The organization of the rat motor cortex: a microstimulation mapping study. *Brain Res. Rev.* **11,** 77–96.

211. Doutrelant-Viltart, M., Sauvage, M., and Sequeira, H. (1997) Expression of c-fos in bulbar nuclei involved in cardiovascular control following electrical stimulation of the sensorimotor cortex in the rat. *Neurosci. Lett.* **227,** 71–74.

212. Ba-M'Hamed, S., Sequeira, H., Poulain, P., Bennis, M., and Roy, J. C. (1993) Sensorimotor cortex projections to the ventrolateral and the dorsomedial medulla oblongata in the rat. *Neurosci. Lett.* **164,** 195–198.

213. Ba-M'Hamed, S., Roy, J. C., Poulain, P., Bennis, M., and Sequeira, H. (1996) Corticospinal collaterals to medullary cardiovascular nuclei in the rat: an anterograde and a retrograde double labeling study. *J. Brain Res.* **37,** 367–375.

214. McGeorge, A. J. and Faull, R. L. M. (1989) The organization of the projection from the cerebral cortex to the striatum in the rat. *Neuroscience* **29,** 503–537.

215. Zilles, K. and Wree, A. (1995) Cortex: areal and laminar structure, in *The Rat Nervous System* (Paxinos, G., ed.), Academic, San Diego, CA, pp. 649–688.

216. Spyer, K. M. (1994) Central nervous mechanisms contributing to cardiovascular control. *J. Physiol.* **474,** 1–19.

217. Roeling, T. A. P. (1993) The neuronal substrate of hypothalamically induced behaviour in the rat: an anatomical and behavioural study, thesis, University Nijmegen, pp. 1–199.

CHAPTER 3

Circadian Organization of the Autonomic Nervous System

Ruud M. Buijs, Michael L.H.J. Hermes,
Jiapei Dai, Frank Scheer, and Andries Kalsbeek

Introduction

Life on our planet is mainly dependent on the presence of our sun, which provides us daily with the energy we need for survival. It is, therefore, not surprising that most organisms have developed a system that allows them to synchronize their (metabolic) activity with the daily appearance of the sun. In more complex organisms, these daily cycles are also responsible for the organization of multiple-day rhythms, such as the weekly, monthly, or yearly reproduction cycles.

More and more evidence has accumulated that, apart from being under the influence of the sun, these cycles also depend on the presence of an internal oscillator. Most organisms (fungi, plants, bacteria, invertebrates, and vertebrates) have developed an internal clock that allows them to anticipate the coming sunrise or sunset (1).

In this chapter, attention will be paid to mammals, including man, and the massive physiological changes that are essential for the organisms' ability to execute very different functions during the day and the night period, often synonyms for the resting period and the active period, or vice

From: *The Nervous System and the Heart*
Ed: G. J. Ter Horst © Humana Press Inc.

versa. Furthermore, attention will be paid to the responsible central nervous system (CNS) processes that are essential to the regulation of these physiological functions. We will review the evidence that the mammalian biological clock is the functional basis for the expression of these activity patterns. Basic mechanisms as revealed by anatomical, physiological, and electrophysiological techniques will be discussed. Furthermore, recent anatomical data will be presented that suggest a high congruence of organization in the rodent hypothalamus as compared with the human. Subsequently, data will be presented that suggest the implication of the biological clock in physiological derangements such as high blood pressure.

2. The Biological Clock

These days much attention is paid to unraveling the molecular mechanisms responsible for the circadian-clock-like function of unicellular or multicellular organisms (1). The present study will not review these developments but will discuss the physiological mechanisms that these daily oscillators use to transmit their clock message to the rest of the organism. In unicellular organisms, a simple protein derived from the clock may suffice. In more complex organisms, such as the fruit fly *Drosophila*, it is suggested that every cell in the body may have clocklike functions (2,3), which would also solve the problem of the transmission of the clock signal to the organism. In mammals, the biological clock is located within the central nervous system and resides within the retina and within a hypothalamic structure, the suprachiasmatic nucleus (SCN). Lesioning the SCN [experiments initially executed in rodents but also confirmed by observations in humans (4)] results in a complete inability of the individual to synchronize its activity to the changing light–dark cycle. Definitive proof that the SCN is the master clock in mammals was provided by an experiment that combined lesioning of the SCN with transplantation of the SCN of a donor animal. The host always adopted the endogenous rhythm of the

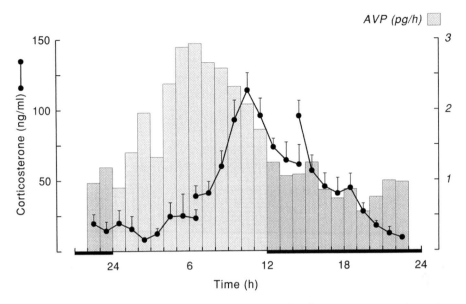

Fig. 1. Phase relation between the diurnal release patterns of corti-costerone as measured in blood samples obtained from free-moving animals, and vasopressin from SCN terminals (shaded bars) as measured by means of microdialysis probes placed within the vicinity of the SCN.

donor animal, even when that rhythm was changed by a mutation (5).

Considering this and the fact that the SCN-lesioned animals suffered a complete disappearance of their endogenous circadian rhythm, it is evident that there must be mechanisms that transfer information from the SCN to the rest of the CNS and the rest of the body.

Interestingly, the daily patterns of electrical activity of the SCN neurons not only result in synchronization of behavioral activity but are also translated in different daily patterns of hormone secretion. Several hormones, such as corticosterone in rodents or cortisol in humans, melatonin, or thyroid hormone, show clear circadian patterns. Each of these patterns is coupled to a particular moment of the light/ dark or activity cycle (Fig. 1). Also, the circadian secretion of these hormones is highly dependent on the presence of the SCN. In SCN-lesioned animals, these circadian hormonal patterns disappear. Each of these hormones has the unique property of being able to pass more or less freely into all body tissues; consequently, this temporal pattern in hormone secretion seems to be an essential feature of the SCN for transmitting its circadian signal to all parts of the body (6).

The question arises, consequently, of how the SCN is able to control these various hormonal rhythms that are associated with the different moments of the light–dark cycle, and whether other mechanisms exist that are utilized by the SCN to impose its rhythm onto the individual.

3. The Suprachiasmatic Nucleus

The SCN is a tiny structure of approximately 10,000 neurons in rodents and 70,000 neurons in humans (7). It is situated bilaterally of the third ventricle, on top of the optic chiasm from which it receives direct information about the light–dark cycle via the retina (8). The unique property of the SCN is that it is able to maintain, without any input—even in vitro—a circadian rhythm in firing frequency that is higher during the subjective day than during the subjective dark period (9–11).

One of the first demonstrations of the endogenous circadian activity changes of the SCN was by means of the uptake of 2-deoxyglucose, which was clearly associated with the subjective light phase. Much more 2-deoxyglucose is taken up by the SCN in the (subjective) light period, which coincides with the period that the SCN shows its highest electrical activity (12,13). These experiments also showed an identical pattern of 2-deoxyglucose uptake, irrespective of whether nocturnal or diurnal animals were examined.

This indicates that activity of the SCN may have a completely different function in day-active animals as compared to night-active ones. In day-active animals, the activity of the SCN transmits the signal to activate behavior, whereas the opposite will be true for night-active animals. For example, recent experiments in our group have demonstrated that exposure to light during the dark period decreases the heart rate in rats, whereas it increases heart rate in humans, independent of behavioral activity *(14)*.

4. SCN Transmitters

In their anatomical analysis of the classical neuroendocrine neurons of the paraventricular nucleus (PVN) and supraoptic nucleus (SON) of the hypothalamus, first, neurophysin and, later, vasopressin were demonstrated to be present in the neurons of the SCN by Swaab et al. *(15)* and Vandesande et al. *(16)*.

Soon after, a host of other peptides was demonstrated inside the neurons of the SCN *(17,18)*, to which only much later were GABA and glutamate added as potential transmitters of the biological clock *(19,20)*.

Interestingly, GABA was found to be colocalized within the peptidergic neurons of the SCN. This colocalization appeared to extend itself to SCN terminals within the SCN, but also in target areas of the SCN. Interestingly, in spite of the claim that GABA is present in all SCN neurons *(21)*, only in approximately 30% of the terminals GABA immunoreactivity could be demonstrated *(19,22)* (Fig. 2).

One of the intriguing questions regarding the colocalization of the various peptidergic transmitters of the SCN with GABA is whether the neuron is able to control which transmitter will be released from its terminal. Numerous studies have appeared that indicated that a peptide is more efficiently released with bursts of activity and at a higher frequency than the classical transmitters released with single neuronal discharges *(23–26)*. This suggests that during the light period, when the SCN neurons are most active *(13,27)*, a larger portion of peptides is secreted by these active neurons, whereas during the dark period, the secretion of GABA prevails. The high level of vasopressin released by the SCN during the (subjective) light period *(28)* seems to support this idea. This suggests that the function of a single SCN neuron containing vasopressin and GABA in its terminal may change, depending on its firing frequency: excitatory during the (subjective)

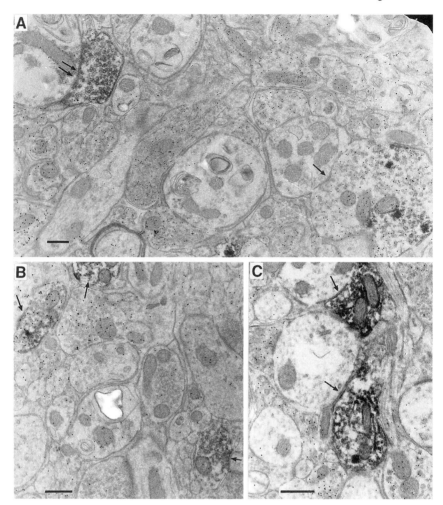

Fig. 2. Ultrastructural micrographs representing a preembedding staining for vasopressin, followed by a postembedding staining for γ-aminobutyric acid (GABA) with 10-nm gold illustrating the differences in staining intensities for GABA. **(A)** Two vasopressin-positive terminals; one has a high staining intensity for GABA (single arrow), whereas the other is very lightly stained (two arrows). Both, however, were classified as vasopressin and GABA positive. **(B)** Two terminals were classified as GABA positive (arrows, upper left), whereas the third (arrow, bottom right) was considered "undecided." Arrows indicate terminals. **(C)** Illustration of two vasopressin terminals (arrows). The complete absence of gold labeling, also over the mitochondria, classifies this terminal as GABA negative. In this way, of the 645 VP terminals that were counted, 14% was clearly GABA positive, 73% was negative, and 13% was undecided. Scale bars = 0.25 μm.

light period, when vasopressin is released [vasopressin is usually found to be excitatory *(29–31)*] and switching to inhibitory during the dark period, when GABA is released.

However, recent experiments by Kalsbeek et al. *(32)* demonstrated that exposing animals to light in the dark phase and, consequently, increasing the firing frequency of SCN neurons to daytime levels resulted in the secretion of GABA at presumed SCN terminals and, consequently, in the inhibition of melatonin secretion. This inhibition of melatonin secretion could be prevented by the infusion of bicuculline in the PVN (Fig. 3). Bicuculline infusion during the dark period did not elevate basal melatonin levels; thus, the assumption that SCN terminals favor the secretion of GABA during the dark phase is not supported. Instead, other mechanisms might be in place that change the reaction of SCN neurons from inhibitory to excitatory, depending on the circadian cycle of these SCN neurons *(33)*.

Interestingly, the first transmitter molecule that was demonstrated in the SCN also appeared to be the first peptide that was demonstrated to have a clearly fluctuating level in the cerebrospinal fluid (CSF) with a circadian rhythm [i.e., high in the light phase and low in the dark phase *(13)*]. Lesioning studies demonstrated that only removal of the SCN resulted in the loss of this circadian pattern in vasopressin levels in the CSF; in addition, it resulted in a drop in vasopressin CSF to an almost undetectable level *(34,35)*. The latter observation indicates that the SCN not only drives the circadian rhythm in vasopressin secretion, but it is also the main source of CSF vasopressin. Later, by means of precisely placed microdialysis probes, Kalsbeek et al. *(36)* were able to demonstrate in vivo that a circadian rhythm in vasopressin secretion could only be measured when the probes were placed in the immediate vicinity of the SCN and not elsewhere. Other studies have demonstrated, in addition, that the concentration of vasopressin mRNA also showed a daily fluctuation, together with a daily change in the length of the poly-A tail of the vasopressin mRNA *(37,38)*. An interesting observation was made in the Brattleboro rat, which is unable

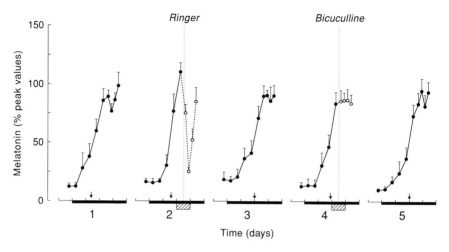

Fig. 3. Mean melatonin-release patterns during the first half of the dark period on 5 subsequent days ($n = 8$), days 1, 3, and 5 being control days, and days 2 and 4 being days of exposure to light. During exposure to light hypothalamic probes were perfused for 2 h with either Ringer or Ringer + BIC (bicuculline), in a staggered order. For reasons of clarity, however, data are presented as if all Ringer perfusions were performed on day 2 and every Ringer + BIC administration on day 4. Days 3 and 5 represent results of the control days following Ringer and Ringer + BIC administration, respectively. The vertical dotted line indicates the time of the 1-min exposure to light. Please note that infusion with the GABA antagonist BIC completely prevented the light-induced inhibition of melatonin. This result was obtained only when the probes were positioned in the dorsal PVN.

to synthetize vasopressin because of a deletion in its vaso-pressin coding part of the DNA. In these rats, this mRNA, transcribed on the mutated DNA, still shows a daily variation in its synthesis (37).

It has been demonstrated that SCN vasopressin levels are affected by the concentration of adrenal steroid hormones. In rats, adrenalectomy as well as dexamethasone treatment affected the levels of vasopressin or vasopressin mRNA in the SCN (39). These data indicate an important role of gluco-corticoids for the SCN. Interestingly, glucocorticoid receptors are only demonstrated in the SCN early in development and disappear after 5 d postnatally (40). This observation could, however, not be reproduced in later studies and was not detectable when we used a highly sensitive antibody to the glucocorticoid receptor *(41)*. For melatonin, no such effects on transmitter levels have been described, although it is certain—by the presence of melatonin receptors in the SCN and their effect on the electrical activity on SCN neurons *(42,43)*—that melatonin will noticeably affect the SCN.

With the evidence that circadian patterns in neuronal activity are indeed reflected in circadian patterns of SCN transmitter secretion, it is essential to identify the CNS structures that may be directly influenced by the biological clock. For this reason, it is essential to determine the exact projections of the SCN.

5. The Suprachiasmatic Nucleus–Hypothalamus Interaction

The discovery of the presence of vasopressin within SCN neurons was followed by the description of the vasopressin pathways emanating from the SCN *(44,45)*. Initially, this was done purely on the basis of following stained fibers, or even on the basis of the size of vasopressin fibers in different brain regions. Both procedures resulted in an assumption of a too extensive pattern of SCN projections. Lesioning the SCN resolved this issue and clarified, by means of the disappearance of vasopressin fibers in several target areas *(46)*, the vasopressin-containing SCN projections. These vasopressin-containing SCN projections were demonstrated to run to the area of the paraventricular nucleus of the hypothalamus (PVN), to the dorsomedial nucleus of the hypothalamus (DMH), to the paraventricular nucleus of the thalamus (PVT), to the medial preoptic nucleus, and to the organum vasculosum of the lamina terminalis. In the meantime, anterograde tracing studies by means of horseradish peroxidase (HRP) were carried out as well, but these did not allow determination of the SCN projections in more detail *(47,48)*.

Finally, by means of precise, localized injections of the anterograde tracer Phaseolus vulgaris leucoagglutinin (Pha-L), it proved possible to determine the general projections of the

SCN *(19,49–51)*. With respect to the different peptides that are located in different regions of the SCN, some small differences in projection patterns and densities were described for vasoactive intestinal peptide (VIP) and vasopressin *(50)*. Especially the Pha-L tracing studies, but also the VIP staining, revealed a more detailed picture of the innervation of the PVN *(50,52)*. Thus, it became clear that SCN projections in general avoid the body of the PVN, except for its ventral periventricular and dorsal borders. In the dorsal part of the PVN, where mostly neurons are situated that project to the spinal cord, many contacts between SCN projections and these so-called autonomic PVN neurons have been demonstrated *(52–54)*.

Taken together, all tracing studies indicate that the observed SCN projections are mainly restricted to target areas situated in the medial hypothalamus, with the exception of its projections to the PVT, and the lateral geniculate nucleus *(49,50)*. On the basis of these general anatomical data alone, it is clear that the medial hypothalamus will play an essential role in the synchronization of homeostatic functions with the daily light–dark cycle. On the basis of what is already known of these hypothalamic targets of the SCN with respect to their own projections, transmitter content, and physiological functions, a further subdivision can be made with respect to specific circadian functions. It seems evident that the SCN projections to the specific sites in the medial hypothalamus will serve to modulate the release of hormones into a pattern that expresses a circadian rhythm. Most pituitary-controlling neuroendocrine neurons are situated in the medial hypothalamus. Closer examination of the precise SCN projections in combination with target identification will have to provide the picture that reveals where exactly the SCN may influence these releasing-factor-containing neurons. In relation to the circadian control of general (motor) activity, it is not apparent yet what target area is involved. It is possible that this message is transmitted to all SCN target areas and that all these target areas together control motor activity to some extent for a particular kind of behavior. On the other hand, it is possible that one or more target areas, such as the PVT or lateral geniculate nucleus (LGN), serve to modulate motor activity *(55,56)*. Consequently, it is of importance to also collect knowledge on the projections and functions of the target sites of the SCN, thus making it possible to draw conclusions on the processes that may be influenced by these target areas.

In order to acquire more insight into the manner in which the SCN influences hormone secretion, considerable attention was paid in our anatomical and physiological studies to elucidating sites and action of SCN transmitters. Initially a great deal of effort was directed to the question of whether the observed anatomical network of SCN terminals in the dorsomedial hypothalamus can, indeed, provide an explanation for the diurnal peak in corticosterone and melatonin.

6. Circadian Control of Corticosterone Secretion

Lesion studies have shown that the SCN has a profound inhibitory influence on corticosterone secretion: A SCN lesion results in highly elevated plasma corticosterone levels after a novel environment stimulus as compared with intact animals, which only show a moderate increase in corticosterone levels irrespective of the circadian time at which they are subjected to a novel environment *(6)*. The corticotropin-releasing hormone (CRH) is produced in neurons in the parvocellular part of the PVN (PVNp) and is released into the portal circulation of the median eminence to largely control the adrenocorticotropin-releasing hormone (ACTH) release from the adenohypophysis, which, in turn, stimulates the adrenal cortex to secrete corticosterone *(57,58)*. Much attention has been directed to the question whether the SCN is able to influence these CRM neurons directly.

Consequently, much attention has been directed to the question whether the SCN is able to influence these CRH neurons directly. Thus far, in spite of the observed circadian rise in CRH mRNA immediately preceding the corticosterone peak *(59)*, there have been no anatomical studies that have indicated any substantial direct projection to CRH neurons *(50,51)*. Instead, Watts et al. *(49)* demonstrated a massive projection of the SCN to an area just ventral of the PVN, which they called the sub-PVN zone. In their article, they suggested that this region may project into the PVN. Furthermore, using Pha-L tracing, Buijs et al. *(50)* showed that not only the subPVN but also the DMH receives a massive SCN input. Subsequently, Roland and Sawchenko *(60)* provided evidence that peri-PVN areas contain GABAergic neurons projecting to parvocellular PVN neurons. This also holds for the DMH, which has an established direct connection with the PVNp; one of the peptide transmitters of this projection is galanin *(61,62)*. Moreover, Kalsbeek et al. *(63)* provided substantial evidence that the DMH is the site, or one of the sites, where vasopressin of SCN origin serves to inhibit ACTH and corticosterone secretion. This corroborates the observation that the SCN projects extensively to the DMH with vasopressin fibers *(46)*.

Because of the lack of direct contacts between SCN efferents and PVN–CRH neurons and in order to investigate which (other) putative sites in the hypothalamus might be influenced by the SCN and may change the hypothalamo-pituitary axis (HPA), we decided to label SCN efferents in combination with the identification of neurons implicated in the stress response by fos immunocytochemistry *(50)*. A 15-min restraint stress resulted in the presence of numerous fos-positive neurons in the medial hypothalamus. Apart from the CRH neurons in the parvocellular part of the PVN (PVNp), fos-positive neurons were also present in the DMH, periventricular PVN (PVNpe), dorsal cap of the PVN (PVNdc), and rostral PVN (PVNr). All these areas with fos-positive neurons receive a dense input from the SCN, except for the PVNp, where only a few Pha-L-labeled SCN efferents could be detected, which suggested no or very limited output to CRH neurons. Similarly, when we employed a CRH-immunocytochemical staining to identify the PVN neurons involved in the control of the ACTH cells of the hypophysis, we were unable to demonstrate extensive interaction between SCN efferents and CRH neurons (Fig. 4). This observation was

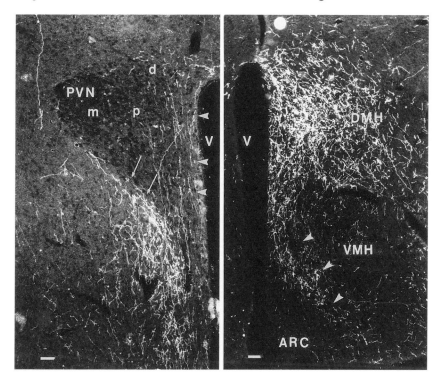

Fig. 4. Dark-field illustration of the projections of the SCN in the rat brain to the region of the paraventricular nucleus (PVN) after an iontophoretic injection of PHA-L into the SCN. Note the absence of fibers in the magnocellular and parvicellular part of the PVN (m, p). Only fibers are present in the periventricular part and dorsal part of the PVN (d). The long arrows indicate the dense innervation in the subparaventricular zone just ventral to the PVN. The arrowheads indicate the area that has been investigated in the electron microscopic study as periventricular PVN. V, ventricle. Scale bar = 50 μm. **(B)** Dark-field illustration of SCN projections to the dorsomedial hypothalamus (DMH), where a dense terminal field can be observed. Note the presence of a concentration of fibers in the region between the ventromedial hypothalamus (VMH) and the arcuate nucleus (ARC; arrowheads). V, ventricle. Scale bar = 50 μm.

corroborated by Vrang et al. *(51)*, who used the same procedure. In view of (1) the elaborate SCN terminals in the DMH region on "after stress fos-positive" neurons and the extensive projections of the DMH to the parvocellular PVN *(62)* and (2) the physiological studies pointing to the DMH as an important target for the SCN to control corticosterone secretion (36,64), all anatomical and physiological evidence so far points to an important indirect action of the SCN onto CRH neurons. The disadvantage of the anatomical approach thus far is that it does not allow the determination of contacts between SCN fibers and dendrites of PVN neurons. Therefore, an in vitro slice preparation and electrophysiological analysis were used to investigate the functional connectivity between SCN and PVN.

7. Functional Connectivity Between Rat SCN and PVN

Our observations indicate that electrical stimulation in SCN influences, in a differential manner, the excitability of all cell categories in PVN (20,65). The majority of neurons, including magnocellular neurosecretory cells, showed a decrease in firing following SCN stimulation. The influence of SCN on these latter neurons is remarkable in view of the very sparse innervation by SCN efferents of the magnocellular subdivision of the PVN, although it may be expected, in view of evidence of circadian rhythmicity, in the activity of the magnocellular neurosecretory system (66).

Resolving issues of functional connectivity between SCN and PVN, this study has raised new questions with respect to the neuropharmacology of SCN–PVN connections. First, short latency inhibition following SCN stimulation suggests that the responses are mediated, directly or indirectly, by GABA. In contrast, late and prolonged excitation following SCN stimulation indicates a sustained membrane depolarization, which can have various underlying mechanisms.

To investigate underlying synaptic mechanisms of PVN responses to SCN stimulation by intracellular recording techniques, an in vitro rat hypothalamic slice preparation was developed that preserves projections from the anteroventrally situated SCN to the dorsocaudally located PVN. Instead of using antidromic activation as a distinguishing criterion for different cell categories in PVN, cell types could be differentiated and partially identified on the basis of their intrinsic

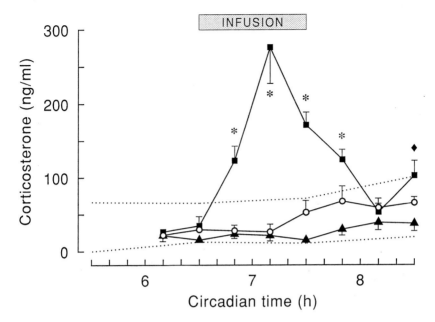

Fig. 5. Effect of Ringer (O—O), vasopressin (▲—▲) and the V1-antago-
nist (■—■) infusions at ZT6.5 to ZT7.5 on plasma corticosterone values.
Drug administration was performed via microdialysis probes in the
DMH. Dotted lines indicate corticosterone levels of control animals
(mean ± SEM). *$p < 0.05$ as compared to Ringer and vasopressin; ♦ $p < 0.05$
as compared to vasopressin.

nomenon is observed in aging humans [i.e., higher basal levels of cortisol *(78–80)*] together with a decreased presence of
vasopressin in the SCN *(81,82)*. In addition, daily and sea-
sonal rhythms of vasopressin activity in SCN neurons may
disappear with increasing age *(83)*, enhancing the deterioration of hormonal rhythms. Although correlative, these data
strongly suggest that degeneration of the SCN (and more
specifically its vasopressin-containing population of neurons)
with aging is an important causal factor for elevated cortisol
levels in elderly people.

8.2 Stimulatory SCN Input to the HPA Axis

The variation in corticosterone responses upon application of the vasopressin antagonist illustrates that the vaso-

pressin rhythm alone cannot explain the complete pattern of corticosterone responses. Therefore, in addition to the inhibitory control by vasopressin, there is also a stimulatory SCN input to the HPA axis (6,63,84), which is active during the second half of the light period. The lack of a pronounced corticosterone secretion at CT2, even if the vasopressinergic inhibition of the SCN is blocked, is thus explained by the simultaneous lack of a stimulatory input to the CRH neuron during the early morning. The decreasing levels of corticosterone during the dark period, in spite of the decline of the inhibitory vasopressin signal, are explained by the concomitant decline of the stimulatory input to the HPA system. Together, both rhythmic inputs from the SCN (i.e., the inhibitory and the stimulatory one) in the presently proposed phase relation (Fig. 6) are able to explain fully the observed rhythm in plasma corticosterone. The presence of an inhibitory as well as a stimulatory signal is also indicated by the fact that the plasma corticosterone levels in SCN-lesioned animals are between the daily trough and the daily peak level. The shape and height of the endogenous corticosterone peak is then defined by the internal synchronization of both rhythms. The importance of this "tuning" of the different circadian rhythms is indicated by the study of Sparrow et al. (85). This prospective study in humans shows that the height of the daily corticosterone peak is inversely related to the annual rate of decline of pulmonary function with aging. Furthermore, a broadening of the diurnal corticosterone peak in aged rats correlates with enhanced cognitive impairments (86).

In previous years, the apparent intact circadian rhythmicity of the vasopressin-deficient Brattleboro rat has frequently been put forward as evidence against the notion that vasopressin serves as an output signal of the circadian timing system (87). The above scenario for the circadian control of basal corticosterone release explains why the Brattleboro rat may still show circadian behavior in general, and a circadian pattern of corticosterone release in particular. Because of the diurnal fluctuation of its stimulatory input to the HPA axis, the SCN will still be able to create a circadian pattern of

(95) and a major target area of the SCN: the dorsomedial hypothalamic nucleus *(96)*. The results demonstrate that the organization pattern of the human hypothalamus is, to a large extent, similar to that of the rat, at least as far as the structures we have investigated are concerned. An anterograde tracer placed in the SCN of a hypothalamic slice obtained within 10 h after death was taken up by neurons and transported over a distance of at least 1.5 cm. This technique allowed us to determine projections of the SCN to target structures within the human hypothalamus. Human SCN projections were revealed to reach identical targets as SCN projections in the rodent brain: the ventral PVN, sub-PVN, and DMH (Figs. 8 and 9). It is demonstrated in the rat that the DMH projects extensively to the PVN. Also, placement of tracer in the human DMH showed similar extensive connections to the PVN, where CRH and vasopressin and oxytocin-containing neurons were shown to be targets of DMH fibers.

These observations illustrated that, as in the rodent, the human SCN utilizes at least two different means to impose its rhythm onto the neuroendocrine PVN neurons: a direct one via monosynaptic connections and an indirect one by connections via intermediate neurons located in the DMH and sub-PVN. In the rodent, a third possibility was demonstrated by which the SCN may influence endocrine organs and that is by direct interaction with the neurons in the PVN that project to the autonomic division in the spinal cord and brainstem. Because of the lack of specific markers for the PVN neurons in the autonomic division, no such information is available for humans. Consequently, it seems possible to apply the data we observed in the rat to human only with certain reservations; one other reservation would be that although the rat is a nocturnal animal, humans are clearly diurnal and will, therefore, organize their activity with a different temporal relationship to the activity of the SCN.

In order to understand how the SCN may affect the organs of the body (for instance, the heart in humans), it is also important to keep these restrictions in mind. In this way,

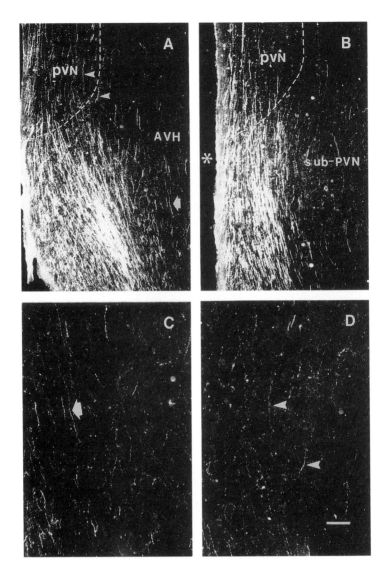

Fig. 8. **(A)** Dark-field photomicrograph showing SCN projection fibers of the human brain at the level just caudal to the suprachiasmatic nucleus (SCN). Many labeled SCN fibers pass through the area and run posteriorly. Some fibers project to the ventral part of the paraventricular nucleus (PVN; arrowheads) or the anteroventral hypothalamic area (AVH; large arrow). **(B)** Projection fibers at the level of sub-PVN. The asterisk indicates the third ventricle. **(C,D)** High magnification of areas in (A), showing branching or terminal bouton fibers in the AVH (arrow in [C]) and ventral part of the PVN (arrowheads in [D]). The dashed lines in (A) and (B) indicate the ventrolateral border of the PVN. Scale bar = 400 μm in (A) and (B), 160 μm in (C) and (D).

for example, it is essential to see that melatonin, which is the hormone of the night, transmits a different signal in night-active animals, such as rodents, or in night-inactive species, such as humans. Melatonin receptors are concentrated in the SCN in most species. Recent electrophysiological research in our laboratory has demonstrated that melatonin serves to hyperpolarize all SCN neurons. This results in a reduction of firing during the day and in a further hyperpolarization of the membrane potential of the already nonfiring night SCN neuron. In this way melatonin serves to enhance the night function of the SCN (i.e., sleep [inactivity] in humans and activity in nocturnal animals).

8.2.4. SCN–Autonomic Nervous System Interaction

We would like to propose that the modulation of the autonomic nervous system by the SCN is not limited to its influence on the pineal and adrenal; in a similar way, SCN control of the ANS might be essential to the heart, kidney, pancreas, and so forth, thus spreading the time-of-day message to the important organs of the body, not only through the action of steroid hormones on these organs but also directly by the autonomic nervous system. Recently, we obtained further physiological evidence for the existence of such a SCN–autonomic system interaction by demonstrating that the human heart as well as that of the rat responds acutely to a change in environmental light. In humans, light increases the heart rate, especially at the end of the dark period, whereas light decreases it in the rat, which demonstrates the reverse effect of light via the SCN on the autonomic system, depending on whether the individual is day active or night active *(14)*.

Consequently, the balance obtained by this hypothalamic PVN system is not only influenced by stress but also by many other environmental and endogenous factors, such as water and food intake, light, time of day, and glucocorticoid feedback. The present study demonstrates that the SCN is one of the structures through which these factors may have their effect. It also puts the SCN in the position of integrator

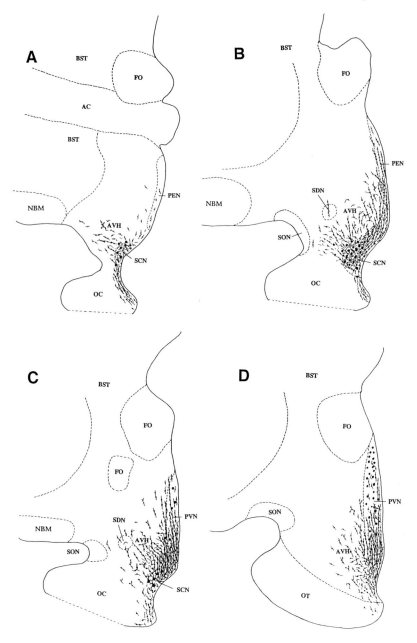

Fig. 9. A series of schematic drawings illustrating the projection of the human SCN arranged from anterior to posterior **(A–H)** in a representative human hypothalamus (case 95-015) to illustrate the distribution of labeled suprachiasmatic nucleus (SCN) fibers, branching fibers with

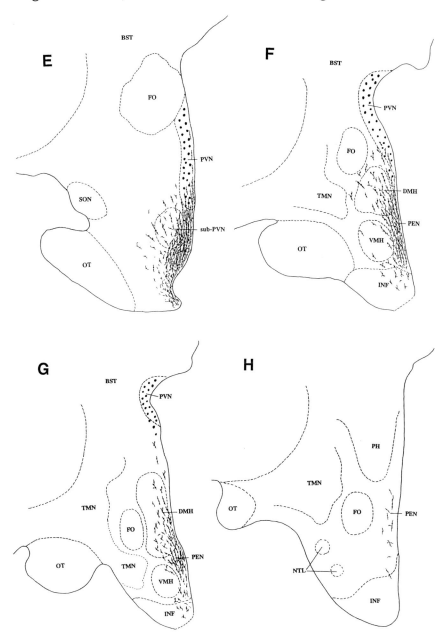

(Fig. 9. continued from opposite page). terminal boutons, and corticotropin-releasing hormone (CRH) cell bodies (dark dots in the PVN). Dark
dots in the SCN represent the area in which labeled neurons can be
detected. (See Section 9 for abbreviations.)

between the periphery and the CNS, adding the time-of-day information to this incoming peripheral information. Together with its multisynaptic pathway to the adrenal cortex, this integrative function of the SCN may form the basis for an explanation of phenomena, such as discrepancies in ACTH and cortisol levels and failing dexamethasone suppression tests during mental depression and Alzheimer's disease (97,98), of which, in the latter disease, a clear-cut deterioration of the SCN is present (81).

The importance of the SCN in maintaining a physiological balance of the body might be further illustrated by the fact that we recently observed dramatic changes in the anatomy of the SCN of persons who died of a circulation problem after a long history of hypertension. In these hypertensive people, postmortem study revealed that in the SCN the number of neurons expressing vasopressin was diminished. In contrast, the PVN was affected in a completely opposite way, as, here, the CRH neurons were present in much higher numbers (99,100).

Interestingly, also in the spontaneously hypertensive rat (SHR), changes of the biological clock are reported, but here it concerns an increase in VIP staining rather than a decrease. The association with the induction of hypertension was clearly demonstrated by transplantation studies of the anterior hypothalamus of SHR into normotensive animals. Such transplantations resulted in the induction of hypertension in the normotensive individual. These observations argue for a causal relationship between hypothalamic changes and the observed hypertension.

Another argument for an important action of the biological clock on circulation is the observed circadian pattern in water resorption by the kidney (101). The presence of the extensive SCN–autonomic connections may explain this phenomenon. In people who underwent a kidney transplantation, this circadian water resorption pattern is lost, which argues for a neuronal regulation of this circadian pattern.

These observations fit the hypothesis that the SCN serves to modulate essential hypothalamic functions. Disturbance of this arrangement may result in disturbances of autonomic functions.

9. Abbreviations

AC	Anterior commissure
AVH	Anteroventral hypothalamic area
BST	Bed nucleus of the stria terminalis
CRH	Corticotropin-releasing hormone
CSF	Cerebrospinal fluid
DMH	Dorsomedial nucleus of the hypothalamus
DMV	Dorsal motor nucleus of the vagus nerve
FO	Fornix
INF	Infundibular nucleus
MB	Mamillary body
NBM	Nucleus basalis of Meynert
NTL	Lateral tuberal nucleus
OC	Optic chiasm
OT	Optic tract
PEN	Periventricular nucleus
PH	Posterior hypothalamic nucleus
PVN	Paraventricular nucleus
PVT	Paraventricular nucleus of thalamus
SCN	Suprachiasmatic nucleus
SCNd	Dorsal part of the suprachiasmatic nucleus
SCNv	Ventral part of the suprachiasmatic nucleus
SDN	Sexually dimorphic nucleus of preoptic area
SON	Supraoptic nucleus
sub-PVN	Area below the paraventricular nucleus
TBS	Tris-buffered saline
TMN	Tuberomamillary nucleus
VMH	Ventromedial nucleus of the hypothalamus
VIP	Vasoactive intestinal polypeptide
VP	Vasopressin
3V	Third ventricle

References

1. Dunlap, J. C., Loros, J. J., Merrow, M., Crosthwaite, S., Bell-Pedersen, D., Garceau, N., et al. (1996) The genetic and molecular dissection of a prototypic circadian system, in *Hypothalamic Integration of Circadian Rhythms. Progress in Brain Research* (Buijs, R. M., Kalsbeek, A.,

Romijn, H. J., Pennarts, C. M., and Mirmiran, M., eds.), Elsevier, Amsterdam, pp. 11–39.

2. Stanewsky, R., Frisch, B., Brandes, C., Hamblencoyle, M. J., Rosbash, M., and Hall, J. C. (1997) Temporal and spatial expression patterns of transgenes containing increasing amounts of the Drosophila clock gene period and a lacZ reporter: mapping elements of the PER protein involved in circadian cycling. *J. Neurosci.* **17,** 676–696.

3. Plautz, J. D., Kaneko, M., Hall, J. C., and Kay, S. A. (1997) Independent photoreceptive circadian clocks throughout drosophila. *Science* **278,** 1632–1635.

4. Cohen, R. A. and Albers, H. E. (1991) Disruption of human circadian and cognitive regulation following a discrete hypothalamic lesion: a case study. *Neurology* **41,** 726–729.

5. Ralph, M. R., Foster, R. G., Davis, F. C., and Menaker, M. (1990) Transplanted suprachiasmatic nucleus determines circadian period. *Science* **247,** 975–978.

6. Buijs, R. M., Wortel, J., Van Heerikhuize, J. J., and Kalsbeek, A. (1997) Novel environment induced inhibition of corticosterone secretion: Physiological evidence for a suprachiasmatic nucleus mediated neuronal hypothalamo-adrenal cortex pathway. *Brain Res.* **758,** 229–236.

7. Swaab, D. F., Van Someren, E. J., Zhou, J. N., and Hofman, M. A. (1996) Biological rhythms in the human life cycle and their relationship to functional changes in the suprachiasmatic nucleus. *Prog. Brain Res.* **111,** 349–368.

8. Dai, J. P. Van der Vliet, J. Swaab, D. F., and Buijs, R. M. (1998) The human retinohypothalamic tract as revealed by in vitro postmortem tracing. *J. Comp. Neurol.* **397,** 357–370.

9. Groos, G., Mason, R., and Meijer, J. (1983) Electrical and pharmacological properties of the suprachiasmatic nuclei. *Fed. Proc.* **42,** 2790–2795.

10 Bos, N. P. A. and Mirmiran, M. (1990) Circadian rhythms in spontaneous neuronal discharges of the cultured suprachiasmatic nucleus. *Brain Res.* **511,** 158–162.

11. Welsh, D. K., Logothetis, D. E., Meister, M., and Reppert, S. M. (1995) Individual neurons dissociated from rat suprachiasmatic nucleus express independently phased circadian firing rhythms. *Neuron.* **14,** 697–706.

12. Schwartz, W. J. and Gainer, H. (1977) Suprachiasmatic nucleus: Use of 14C-labeled deoxyglucose uptake as a functional marker. *Science* **197,** 1089–1091.

13. Gillette, M. U. and Reppert, S. M. (1987) The hypothalamic suprachiasmatic nuclei: circadian patterns of vasopressin secretion and neuronal activity *in vitro*. *Brain Res. Bull.* **19,** 135–139.

14. Scheer, F. A. J. L., van Doornen, L. J. P., and Buijs, R. M. (1999) Light and diurnal cycle affect human heart rate: possible role for the circadian pacemaker. *J. Biol. Rhythms,* **14,** 202–212.

15. Swaab, D. F., Pool, C. W., and Nijveldt, F. (1975) Immunofluorescence of vasopressin and oxytocin in the rat hypothalamo-neurohypophyseal system. *J. Neural Transm.* **36,** 195–215.
16. Vandesande, F., Dierickx, K., and De Mey, J. (1975) Identification of the vasopressin–neurophysin producing neurons of the rat suprachiasmatic nuclei. *Cell Tissue Res.* **156,** 377–380.
17. Vandenpol, A. N. and Gorcs, T. (1986) Synaptic relationships between neurons containing vasopressin, gastrin-releasing peptide, vasoactive intestinal polypeptide, and glutamate–decarboxylase immunoreactivity in the rat suprachiasmatic nucleus. *J. Comp. Neurol.* **252,** 507–521.
18. Card, J. P., Brecha, N., Karten, H. J., and Moore, R. Y. (1981) Immunocytochemical localization of vasoactive intestinal polypeptide-containing cells and processes in the suprachiasmatic nucleus of the rat: light and electron microscopic analysis. *J. Neurosci.* **11,** 1289–1303.
19. Buijs, R. M., Hou, Y. X., Shinn, S., and Renaud, L. P. (1994) Ultrastructural evidence for intra- and extranuclear projections of GABAergic neurons of the suprachiasmatic nucleus. *J. Comp. Neurol.* **335,** 42–54.
20. Hermes, M. L. H. J., Coderre, E. M., Buijs, R. M., and Renaud, L. P. (1996) GABA and glutamate mediate rapid neurotransmission from suprachiasmatic nucleus to hypothalamic paraventricular nucleus in rat. *J. Physiol. London* **496,** 749–757.
21. Moore, R. Y. and Speh, J. C. (1993) GABA is the principal neurotransmitter of the circadian system. *Neurosci. Lett.* **150,** 112–116.
22. Buijs, R. M., Wortel, J., and Hou, Y. X. (1995) Colocalization of gamma-aminobutyric acid with vasopressin, vasoactive intestinal peptide, and somatostatin in the rat suprachiasmatic nucleus. *J. Comp. Neurol.* **358,** 343–352.
23. Lundberg, J. M., Änggård, A., and Fahrenkrug, J. (1981) Complementary role of vasoactive intestinal polypeptide (VIP) and acetylcholine for cat submandibular gland blood flow and secretion. II. Effects of cholinergic antagonists and VIP antiserum. *Acta Physiol. Scand.* **113,** 329–336.
24. Lundberg, J. M., Francocereceda, A., Lou, Y. P., Modin, A., and Pernow, J. (1994) Differential release of classical transmitters and peptides. *Molecular and Cellular Mechanisms of Neurotransmitter of Meurotransmitter Release,* vol. 29 (Stjarne, L., Grillner, S. E., and Greengard, P., eds.), Raven Press, New York.
25. Whim, M. D. and Lloyd, P. E. (1989) Frequency-dependent release of peptide cotransmitters from identified cholinergic motor neurons in aplysia. *Proc. Natl. Acad. Sci. USA* **86,** 9034–9038.
26. Cropper, E. C. M., Miller, M. W., Villm, F. S., Tenenbaum, R., Kupferman, I., and Weiss, K. R. (1990) Release of peptide cotransmitters

from a cholinergic motor neuron under physiological conditions. *Proc. Natl. Acad. Sci. USA* **87,** 933–937.

27. Inouye, S. T. and Kawamura, H. (1979) Persistence of circadian rhythmicity in a mammalian hypothalamic "island" containing the suprachiasmatic nucleus. *Proc. Natl. Acad. Sci. USA* **76,** 5962–5966.
28. Earnest, D. J. and Sladek, C. D. (1986) Circadian rhythms of vasopressin release from individual rat suprachiasmatic explants in vitro. *Brain Res.* **382,** 129–133.
29. Joëls, M. and Urban, I. J. A. (1982) The effect of microiontophoretically applied vasopressin and oxytocin on single neurones in the septum and dorsal hippocampus of the rat. *Neurosci. Lett.* **33,** 79–84.
30. Van Den Hooff, P. and Urban, I. J. A. (1990) Vasopressin facilitates excitatory transmission in slices of the rat dorso-lateral septum. *Synapse* **5,** 201–206.
31. Raggenbass, M., Tribollet, E., Dubois-Dauphin, M., and Dreifuss, J. J. (1989) Vasopressin receptors of the vasopressor (V1) type in the nucleus of the solitary tract of the rat mediate direct neuronal excitation. *J. Neurosci.* **9,** 3929–3936.
32. Kalsbeek, A., Cutrera, R. A., Van Heerikhuize, J. J., Van der Vliet, J., and Buijs, R. M. (1999) GABA release from SCN terminals is necessary for the light-induced inhibition of nocturnal melatonin release in the rat. *Neuroscience* **91,** 453–461.
33. Wagner, S., Castel, M., Gainer, H., and Yarom, Y. (1997) GABA in the mammalian suprachiasmatic nucleus and Its role in diurnal rhythmicity. *Nature* **387,** 598–603.
34. Schwartz, W. J. and Reppert, S. M. (1985) Neural regulation of the circadian vasopressin rhythm in cerebrospinal fluid: a pre-eminent role for the suprachiasmatic nuclei. *J. Neurosci.* **5,** 2771–2778.
35. Jolkonen, J., Tuomisto, L., Van Wimersma Greidanus, T. B., and Riekkinen, P. J. (1988) Vasopressin levels in the cerebrospinal fluid of rats with lesions of the paraventricular and suprachiasmatic nuclei. *Neurosci. Lett.* **86,** 184–188.
36. Kalsbeek, A., Van der Vliet, J., and Buijs, R. M. (1996) Decrease of endogenous vasopressin release necessary for expression of the circadian rise in plasma corticosterone: a reverse microdialysis study. *J. Neuroendocrinol.* **8,** 299–307.
37. Uhl, G. R. and Reppert, S. M. (1986) Suprachiasmatic nucleus vasopressin messenger RNA: circadian variation in normal and Brattleboro rats. *Science* **232,** 390–393.
38. Robinson, B. G., Frim, D. M., Schwartz, W. J., and Majzoub, J. A. (1988) Vasopressin mRNA in the suprachiasmatic nuclei: daily regulation of polyadenylate tail length. *Science* **241,** 342–344.
39. Larsen, P. J., Vrang, N., Moller, M., Jessop, D. S., Lightman, S. L., Chowdrey, H. S., et al. (1994) The diurnal expression of genes encoding vasopressin and vasoactive intestinal peptide within the

rat suprachiasmatic nucleus is influenced by circulating glucocorticoids. *Mol. Brain Res.* **27,** 342–346.

40. Rosenfeld, P., Vaneekelen, J. A. M., Levine, S., and De Kloet, E. R. (1993) Ontogeny of corticosteroid receptors in the brain. *Cell. Mol. Neurobiol.* **13,** 295–319.

41. Visser, D. T. M., Hu, Z. T., Pasterkamp, R. J., Morimoto, M., and Kawata, M. (1996) The alteration of glucocorticoid receptor-immunoreactivity in the rat forebrain following short-term and long-term adrenalectomy. *Brain Res.* **729,** 216–222.

42. Reppert, S. M., Weaver, D. R., and Ebisawa, T. (1994) Cloning and characterization of a mammalian melatonin receptor that mediates reproductive and circadian responses. *Neuron* **13,** 1177–1185.

43. Liu, C., Weaver, D. R., Jin, X. W., Shearman, L. P., Pieschl, R. L., Gribkoff, V. K., and Reppert, S. M. (1997) Molecular dissection of two distinct actions of melatonin on the suprachiasmatic circadian clock. *Neuron* **19,** 91–102.

44. Buijs, R. M. (1978) Intra- and extrahypothalamic vasopressin and oxytocin pathways in the rat. Pathways to the limbic system, medulla oblongata and spinal cord. *Cell Tissue Res.* **192,** 423–435.

45. Sofroniew, M. V. and Weindl, A. (1978) Extrahypothalamic neurophysin-containing perikarya, fiber pathways and fiber clusters in the rat brain. *Endocrinology* **102,** 334–337.

46. Hoorneman, E. M. D. and Buijs, R. M. (1982) Vasopressin fiber pathways in the rat brain following suprachiasmatic nucleus lesioning. *Brain Res.* **243,** 235–241.

47. Berk, M. L. and Finkelstein, J. A. (1981) An autoradiographic determination of the efferent projections of the suprachiasmatic nucleus of the hypothalamus. *Brain Res.* **226,** 1–13.

48. Stephan, F. K., Berkley, K. J., and Moss, R. L. (1981) Efferent connections of the rat suprachiasmatic nucleus. *Neuroscience* **6,** 2625–2641.

49. Watts, A. G., Swanson, L. W., and Sanchez-Watts, G. (1987) Efferent projections of the suprachiasmatic nucleus: I. Studies using anterograde transport of Phaseolus vulgaris leucoagglutinin in the rat. *J. Comp. Neurol.* **258,** 204–229.

50. Buijs, R. M., Markman, M., Nunes-Cardoso, B., Hou, Y. X., and Shinn, S. (1993) Projections of the suprachiasmatic nucleus to stress-related areas in the rat hypothalamus: a light and electronmicroscopic study. *J. Comp. Neurol.* **335,** 42–54.

51. Vrang, N., Larsen, P. J., Moller, M., and Mikkelsen, J. D. (1995) Topographical organization of the rat suprachiasmatic–paraventricular projection. *J. Comp. Neurol.* **353,** 585–603.

52. Teclemariam-Mesbah, R., Kalsbeek, A., Pevet, P., and Buijs, R. M. (1997) Direct vasoactive intestinal polypeptide-containing projection from the suprachiasmatic nucleus to spinal projecting hypothalamic paraventricular neurons. *Brain Res.* **748,** 71–76.

53. Teclemariam-Mesbah, R., Kalsbeek, A., Buijs, R. M., and Pevet, P. (1997) Oxytocin innervation of spinal preganglionic neurons projecting to the superior cervical ganglion in the rat. *Cell Tissue Res.* **287,** 481–486.
54. Teclemariam-Mesbah, R., Ter Horst, G. J., Postema, F., Wortel, J., and Buijs, R. M. (1999) Anatomical demonstration of the suprachiasmatic nucleus-pineal pathway. *J. Comp. Neurol.* **406,** 171–182.
55. Johnson, R. F., Morin, L. P., and Moore, R. Y. (1988) Retinohypothalamic projections in the hamster and rat demonstrated using cholera toxin. *Brain Res.* **462,** 301–312.
56. Berendse, H. W., Voorn, P., te Kortschot, A., and Groenewegen, H. J. (1988) Nuclear origin of thalamic afferents of the ventral striatum determines their relation to patch/matrix configurations in enkephalin-immunoreactivity in the rat. *J. Chem. Neuroanat.* **1,** 3–10.
57. Dallman, M. F., Akana, S. F., Scribner, K. A., Bradbury, M. J., Walker, C. D., Strack, A. M., and Cascio, C. S. (1992) Stress, feedback and facilitation in the hypothalamo–pituitary–adrenal axis. *J. Neuroendocrinol.* **4,** 517–526.
58. Swanson, L. W. and Simmons, D. M. (1989) Differential steroid hormone and neural influences on peptide mRNA levels in CRH cells of the paraventricular nucleus: a hybridization histochemical study in the rat. *J. Comp. Neurol.* **285,** 413–435.
59. Kwak, S. P., Morano, M. I., Young, E. A., Watson, S. J., and Akil, H. (1993) Diurnal CRH messenger RNA rhythm in the hypothalamus–decreased expression in the evening is not dependent on endogenous glucocorticoids. *Neuroendocrinology* **57,** 96–105.
60. Roland, B. L. and Sawchenko, P. E. (1993) Local origins of some GABAergic projections to the paraventricular and supraoptic nuclei of the hypothalamus in the rat. *J. Comp. Neurol.* **332,** 123–143.
61. Levin, M. C., Sawchenko, P. E., Howe, P. R. C., Bloom, S. R., and Polak, J. M. (1987) Organization of galanin-immunoreactive inputs to the paraventricular nucleus with special reference to their relationship to catecholaminergic afferents. *J. Comp. Neurol.* **261,** 562–582.
62. Ter Horst, G. J. and Luiten, P. G. M. (1986) The projections of the dorsomedial hypothalamic nucleus in the rat. *Brain Res. Bull.* **16,** 231–248.
63. Kalsbeek, A., Buijs, R. M., Van Heerikhuize, J. J., Arts, M., and Van Der Woude, T. P. (1992) Vasopressin-containing neurons of the suprachiasmatic nuclei inhibit corticosterone release. *Brain Res.* **580,** 62–67.
64. Kalsbeek, A., Van Heerikhuize, J. J., Wortel, J., and Buijs, R. M. (1996) A diurnal rhythm of stimulatory input to the hypothalamo–pituitary–adrenal system as revealed by timed intrahypothalamic administration of the vasopressin V-1 antagonist. *J. Neurosci.* **16,** 5555–5565.

frontal cortex also interfere with the conditioned heart rate response *(77–79)*. It was demonstrated that lesions of the medial prefrontal cortex, which included the infralimbic cortex, significantly reduce the sympathetic but not the parasympathetic component of the heart rate change evoked by a conditioned stimulus *(79)*.

The infralimbic cortex has extensive connections with both the limbic and autonomic systems of the brain. It receives inputs from the insular and entorhinal cortices, the hippocampus amygdala (particularly the basal lateral nucleus), the visceral relay nuclei of the thalamus, the paraventricular nucleus of the thalamus, the parabrachial nucleus, and the nucleus of the solitary tract *(39,42,80–86)*. The infralimbic cortex has descending projections to a number of autonomic sites, including the insular cortex, the central nucleus of the amygdala, the visceral relay nuclei of the thalamus, anterior hypothalamus, lateral hypothalamic area, parabrachial nucleus, nucleus of the solitary tract, and spinal cord *(86–90)*. The comprehensive study of the infralimbic cortex by Takagishi and Chiba *(90)* support the concept that the infralimbic cortex can be considered the "visceral motor cortex." Recent evidence, in anesthetized rats, has indicated that the cardiovascular responses originating in the infralimbic cortex is relayed through the lateral hypothalamic area *(91)*. In addition, the decrease in blood pressure elicited by the infralimbic cortex is mediated by a glutamatergic input onto local GABA neurons in the lateral hypothalamic area (unpublished results). Thus, the infralimbic connectivity provides the anatomical substrate for a critical role in autonomic control, even though the complete function of these pathways is unknown.

5. Amygdala

The amygdala plays an important role in the expression of emotional behaviors *(92–94)* and integrates the autonomic responses to emotional stimuli under certain conditions, particularly those related to fear and anxiety *(95)*. The amygdala in humans has been shown to be activated by emotional response *(96)*. In rabbits, lesions or β-adrenergic antagonist or opiate agonist injections into the amygdala attenuate the bradycardia response induced by a conditioned fear response *(97–99)*. Furthermore, both the behavioral and autonomic concomitants of classical conditioning of fear to an acoustic stimulus sequentially involve the primary auditory sites in the brainstem, the auditory receptive region of the thalamus, and, finally, the amygdala *(93,100–102)*.

Many cardiovascular investigations involving stimulation of the amygdala have been difficult to interpret because of the use of anesthetics or electrical stimulation [reviewed by Iwata et al. *94)*]. Investigations utilizing electrical stimulation have observed an increase in blood pressure and heart rate in awake rat preparations, whereas a decrease in pressure is obtained in anesthetized animals *(103,104)*. Similar changes in arterial blood pressure and heart rate have also been demonstrated using microinjections of glutamate, which activate cell bodies only and not fibers of passage *(94)*. This dependence on the state of the animal was further indicated by the demonstration that the pressor response evoked by amygdalar stimulation is greatly attenuated during sleep states *(105)*.

The amygdala receives cardiopulmonary information and has direct projections to autonomic control sites, such as the hypothalamus, parabrachial nucleus, nucleus of the solitary tract, and dorsal motor nucleus of the vagus, which may be the anatomical substrate for descending control over the autonomic nervous system *(106–120)*. In addition, the amygdala has intense reciprocal connections with the infralimbic cortex. The afferents to the infralimbic cortex are ipsilateral and arise primarily from the basal lateral nucleus *(80)*, whereas the efferents from the infralimbic cortex terminate primarily in the central and medial nuclei of the amygdala *(87)*. Thus, the amygdala is a critical site for mediating emotional behaviors with major inputs to and projections from the infralimbic cortex.

A number of lines of evidence have contributed to our understanding of the interrelationships of the insular cortex

and the amygdala in mediating the cardiovascular consequences of stress and stroke. First, as indicated, the amygdala
is an important cardiovascular control center within the limbic system with reciprocal connections with the insular cortex and direct projections to other autonomic control centers
in the hypothalamus, pons, and medulla, and studies on fear
and anxiety reactions demonstrate that the amygdala is central in integrating autonomic responses to emotional stimuli.
Second, the startle response, with its accompanying autonomic and behavioral changes to an acoustic stimulus, is
mediated through the subcortical auditory centers directly
to the amygdala *(94,100–102,121–124)*. Third, there is evidence that lesion of the insular cortex, such as is observed in
the MCAO stroke model from our laboratory, can elicit
changes in arterial pressure and heart rate, in response to
stressful stimuli, which are greater in MCAO rats than a
sham-operated control group *(125)*. In addition, power spectral analysis of heart rate variability indicated that the exaggerated responses to the stressful stimuli were mediated by
increases in sympathetic activity. The stressful stimuli used
in these experiments included intermittent and continuous
noise and air-jet stimulation of the face. Cardiovascular
responses to these stimuli were examined on d 2, and 5–10
after MCAO or sham MCAO. The peak of the enhanced cardiovascular responses occurred on d 5–7 and had recovered
by d 10. This time-course of events was very similar to that
observed for the neurochemical (dynorphin and neurotensin)
changes in the central nucleus of the amygdala *(126–128)* and
provides further support that there are functional changes
in the amygdala, as evidenced by the neurochemical changes,
that may be mediating the cardiovascular complications of
stroke. Finally, we have recently obtained preliminary evidence that one of these neurochemical changes (dynorphin)
is directly involved in the generation of exaggerated cardiovascular responses to acoustic stress. In anesthetized rats, the
acoustic-stress pathway was electrically stimulated and the
cardiovascular responses monitored before and after microinjection of dynorphin into the amygdala. Administration of

dynorphin into the amygdala significantly enhanced the cardiovascular responses to stimulation of the acoustic-stress pathway. Thus, the results suggest that a lesion of the insular cortex, as occurs in hemispheric stroke, through its direct connections, can alter the neurochemical components of the central nucleus of the amygdala, which, in turn, is involved in modulating the cardiovascular consequences of stress via increases in dynorphin.

6. Summary

Three regions of the forebrain have been described that are intimately involved in central control of the cardiovascular system and are the mediators of the cardiovascular consequences of stroke and stress and likely play a significant role in the pathologies such as sudden cardiac death. The insular cortex can generate substantial cardiovascular responses via a pathway that includes synapses in the lateral hypothalamic area and the rostral–ventral lateral medulla. The responses can be a severe disruption of the cardiac control to the point of complete asystole. The insular cortex also receives topographically organized visceral inputs. It has intimate connections with the adjacent somatosensory areas and other cortical and subcortical cardiovascular control centers, such as the infralimbic cortex, amygdala, which suggest its important role in the integration of somatic and visceral functions in response to physical activities, behavioral changes, and different emotional states. The infralimbic cortex, visceral motor cortex, can also generate substantial cardiovascular changes, primarily inhibition of autonomic tone. It has considerable interconnections with autonomic and limbic structures, particularly the insular cortex and the amygdala and a direct pathway to the sympathetic preganglionics neurons in the spinal cord. Finally, the amygdala appears to be the primary subcortical structure in the basal forebrain that interrelates the insular cortex and the infralimbic cortex. The amygdala plays a major role in integrating autonomic responses to emotional stimuli and

62. Oppenheimer, S. M., Gelb, A., Girvan, J. P., and Hachinski, V. C. (1992) Cardiovascular effects of human insular cortex stimulation. *Neurology* **42,** 1727–1732.
63. Sander, D. and Klingelhofer, J. (1995) Stroke-associated pathological sympathetic activation related to size of infarction and extent of insular damage. *Cerebrovasc. Dis.* **5,** 381–385.
64. Sander, D. and Klingelhofer, J. (1995) Changes of circadian blood pressure patterns and cardiovascular parameters indicate lateralization of sympathetic activation following hemispheric brain infarction. *J. Neurol.* **242,** 313–318.
65. Oppenheimer, S. M., Kedem, G., and Martin, W. M. (1996) Left-insular cortex lesions perturb cardiac autonomic tone in humans. *Clin. Autonom. Res.* **6,** 1–4.
66. Cechetto, D. F. and Saper, C. B. (1990) Role of the cerebral cortex in autonomic function, in *The Autonomic Nervous System: Central Regulation of Autonomic Functions* (Loewy, A. D. and Spyer, K. M., eds.), Oxford University Press, New York, pp. 208–223.
67. Smith, W. K. J. (1945) The functional significance of the rostral cingular cortex as revealed by its response to electrical stimulation. *Neurophysiology* **8,** 241–255.
68. Ward, A. A. (1948) The cingular gyrus: area 24. *J. Neurophysiol.* **11,** 13–23.
69. Lofving, B. (1961) Cardiovascular adjustments induced from the rostral cingulate gyrus. *Acta Physiol. Scand.* **53(Suppl. 184),** 1–82.
70. Buchanan, S. L., Powell, D. A., and Buggy, J. (1984) 3H-2-Deoxyglucose uptake after electrical stimulation of cardioactive sites in anterior medial cortex in rabbits. *Brain Res. Bull.* **13,** 371–382.
71. Buchanan, S. L., Valentine, J., and Powell, D. A. (1985) Autonomic responses are elicited by electrical stimulation of the medial but not lateral frontal cortex in rabbits. *Behav. Brain Res.* **18,** 51–62.
72. Burns, S. M. and Wyss, J. M. (1985) The involvement of the anterior cingulate cortex in blood pressure control. *Brain Res.* **340,** 71–77.
73. Hurley-Guis, K. M. and Neafsey, E. J. (1986) The medial frontal cortex and gastric motility: microstimulation results and their possible significance for the overall pattern of organization of rat frontal and parietal cortex. *Brain Res.* **365,** 241–248.
74. Verberne, A. J. M. (1996) Medullary sympathoexcitatory neurons are inhibited by activation of the medial prefrontal cortex in the rat. *Am. J. Physiol.* **270,** R713–R719.
75. Verberne, A. J. M., Lewis, S. J., Worland, P. J., Beart, P. M., Jarrott, B., Christie, M. J., et al. (1987) Medial prefrontal cortical lesions modulate baroreflex sensitivity in the rat. *Brain Res.* **426,** 243–249.
76. Szilagyi, J. E., Taylor, A. A., and Skinner, J. E. (1987) Cryoblockade of the ventromedial frontal cortex reverses hypertension in the rat. *Hypertension* **9,** 576–581.

77. Buchanan, S. L. and Powell, D. A. (1982) Cingulate damage attenuates conditioned bradycardia. *Neurosci. Lett.* **29,** 261–268.
78. Buchanan, S. L. and Powell, D. A. (1982) Cingulate cortex: its role in Pavlovian conditioning. *J. Comp. Physiol. Psychol.* **96,** 755–774.
79. Frysztak, R. J. and Neafsey, E. J. (1994) The effect of medial frontal cortex lesions on cardiovascular conditioned emotional responses in the rat. *Brain Res.* **643,** 181–193.
80. Condé, F., Marie-Lepoivre, E., Audinat, E., and Crêpel, F. (1995) Afferent connections of the medial frontal cortex of the rat. II. Cortical and subcortical afferents. *J. Comp. Neurol.* **352,** 567–593.
81. Fulwiler, C. E. and Saper, C. B. (1984) Subnuclear organization of the efferent connections of the parabrachial nucleus in the rat. *Brain Res. Rev.* **7,** 229–259.
82. Rosene, D. L. and van Hoesen, G. W. (1977) Hippocampal efferents reach widespread areas of cerebral cortex and amygdala in the rhesus monkey. *Science* **198,** 315–317.
83. Saper, C. B. (1985) Organization of cerebral cortical afferent systems in the rat. II. Hypothalamocortical projections. *J. Comp. Neurol.* **237,** 21–46.
84. Swanson, L. W. (1981) A direct projection from Ammon's horn to prefrontal cortex in the rat. *Brain Res.* **217,** 150–154.
85. van der Kooy, D., Koda, L. Y., McGinty, J. F., Gerfen, C. R., and Bloom, F. E. (1984) The organization of projections from the cortex, amygdala, and hypothalamus to the nucleus of the solitary tract in rat. *J. Comp. Neurol.* **224,** 1–24.
86. Yasui, Y., Itoh, K., Kaneko, T., Sugimoto, T., and Mizuno, N. (1986) Direct projections from the parvocellular part of the posteromedial ventral nucleus of the thalamus to the infralimbic cortex in the cat. *Brain Res.* **368,** 384–388.
87. Hurley, K. M., Herbert, H., Moga, M. M., and Saper, C. B. (1991) Efferent projections of the infralimbic cortex of the rat. *J. Comp. Neurol.* **308,** 249–276.
88. Room, P., Russchen, F. T., Groenwegen, H. J., and Lohman, A. H. M. (1985) Efferent connections of the prelimbic (area 32) and the infralimbic (area 25) cortices: an anterograde tracing study in the cat. *J. Comp. Neurol.* **242,** 40–55.
89. Terreberry, R. R. and Neafsey, E. J. (1983) Rat medial frontal cortex: a visceral motor region with a direct projection to the solitary nucleus. *Brain Res.* **278,** 245–249.
90. Takagisha, M. and Chiba, T. (1991) Efferent projections of the infralimbic (area 25) region of the medial prefrontal cortex in the rat: an anterograde tracer PHA-L study. *Brain Res.* **566,** 26–39.
91. Way, M. and Cechetto, D. F. (1996) Neurotransmitters in the lateral hypothalamic area mediating cardiovascular responses from the infralimbic cortex. *Soc. Neurosci. Abstr.* **22,** 391.

92. Folkow, B., Hallback-Nordlander, M., Martner, J., and Nordberg, C. (1982) Influence of amygdala lesions on cardiovascular responses to alerting stimuli, on behaviour and on blood pressure development in spontaneously hypertensive rats. *Acta Physiol. Scand.* **116,** 133–139.

93. Iwata, J., LeDoux, J. E., Meeley, M. P., Arneric, S., and Reis, D. J. (1986) Intrinsic neurons in the amygdaloid field projected to by the medial geniculate body mediate emotional responses conditioned to acoustic stimuli. *Brain Res.* **383,** 195–214.

94. Iwata, J., Chida, K., and LeDoux, J. E. (1987) Cardiovascular responses elicited by stimulation of neurons in the central amygdaloid nucleus in awake by not anesthetized rats resemble conditioned emotional responses. *Brain Res.* **418,** 183–188.

95. Davis, M. (1992) The role of the amygdala in fear and anxiety. *Annu. Rev. Neurosci.* **15,** 353– 375.

96. Irwin, W., Davidson, R. J., Lowe, M. J., Mock, B. J., Sorenson, J. A., and Turski, P. A. (1996) Human amygdala activation detected with echo-planar functional magnetic resonance imaging. *NeuroReport* **7,** 1765–1769.

97. Gallagher, M., Kapp, B. S., Frysinger, R. C., and Rapp, P. R. (1980) Beta-adrenergic manipulation in amygdala central n. alters rabbit heart rate conditioning. *Pharmacol. Biochem. Behav.* **12,** 419–426.

98. Gallagher, M., Kapp, B. S., and Pascoe, J. P. (1982) Enkephalin analogue effects in the amygdala central nucleus on conditioned heart rate. *Pharmacol. Biochem. Behav.* **17,** 217–222.

99. Kapp, B. S., Frysinger, R. C., Gallagher, M., and Haselton, J. R. (1979) Amygdala central nucleus lesions: effect on heart rate conditioning in the rabbit. *Physiol. Behav.* **23,** 1109–1117.

100. LeDoux, J. E., Delbo, A., Tucker, L. W., Harshfield, G., Talman. W. T., and Reis, D. J. (1982) Hierarchic organization of blood pressure responses during the expression of natural behaviors in rat: mediation by sympathetic nerves. *Exp. Neurol.* **78,** 121–133.

101. LeDoux, J. E., Sakaguchi, A., Iwata, J., and Reis, D. J. (1986) Interruption of projections from the medial geniculate body to an archineostriatal field disrupts the classical conditioning of emotional responses to acoustic stimuli. *Neuroscience* **17,** 615–627.

102. LeDoux, J. E., Ruggiero, D. A., Forest, R., Stornetta, R., and Reis, D. J. (1987) Topographic organization of convergent projections to the thalamus from the inferior colliculus and spinal cord in the rat. *J. Comp. Neurol.* **264,** 123–146.

103. Galeno, T. M. and Brody, M. J. (1983) Hemodynamic responses to amygdaloid stimulation in spontaneously hypertensive rats. *Am. J. Physiol.* **245,** R281–R286.

104. Gelsema, A. J., McKittrick, D. J., and Calaresu, F. R. (1987) Cardiovascular responses to chemical and electrical stimulation of amygdala in rats. *Am. J. Physiol.* **253,** R712–R718.

105. Frysinger, R. C. and Harper, R. M. (1984) Sleep states attenuate the pressor response to central amygdala stimulation. *Exp. Neurol.* **83,** 604–617.
106. Allen, G. V., Saper, C. B., Hurley, K. M., and Cechetto, D. F. (1991) Organization of visceral and limbic connections in the insular cortex of the rat. *J. Comp. Neurol.* **311,** 1–16.
107. Cechetto, D. F. and Calaresu, F. R. (1983) Response of single units in the amygdala to stimulation of buffer nerves in cat. *Am. J. Physiol.* **244,** R646–R651.
108. Cechetto, D. F., Ciriello, J., and Calaresu, F. R. (1983) Afferent connections to cardiovascular sites in the amygdala: a horseradish peroxidase study in the cat. *J. Auton. Nerv. Syst.* **8,** 97–110.
109. Cechetto, D. F. and Calaresu, F. R. (1983) Parabrachial units responding to stimulation of buffer nerves and forebrain in the cat. *Am. J. Physiol.* **245,** R811–R819.
110. Cechetto, D. F. and Calaresu, F. R. (1984) Units in the amygdala responding to activation of carotid baro- and chemoreceptors. *Am. J. Physiol.* **246,** R832–R836.
111. Cechetto, D. F. and Calaresu, F. R. (1985) Central pathways relaying cardiovascular afferent information to amygdala. *Am. J. Physiol.* **248,** R38–R45.
112. Cechetto, D. F. (1987) Central representation of visceral function. *Fed. Proc.* **46,** 17–230.
113. Cechetto, D. F. (1995) Supraspinal mechanisms of visceral representation, in *Visceral Pain,* Progress in Pain Research and Management, Vol. 5 (Gebhart, G. F., ed.), IASP, Seattle, WA, pp. 261–289.
114. Danielsen, E. H., Magnuson, D. J., and Gray, T. S. (1989) The central amygdaloid nucleus innervation of the dorsal vagal complex in rat: a Phaseolus vulgaris leucoagglutinin lectin anterograde tracing study. *Brain Res. Bull.* **22,** 705–715.
115. Hopkins, D. A. and Holstege, G. (1978) Amygdaloid projections to the mesencephalon, pons and medulla oblongata in the cat. *Exp. Brain Res.* **32,** 529–547.
116. Mizuno, M., Takahashi, O., Satoda, T., and Matsushima, R. (1985) Amygdalospinal projections in the macaque monkey. *Neurosci. Lett.* **53,** 327–330.
117. Moga, M. M., Herbert, H., Hurley, K. M., Yasui, Y., Gray, T. S., and Saper, C. B. (1990) Organization of cortical, basal forebrain, and hypothalamic afferents to the parabrachial nucleus in the rat. *J. Comp. Neurol.* **295,** 624–661.
118. Price, J. L. and Amaral, D. G. (1981) An autoradiographic study of the projections of the central nucleus of the monkey amygdala. *J. Neurosci.* **1,** 1242–1259.
119. Sandrew, B. B., Edwards, D. L., Poletti, C. E., and Foot, W. E. (1986) Amygdalospinal projections in the cat. *Brain Res.* **373,** 235–239.

120. Schwaber, J. S., Kapp, B. S., Higgins, G. A., and Rapp, P. R. (1982) Amygdaloid and basal forebrain direct connections with the nucleus of the solitary tract and the dorsal motor nucleus. *J. Neurosci.* **2,** 1424–1438.
121. Koch, M. and Ebert, U. (1993) Enhancement of the acoustic startle response by stimulatin of an excitatory pathway from the central amygdala/basal nucleus of meynert to the pontine reticular formation. *Exp. Brain Res.* **93,** 231–241.
122. LeDoux, J. E., Iwata, J., Cicchetti, P., and Reis, D. J. (1988) Different projections of the central amygdaloid nucleus mediate autonomic and behavioral correlates of conditioned fear. *J. Neurosci.* **8,** 2517–2529.
123. LeDoux, J. E., Farb, C. R., and Romanski, L. M. (1991) Overlapping projections of the amygdala and striatum from auditory processing areas of the thalamus and cortex. *Neurosci. Lett.* **134,** 139–144.
124. LeDoux, J. E., Ruggiero, D. A., and Reis, D. J. (1985) Projections to the subcortical forebrain from anatomically defined regions of the medial geniculate body in the rat. *J. Comp. Neurol.* **242,** 182–213.
125. Cheung, R. T. F., Hachinski, V. C., Cechetto, D. F. (1997) Cardiovascular responses to stress following middle cerebral artery occlusion in the rat. *Brain Res.* **747,** 181–188.
126. Allen, G. V., Cheung, R. T. F., and Cechetto, D. F. (1995) Neurochemical changes following occlusion of the middle cerebral artery in rats. *Neuroscience* **68,** 1037–1050.
127. Cheung, R. T. F., Diab, T., and Cechetto, D. F. (1994) Time-course of neuropeptide changes in the peri- infarct area and amygdala following focal ischemia in rats. *J. Comp. Neurol.* **360,** 101–120.
128. Cheung, R. T. F. and Cechetto, D. F. (1995) Neuropeptide changes following excitotoxic lesion of the insular cortex in rats. *J. Comp. Neurol.* **362,** 535–550.

CHAPTER 5

Neuropathology and Cardiovascular Regulation

Clinical Aspects

Vilho V. Myllylä, Juha T. Korpelainen,
Uolevi Tolonen, Hannele Havanka, and Anne Saari

1. Clinical Relevance of Studying Cardiovascular Regulation in Neurological Diseases

The most important physiological role of the autonomic nervous system (ANS) is to regulate the functions of various organs, which means it aims to adapt and modulate the somatic behavior to the changing circumstances of endogenous or environmental origin. Therefore, reactions of ANS are linked to almost all the physiological and pathological conditions of the human body. In addition, there are diseases that may primarily or secondarily affect ANS. However, we have to admit that, at the moment, our knowledge of the frequency and severity of the diseases of ANS is inadequate and contradictory, which may be explained by the limited number and reliability of the diagnostic methods, but the situation is rapidly improving, and in the near future, these problems are certainly overcome.

Disturbances of ANS are seen as secondary to the diseases of the peripheral nervous system (PNS) and to those of the central nervous system (CNS) as well as a primary, selective disease involving only ANS, that is often called the pro-

From: *The Nervous System and the Heart*
Ed: G. J. Ter Horst © Humana Press Inc.

gressive autonomic failure (PAF) *(1)*. The most frequently seen diseases of PNS that may be associated with secondary autonomic neuropathy are diabetes, rheumatoid arthritis, amyloidosis, acute polyradiculitis or Guillain–Barré syndrome, uremia and porphyria *(1–4)*. Besides these conditions, we know that autonomic failure may be encountered after toxic exposures, especially after excessive use of alcohol. According to Bannister *(1)*, PAF can be seen as an independent disease or in combination with degenerative CNS diseases, such as Parkinson's disease (PD) and multiple system atrophy (MSA). During the past few years, lots of studies on ANS function in cardiovascular diseases have been performed.

In diabetic patients, the manifestation of autonomic neuropathy generally worsens the prognosis and the life expectancy of the patients, the mortality of the patients being more than 50% within the subsequent 5 yr from the detection of autonomic neuropathy *(5,6)*. Excessive mortality has been explained by increased frequency of cardiac sudden deaths induced by the autonomic neuropathy *(7,8)*. There are some reported cases with total denervation of the heart in diabetics *(9)*, which may lead to circumstances in which the heart does not react at all to external stimuli (e.g., exercise). Silent myocardial infarcts seem to be more prevalent among diabetics than in the normal population *(10)*. Correspondingly, it has been shown that chronic alcoholism associated with autonomic neuropathy markedly worsens the life expectancy of the affected individuals *(11)*.

Recent studies suggest that diminished heart rate (HR) variability and especially a loss of its circadian oscillation are associated with an increased risk of cardiac arrhythmia and sudden death in coronary heart disease *(12–14)*. It is particularly the suppressed vagal activity that during the night seems to be an unfavorable phenomenon leading to unopposed sympathetic activity and an imbalance between the sympathetic and parasympathetic regulatory systems *(12–14)*. On the other hand, it is interesting that also acute cerebrovascular diseases cause prognostically unfavorable suppression of HR variability similar to that observed in coronary heart disease *(15–20)*.

Autonomic disturbances can also lead to serious complications of other CNS diseases (e.g., of syringobulbia clearly increasing the risk of sudden death) *(21)*. Many further reports indicate that autonomic dysfunction is a common phenomenon in the group of degenerative CNS disorders [e.g., a majority of PD patients do suffer from vegetative symptoms *(22)*] and the disturbances can be objectively verified by the bedside methods commonly used. However, the exact clinical significance of these findings still remains to be shown.

Because of the serious complications induced by the diseases of ANS and their prognostic implications, it is important that scientific research work will continue providing us with new sophisticated methods and new data on the role of ANS in healthy and diseased individuals. As it is known that there are wide individual and interindividual variations of the autonomic responses, it is important that objective recording methods be developed. At the moment, the physiology and pathology of HR variability are best known. It is probable that the nonlinear methods applying long-term registrations will be developed and utilized more in the near future. The function of the heart can be approached as a target of autonomic innervation, which, as we know, can be disturbed by many neurological diseases. Analogously, the function of ANS can be seen to be dependent on the condition and diseases of other organs, especially of the heart. It is also obvious that these interactions between ANS and other systems will deserve much future research, including the interactions with endocrinological as well as immunological systems. These studies will certainly be helpful also to individual patients suffering from autonomic dysfunction, providing methods for a careful examination in order to assess the extent and severity of ANS disturbances and, finally, even the specific therapy.

2. Methods for Assessing Cardiovascular Autonomic Function

Clinical evaluation of autonomic dysfunction is laborious. Objective and quantitative methods are needed. During the last few years, various methods of analyzing HR and blood pressure (BP) variability for testing and quantifying of the ANS function are increasingly used *(23)*.

Parasympathetic and sympathetic neural mechanisms that control cardiovascular system generate different low-frequency and high-frequency rhythms in HR variability (HRV) and arterial BP *(24)*. Vagal nerve traffic cannot be measured directly in humans. The measurement of HR variability has become the most widely used indirect measure of vagal nerve function *(23)*. Muscle and skin sympathetic activity can be directly measured in humans, but these techniques are not applicable for clinical studies *(25)*. Surveying of HR variability at rest and HR and arterial BP responses to certain tests such as deep breathing, Valsalva maneuvre, and standing provide a golden standard for bedside assessing of the cardiovascular autonomic function *(23)*.

Other tests suited to assess neural and vascular autonomic functions are the thermoregulatory sweating test, the quantitative sudomotor axon reflex test, the sympathetic skin response (SSR), and the laser Doppler flowmetry of skin vasomotor reflexes.

3. Evaluation of Orthostatic Hypotension

Orthostatic hypotension (OH) is defined as a reduction of systolic BP of at least 20 mm-Hg or diastolic BP of at least 10 mm Hg within 3 min of standing or head-up tilting at an angle of at least 60° *(26)*. It is a physical sign but not a disease. It may be symptomatic or asymptomatic. Symptoms of OH are those that develop upon assuming the erect position or following head-up tilt and usually resolve on resuming the recumbent position. They include light-headedness, dizziness, blurred vision, weakness, fatigue, cognitive impairment, nausea, palpitations, tremulousness, headache, and neck pain. OH may be idiopathic or it may be connected to pure autonomic failure (PAF), Parkinson's disease (PD), or multiple system atrophy (MSA) *(26)*.

When OH is part of a more widespread autonomic failure as in PAF, reduced supine plasma norepinephrine levels are characteristic, in addition to BP reduction upon standing or head-up tilt, and measurement of plasma norepinephrine concentration should be performed.

Spectral estimation of HRV may enhance diagnosing of OH *(27)*: Disappearance of slow oscillations in HRV spectrum after tilting might reflect withdrawal of effect sympathetic drive and initiation of central inhibitory vasodepressor reflex as an early trigger of syncope.

4. Cardiovascular Reflexes

The most commonly used cardiovascular reflex tests are as follows:

- Evaluation of respiratory sinus arrhythmia at rest
- Evaluation of respiratory sinus arrhythmia during deep breathing
- HR and BP responses to Valsalva maneuvre
- HR and BP responses to standing or tilting
- BP changes evoked by isometric handwork

4.1. Investigation Procedure

Cardiovascular autonomic function tests are performed under standardized environmental conditions: in a warm and silent room at a comfortable bed (seldom on a chair). Anxiety by increasing sympathetic drive especially in children may attenuate, for example, deep breathing HR variability reaction. Because many things can affect ANS balance, the tests should be performed after a normal night's sleep, without drinking of coffee or ingesting food during the last few hours (for 3 h in our laboratory) before the test. Alcohol is not permitted for 12–14 h prior to testing. Drugs affecting ANS are discontinued before testing: anticholinergics, 9-α-fludrocortisone, diuretics, sympathomimetic and parasympathomimetic agents, as well as α- and β-antagonists. According to Braune et al. *(28)*, the registration time in the morning or afternoon did not affect results.

The signals are registered to a computer. In addition to an electrocardiogram (ECG), a breathing signal often using nasal thermistore is conveyed to a computer. In addition to routine BP measurement, the continuous BP pressure monitoring with such a pletysmographic instrument as a Finapress (Ohmeda, Englewood, Colorado, USA) should be used. The optimal sampling frequency is 250 Hz and a sufficiently broad frequency band including a cutoff frequency > 0.02 Hz should be used (29). During analysis, it should be possible to visualize the raw signals (artifact rejection) and it should be possible to check on the performances of Valsalva blowing, breathing, and isometric handgrip; missed tests must be abolished.

Usually during the same session, several subtests are performed. The interval between the subtests must be standardized: In our laboratory, the next test is not begun until HR and BP return to the rest levels. Before the tests, a patient's maximum contracting power (handgrip) of the dominant or healthy hand is measured with a dynamometer for the isometric work test. Thereafter, the maximum blowing power is also tested for the Valsalva maneuvre. A few elderly people cannot blow with a power of 40 mm-Hg, which is often used in the Valsalva test. The patients then rest for 30 min. Thereafter, the cardiovascular reflex tests are performed in the following order:

1. In the normal breathing test, consecutive R–R intervals for a period of 5–10 min are recorded. The standard deviation of consecutive R–R intervals is a simple and useful parasympathetically mediated time-domain indicator of HR variability. It is one of the acceptable parameters for the evaluation of HR variability defined by the Task Force of the European Society of Cardiology and the North American Society of Pacing and Electrophysiology 1996 (29). Frequency-domain analysis is often performed using either fast Fourier transform (FTT) or autoregressive frequency analyses. Mainly a sympathetically mediated very low-frequency peak (VLF) < 0.04 Hz and a low-frequency peak (LF) of 0.04–0.15 Hz, as well as the parasympathetically mediated high-frequency peak (HF) correspond-

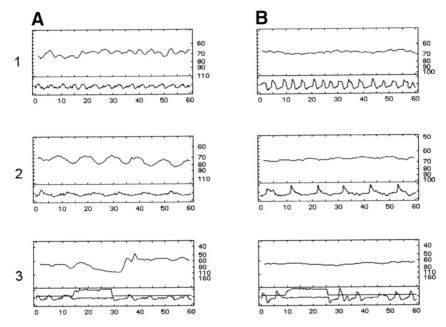

Fig. 1. The normal pulse variation of a healthy subject of 56 yr of age **(A)** and the attenuated pulse variation of a patient of 54 yr of age with autonomic nervous system deficit **(B)**. 1 = normal breathing, 2 = deep breathing, and 3 = the Valsalva maneuvre. Pulse rate on *y* axis (upper rectangles) and time (seconds) on *x* axis. Respiration signal (1–3) and blowing profiles in the Valsalva maneuvers (3) in lower rectangles. (Courtesy of U. Tolonen, unpublished data.)

ing respiratory frequency (0.15–0.4 Hz) can be detected.

2. In the deep-breathing test, the patient is breathing 6 cycles/min following verbal commands for inspiration and expiration (Fig. 1). The ratio (the mean, median, or highest) of the longest (expiration) to the shortest (inspiration) R–R interval is used as a test indicator (E : I ratio). Arterial BP variations significantly influence the amplitude of the HR variations in deep breathing, and continuous BP monitoring during deep breathing is suggested *(30)*.

3. In the Valsalva maneuvre, the patient maintains 50% of the individual maximum expiratory pressure for 15 s (40 mm-Hg is often used, but it may be too high for some elderly people to perform) (Fig. 1). A small leak in the

tube ensures that the epiglottis is not closed. The Valsalva ratio (the longest R–R interval after blowing to the shortest one during blowing or immediately after it) is the test parameter used. The sympathetically mediated tachycardia ratio (pulse increase during blowing) is often calculated, too. In people over 65 yr of age, it may be more useful than the usual Valsalva ratio *(28)*. Continuous BP monitoring increases the sensitivity of the test: Especially in early and mild adrenergic failure, HR ratios may be normal although BP changes occur *(23)*.

4. In tilt-table test, the duration of standing should be at least 5 min, but if most of neurally mediated syncopes and orthostatic tachycardia plus syndromes must be documented, the duration must be 10 min *(31)*. The angle used in tilting may be from 60° to 90° *(31)*. The parasympathetically mediated ratio of longest R–R interval around beat 30 to the shortest one around beat 15 is calculated as the "30 : 15 ratio." This pulse reaction may be missed after passive tilting. According to our own experiences, if tilting is quick and up to 90°, a reaction is often seen, as shown earlier by Sundqvist et al. *(32)*. The BP response is quantified as the largest drop (or lowest increase) in systolic and diastolic pressures. LF activity in HR variability spectra remains after tilting or standing, but the HF peak clearly attenuates. A dynamic autoregressive model is more suitable for spectral analysis of the rapid changes in measured signals than FFT *(33)*.

5. In the isometric work test, the patient grips a dynamometer at 30% of the maximum voluntary force for 5 min. The time from 4 to 5 min is the most important time for diagnosing abnormalities *(34)*. The largest increase in systolic and diastolic pressure is used as the test indicator.

Cardiovascular HRV parameters have been shown to be dependent on age and heart rate *(35–37)*. Therefore, the values of HR must be adjusted for age and baseline HR (after logarithmic transformation in HR responses). BP responses are not age dependent *(36)*. For the isometric work responses,

bradykinesia and rigidity (39%). These symptoms included increased perspiration and salivation, oily skin, bladder disturbances, decreased potency and libido, lachrymation, and cardiovascular and gastrointestinal disturbances. These results were later confirmed by Marttila *(73)*. In the study by Turkka *(22)*, a clinical rating scale for scoring the main autonomic symptoms and signs was developed. He found that in a great majority (93%) of the 47 PD patients with varying durations of the disease suffered from symptoms of autonomic dysfunction. The most frequent complaint was postural dizziness (73%). This is analogous to previous studies in which the most commonly reported disturbances of ANS function in PD patients were OH and postural dizziness *(74–78)*. The duration and severity of PD correlated with the grade of dysautonomia estimated with the rating scale *(22)*.

It is a general clinical assumption that BP values of PD patients tend to be low *(79,80)*, which has been suggested as the reason for the reduced incidence of myocardial infarction and ischemic stroke among PD patients *(79,81)*. There are, however, contradictory results not supporting this statement. Aminoff et al. *(82)* compared the casual systolic and diastolic BP of a large sample of PD patients not receiving dopaminergic medication with a representative sample of general population. They could not find any differences in BP between PD patients and the normal population. Even today, the prevalence of hypotension in PD is unclear. One further reason that makes reliable assessment of the matter complicated is that during lifetime, it may be difficult to definitely make difference between PD and Parkinson plus syndromes with typical ANS disturbances.

On the other hand, there has been a long discussion of whether antiparkinsonian drugs could be the cause of OH in PD patients. Several studies have shown that levodopa may produce OH at least in some patients, especially in the beginning of the treatment *(74,75,78)*, whereas others have not been able to confirm such an effect *(37,83–85)*. In a recent report by Churchyard et al. *(86)*, based on a small selected patient group, antiparkinsonian therapy with selegiline combined with levodopa was reported to be associated with severe OH that is not attributable to levodopa alone. A standard pattern of autonomic cardiovascular responses to physiological stimuli was used for assessing the ANS functions. These results were quite contradictory to the prospective long-term, placebo-controlled trial of Turkka et al. *(37)* in which selegiline was shown to diminish sympathetic autonomic responses, but no patient had clinically significant orthostatic hypotension. On the contrary, the mild sympatholytic effect of selegiline might afford protection against consequences of increased sympathetic tone. Anyhow, in PD patients with verified symptomatic postural hypotension, with greater than a 20 mm-Hg fall of systolic BP, it seems prudent to withdraw selegiline treatment and to carry out retitration of the other antiparkinsonian medication.

Although the frequency and severity of OH in PD seems to be far from clear at the moment, we have a lot of evidence suggesting mild disturbances of ANS, both sympathetic and parasympathetic hypofunctions in PD, that have been shown with sophisticated methods. The responses of serum/plasma noradrenaline (NA) levels to a standing-up stimulus are obviously important indicators of normal regulation of the cardiovascular system (e.g., regulation of BP). Thus, it is important to find out that the NA responses to standing up were found to be significantly diminished in PD patients compared to healthy controls (Fig. 4), suggesting a clear deficit of sympathetic ANS function *(87)*. The correlation between the clinical severity of ANS dysfunction and cerebrospinal fluid 3-methoxy-4-hydroxyphenyl glycol (MHPG) levels further suggests that central noradrenergic system is also involved in PD *(87)*. MHPG is the main brain metabolite of neurotransmitter NA, and its cerebropsinal fluid (CSF) levels may reflect activity of the central parts of ANS.

Cardiovascular autonomic responses have been measured in a number of studies on PD patients. The measured responses to standard provocations have been shown to be diminished in PD patients *(85–90)* compared to healthy controls, indicating a deficit of both sympathetic and parasym-

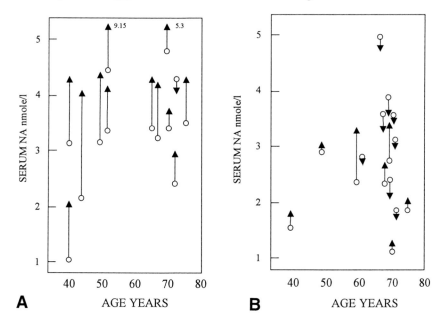

Fig. 4. The effect of standing up on serum Na concentrations in controls **(A)** and in the patients with PD **(B)**. ○ = recording before standing up (levodopa treated and controls); ▲ = recording immediately after standing up. (From ref. 22).

pathetic ANS functions (Fig. 5). Furthermore, the attenuated responses in the R–R variation has been reported to correlate with the clinical severity of dysautonomia and also with the duration of PD *(87,89)*. A recent study of Murata et al. *(91)* further showed that the autonomic dysfunction in PD patients as well as in patients with vascular parkinsonism is linked to a loss of the BP–HR relationship (e.g., while standing up). According to the study of Mesec et al. *(89)*, sympathetic impairment is more pronounced in akinetic–rigid than tremor–akinetic–rigid patients and, furthermore, sympathetic impairment occurs early and parasympathetic impairment develops later during the course of the disease. It is likely that chronic levodopa and anticholinergic medications do not modify cardiovascular autonomic responses *(87,89,91)*. Although these studies suggest a reduction of cardiovascular responses in PD patients, it should be emphasized that

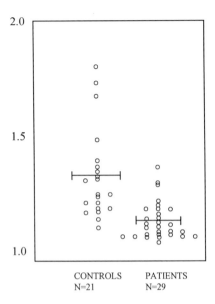

Fig. 5. R–R variation in deep breathing in PD patients and controls. The ratio between the longest R–R interval expirium and shortest one inspirium. The mean value is marked with a horizontal line. (From ref. *83*).

the disturbances are usually mild and cardiovascular reflexes are generally preserved.

On the other hand, it has been suggested that the BP response to ingestion of food could be used to reveal even a latent autonomic deficit. Based on this idea, Thomaides et al. *(92)* recently investigated the effect of a balanced liquid meal on BP and HR both in the supine position and after tilting in patients with PD, multiple system atrophy (MSA), pure autonomic failure (PAF) and in healthy controls. There was a postprandial fall in supine BP in all the patient groups, but not in the controls. Interestingly, tilting did not lower the BP in PD patients and controls, but lowered it in MSA and PAF patients. Thus, there was no postural postprandial hypotension in PD patients and, furthermore, the plasma adrenaline responses to tilting as well as other autonomic tests were within normal limits. These results differ to some extent from those of Micieli et al. *(93)*. They studied the 24-h pattern of BP, HR, and urinary catecholamine excretion and the responses of BP and plasma catecholamines to tilting in 13 untreated PD patients and age-matched controls. Seven of the 13 PD patients showed a postprandial fall of supine systolic BP greater than in controls. The degree of postprandial hypotension was related to the 24-h urinary excretion of dopamine. Eight of the PD patients also showed OH during the tilt test, both in the morning and postprandially. Based on their data, they suggested the existence of a subtype of PD patients who have a widespread impairment of cardiovascular responsiveness that may border on the specific syndromes of ANS failure.

As can be seen from the above-mentioned studies, there is no generally accepted concept concerning the extent of ANS involvement in PD, but it is certainly true that there is impairment of cardiovascular autonomic responses, at least in a noticeable number of PD patients.

Histopathological studies in PD patients have been carried out to find the lesions responsible for the autonomic symptoms linked to the disease. Lewy bodies, histological hallmarks of PD associated with loss and degeneration of neurons, have been found both in central and peripheral ANS, such as hypothalamus, locus ceruleus, dorsal vagal nucleus, nucleus ambiguus, intermediolateral nuclei of the spinal cord, and peripheral sympathetic ganglia *(94)*. Wakabayashi et al. *(95)* examined systematically the distribution of Lewy bodies in visceral ANS of autopsied 12 PD patients. Lewy bodies were found in the enteric nervous system of alimentary tract in all cases and they were distributed widely in the Auerbach's and Meissner's plexuses from the upper esophagus to the rectum. In 6 of the 12 patients, Lewy bodies were found in the cardiac plexus. In the pelvic plexus, Lewy bodies were found in five patients and they were in the ganglia near the urinary bladder and male genitalia. Finally, there were Lewy bodies in the sympathetic ganglion cells of adrenal medulla in four patients.

On theoretical grounds, dysautonomia in PD could relate to a central or peripheral disorder or both of them. Although in most of the earlier studies the importance of a central lesion as an etiological factor has been emphasized, recent data suggest an essential role for peripheral ANS damage.

5.2.2. Other Degenerative Central Nervous System Diseases

The history of multiple system atrophy (MSA) derives from the beginning of this century, when Dejerine and Thomas *(96)* introduced the term "olivopontocerebellar atrophy" (OPCA) and, at the same time, described the main features of MSA patients with a sporadic, late-onset, predominantly cerebellar syndrome combined with parkinsonism and dysautonomia. Shy and Drager *(97)* emphasized neurogenic central dysautonomia in their patients, who also had parkinsonism and cerebellar signs. The pathology of the syndrome was first described by Adams et al. *(98)*. But it was Graham and Oppenheimer *(99)* who first introduced the umbrella term MSA for these conditions.

Multiple system atrophy includes syndromes of striatonigral degeneration, OPCA, and autonomic failure in several combinations. Wenning et al. *(100)* have published an extensive series of 100 patients with MSA. In 14 of the cases, a postmortem examination of the brain was undertaken and diagnosis was confirmed pathologically. Autonomic symptoms were the initial feature in 41% of the patients, but they subsequently developed in 97% at latest follow-up. The most frequent autonomic symptom in men was impotence, and urinary incontinence in women. Symptomatic OH was present in 68% of the patients, but it was severe only in 15%. Parkinsonism was the initial feature in 46%, but it had subsequently developed in 91% of subjects at latest follow-up. Progression of the disease was faster than in PD, so that more than 40% of the patients were markedly disabled or wheelchair bound within 5 yr of the onset of motor symptoms.

The diagnosis of MSA is based on the presence of autonomic failure *(101)*. As mentioned earlier, orthostatic hypotension is the main finding, and it is usually present at first evaluation or within 1 yr from the development of parkinsonism. Symptoms of orthostatic hypotension include lightheadedness, tiredness, ataxia, blurred vision, and retrocollic aching *(101)*. Recently, special emphasis has been placed on orthostatic impairment of mentation reported to be found in about half of the patients with MSA *(102)*. Symptoms of orthostatic hypotension may often arise after excessive nocturia or after a meal *(103)*. It is also typical that symptoms of orthostatic hypotension may worsen during exercise or during standing *(104)*. It is, however, important to remember that patients with orthostatic hypotension usually are very tolerant of low blood pressures, especially when the condition has become chronic.

The deficient ANS function of MSA patients can be demonstrated by recording autonomic function tests. Cardiovascular reflex responses to standing and the Valsalva maneuvre are typically preserved in PD patients but are markedly defective or absent in MSA patients *(105)*. This is combined with severely disturbed thermoregulation in many patients. Cohen et al. *(106)* reported a severe and widespread anhydrosis in both MSA and PAF patients, 91% and 97% of the body surface was anhydrotic. The sympathetic deficit of MSA and PAF patients is also reflected as low levels of plasma noradrenaline that do not increase after head-up tilting because of the block of the baroreceptor pathway *(106)*.

Recently, Wenning et al. *(107)* reported the clinicopathological features of 203 cases of pathologically proven MSA from 108 publications, starting with Schultze in 1887 *(108)*. They found many interesting correlations between the pathological and clinical findings. As for ANS dysfunction, the authors could confirm the association of postural hypotension with intermediolateral cell column degeneration. This is in agreement with the classical concept that depletion of sympathetic preganglionic neurons in the intermediolateral cell column of the spinal cord is thought to be the main substrate of sympathetic failure in MSA, as suggested by Bannister and Oppenheimer in 1972 *(109)*. Depletion of catecholaminergic neurons of the rostral–ventromedial medulla was also recently demonstrated in an autopsy study on patients with MSA who had suffered from autonomic failure *(110)*. There was a significant reduction of tyrosine hydroxylase (TH)-positive neurons in the caudal ventrolateral medulla in three MSA patients. Also, in two of these MSA patients, thoracic spinal cord could be examined and the depletion of TH fibers and sympathetic preganglionic fibers could be found there as well. However, other features of MSA, such as impairment of hypothalamic responses to hemodynamic and other stresses (111–113), baroreflex dysfunction (109), and abnormal cardiorespiratory control, especially during sleep (114), indicate an involvement of brainstem autonomic centers in these patients.

The autonomic nervous system function has been assessed in other degenerative diseases of CNS also. There are already some reports on ANS function in Friedreich's ataxia, Huntington's disease, and progressive supranuclear palsy, as well as in Alzheimer's disease. Further studies are needed to evaluate the clinical significance of the observed abnormalities.

5.3. Multiple sclerosis

Multiple sclerosis (MS) is a chronic inflammatory demyelinating disease of unknown cause. It can affect any part of the central nervous system and, therefore, produce a multiplicity of symptoms. The clinical course of MS may follow a variable pattern over time, but it usually can be characterized by either episodic acute periods of worsening, gradual progressive deterioration of neurologic function, or combinations of both. There is, however, a tendency to develop progressive disability. Magnetic resonance imaging (MRI) is sensitive in detecting brain abnormalities in MS (115).

It is well known that MS can lead to dysfunction of the autonomic nervous system. Some sympathetic and parasympathetic responses may be deficient in MS whereas others are spared. Bladder dysfunction (116,117) and sexual dysfunction (118,119) are relatively common clinical features in MS. There is also evidence of diminished thermoregulatory sweating responses in MS patients (120). Moreover, some recent studies have shown abnormal sympathetic skin

monitored BP reactions and HR by polygraphic recordings before, during, and after migraine attack.

Evidence of sympathetic hypofunction in migraine has been collected during the last 10 yr by many study groups *(154–158)*. Contrasting with these reports in the study by Cortelli et al. *(159)*, sympathetic hyperfunction in migraine patients was suggested to exist, as also in some earlier studies, for example, by Steiner et al, *(143,160)*. The knowledge concerning the effects of migraine on the nervous function is still more controversial, the results of our own study group suggesting hypofunction and the results of Gotoh et al. *(144)* suggesting hyperfunction to be present in migraine.

Hsu et al. *(161,162)* reported a rise in mean plasma levels of NA during the 3 h before wakening in patients with early-morning migraine. Fog-Moller et al. *(163)* reported a fall in plasma NA levels in the beginning of a migraine attack, followed by an increase later during the same attack. Anthony's *(164)* results were in accordance with those of Hsu et al. *(161,162)*. Plasma NA levels were also demonstrated to be higher in migraine patients than in control subjects during headache-free intervals. The control subjects in the study were, however, patients with tension-type headaches; a comparison with healthy subjects was not carried out *(165)*. Anyhow, reduced NA levels in 21 migraine patients during headache-free intervals by were reported Gotoh et al. *(144)*. The finding was the same both in migraine patients with and without aura, and in this study, the results of plasma NA determinations were compared with those of 30 healthy volunteers, not with those of other headache patients.

Interestingly, as early as 1963, Wolff *(165)* published his findings on intravenous NA infusion in headache patients. During headache-free intervals, the infusion did not cause any headache (four patients), and during migraine attacks, NA infusion diminished or abolished the headache pain in 93 of 116 attacks in 35 migraine patients.

The objective verification of autonomic failure has proved difficult. There is a wide normal variation in the reactions of ANS, both interindividually and intraindividually. The most often utilized methods for the clarification of the functions of the ANS are the registration of cardiovascular reflex responses and NA determinations. Other methods (i.e., pupillometric studies, sweating, lachrymation, and salivation studies) have also been utilized. For the evaluation of the ANS function, cardiovascular reflex response registration and NA determination are both simple methods, easy to perform, easy to repeat, and quite painless for the patients.

5.2.4. Cluster Headache

During cluster-headache attacks, bradycardia *(166–170)* as well as tachycardia *(153,170)* and rhythm disturbances *(153,168,170–172)* have been reported.

Various patterns of changes in arterial BP have been described in cluster headache. Some authors have found that BP does not change during spontaneous attacks *(166)*, but others have observed BP instability consisting of a mild increase associated with frequent hypertensive peaks *(153)*. Most authors, however, have reported an increase in BP during spontaneous and provoked attacks *(169,170,173,174)*.

In the study of De Marinis et al. *(175)*, patients with cluster headache underwent head-up tilt and 24-h ECG Holter and automatic BP monitoring. Spectral analysis of HR fluctuation was used to assess the autonomic balance under basal conditions, after sympathetic activation obtained with head-up tilt, and during a spontaneous attack of headache. Normal autonomic balance was found at rest and during sympathetic activation obtained with head-up tilt in the interictal period. Significant differences were found when comparing the spectral parameters obtained before, during, and after headache. During the attack, the BP increased and HR decreased in all subjects. Nevertheless, the possibility that BP was influenced by pain cannot be excluded.

In cluster-headache patients, lachrymation is the most common local sign of autonomic involvement, followed by injection of the conjunctiva on the side of pain. A slight ipsilateral ptosis and/or miosis is often present during attacks and may also persist between attacks. Other symptoms suggesting autonomic nervous system involvement are nasal stuffiness or rhinorrhea and increased forehead sweating. Tear, salivation, and nasal secretion have been studied by Saunte et al. *(176,177)*, and the sweating pattern associated with cluster headache by Sjaastad et al. *(178)* and by Saunte et al *(176)*.

5.4.3. Tension-Type Headache

Reports on ANS function in tension-type headache have rarely been published. Mikamo et al. *(155)* recorded the cardiovascular reflex responses by the orthostatic test, the isometric work test, and the HR variation in patients with a "chronic muscular headache" during headache-free intervals. The plasma NA levels were also measured during the orthostatic tests. In patients with "chronic muscular headache," the BP immediately after standing up decreased more significantly than in the control group. The blood NA level was significantly low. According to the authors, these patients showed cardiovascular sympathetic hypofunction. In 1993, Pogacnik et al *(155)* reported autonomic function testing in 51 patients with tension-type headache. The Valsalva maneuvre, deep-breathing test, sustained handgrip test, orthostatic test, and spectral analysis of HR variability in supine and standing positions were performed. Diastolic BP increase and, particularly, HR increase during sustained handgrip were significantly reduced in the headache group, when compared to the control group. These results suggest sympathetic hypofunction in tension-type headache also.

5.5. Spinal Cord Lesions

Spinal cord lesions are frequently manifested as various symptoms and signs of autonomic dysfunction affecting cardiovascular, gastrointestinal, thermoregulatory, urinary, and genital systems. The autonomic involvement associated with spinal lesion is mainly determined by the site and the extent of the lesion, and there are also certain differences between recently injured patients and those in the chronic spinal stage.

In patients with complete cervical cord transection, the entire sympathetic and sacral parasympathetic ouflow is separated from cerebral control as a result of an interruption of the autonomic pathways from the brain to the intermediolateral column of the spinal cord. The major clinical problems related to autonomic dysfunction are found in patients with cervical and high thoracic spinal cord lesions. Autonomic disorders associated with spinal diseases resemble those found in spinal injuries, but are usually milder and not so frequent.

5.5.1. Recent Injures

Immediately following an acute spinal cord lesion, there is a transient period of hypoexcitability of the isolated cord called "spinal shock," which is characterized by flaccid, areflexic paralysis of skeletal and smooth muscles (179). The pathogenesis of the spinal shock is still poorly outlined and its biochemical and molecular bases are not known. During this stage, spinal autonomic functions and reflexes are impaired below the level of the lesion manifested as atonic bladder and large bowel and various abnormalities in cardiovascular regulation. The basal supine systolic and diastolic blood pressures in recently injured tetraplegics are usually lower (often below 90/50 mm-Hg) than normal, likely the result of diminution in sympathetic nervous activity (180). Because BP is mainly regulated by posture and blood volume without supraspinal control in patients with recent spinal cord injury, postural hypotension is found in a majority of these patients (181,182).

Bradycardia is another commonly found manifestation of cardiovascular autonomic dysfunction in patients with recent spinal cord lesion. In tetraplegics, the maximum HR is usually below 100 beats/min, whereas tachycardia is often encountered in patients with acute low spinal cord lesions (180). This phenomenon is suggested to be related to a reduction in neural and hormonal sympathetically mediated chronotropic influences in tetraplegics, but it may also be contributed to vagal overactivity caused by intact parasympathetic efferent cardiac nerve pathways (180). In a few patients, reflex bradycardia may even lead to cardiac arrest as a consequence of a parasympathetic stimulation, such as intubation or tracheal suction *(183,184)*.

5.5.2. Chronic Injuries

The spinal shock normally lasts from a few days to a few weeks, after which the activity of the isolated spinal cord gradually returns, leading a variety of autonomic disorders caused by an uncontrolled reflex activity at the spinal level. The basal levels of both systolic and diastolic BPs in high spinal cord lesions are still lower than in healthy subjects *(184,185)*, but the basal HR usually returns to normal or remains only slightly lower than in normal subjects *(180)*. Similarly, the basal levels of plasma NA and adrenaline remain low as during the spinal shock reflecting absent tonic supraspinal sympathetic impulses and diminished peripheral sympathetic activity *(180,186)*.

Although OH is particularly severe in recently injured spinal patients, it commonly occurs in chronically injured patients as well *(180,187)*. Impaired cerebral autoregulation may manifest as various clinical symptoms like syncope, dizziness, and acoustic or visual abnormalities. Moreover, tetraplegics are particularly sensitive to certain drugs interfering with the cardiovascular regulatory system despite gradually developing compensational mechanisms, such as the renin–angiotensin–aldosterone system and activation of spinal and local sympathetic reflexes, to maintain BP. Even small doses of diuretics or angiotensin-converting enzyme inhibitors may cause a catastrophic fall in supine BP *(180)*. In chronic tetraplegics, the fall in blood pressure is accompanied by a reduction in central venous pressure, stroke volume, and cardiac output, which is probably a result of venous pooling, diminished venous return, and the inability to increase sympathetic cardiac inotrophic activity *(180)*.

Cardiovascular as well as thermal responses to exercise are abnormal in subjects with high-level spinal lesion, causing problems especially for wheelchair athletes as a form of exercise intolerance and hyperthermia. As a result of venous pooling accompanied by reduced end-diastolic ventricular volume or stroke volume, and of the incomplete ability to increase HR, an exercise-induced hypotension with subsequent exercise intolerance may develop *(188,189)*. BP and HR responses to the Valsalva maneuvre, cutaneous stimulation by either pain or cold, and cognitive stimulation such as mental arithmetics are also impaired in spinal subjects as a reflection of abnormal cardiovascular regulation. Moreover, a recent study *(190)* has shown that the circadian rhythm of BP is abolished in completely tetraplegic patients, whereas it is preserved in subjects with incomplete tetraplegia or paraplegia. Furthermore, another recent study *(191)* showed significantly suppressed HR variability as measured by using spectral analysis techniques both in quadriplegic and paraplegic subjects in comparison with healthy subjects.

5.5.3. Autonomic Dysreflexia

Autonomic dysreflexia is an important complication of spinal cord injury, appearing usually a few months after the lesion *(180,192,193)*. It occurs in up to 85% of individuals with spinal cord injury above the major splanchnic sympathetic outflow (fifth thoracic segment) and is defined as a massive paroxysmal reflex sympathetic activity developing in response to noxious stimuli below the level of the neurologic lesion. The typical clinical presentation of autonomic dysreflexia consists of sudden and paroxysmal headache, hypertension, bradycardia, hyperhidrosis, and piloerection. Although a variety of stimuli can provoke this phenomenon of variable magnitude, bladder and bowel distensions account for most episodes.

The entire pathophysiologic mechanism of the autonomic dysreflexia is incompletely understood. At least a loss of supraspinal inhibitory control and denervation hypersensitivity of sympathetic spinal, ganglionic or peripheral receptor sites, and possibly also a formation of abnormal synaptic connections resulting from axonal sprouting contribute to the pathophysiology of the autonomic dysreflexia *(194,195)*. Nevertheless, the phenomenon is of clinical relevance. Mild

ric work, is recognized very early, and its prevalence even among asymptomatic DM patients is high *(5,102)*. Although these conventional cardiovascular reflex tests still remain the cornerstone for investigation of diabetic autonomic neuropathy, analysis of HR variability has provided new insights into its mechanisms.

Heart rate variability has shown to be reduced in DM patients both using the time-domain and frequency-domain (spectral) analyzing techniques *(215–219)*. The impairment includes all the spectral components of HR variability, and its prevalence seems to be high. Ewing et al. *(215)* assessed HR variability from 24-h ambulatory ECG recordings in 343 DM patients and found that nearly half (146) of the patients had significantly decreased HR variability compared with healthy age- and sex-matched control subjects.

Other peripheral neuropathies, which frequently cause clinically significant autonomic cardiovascular dysfunction, are amyloidosis, porphyry, and familial dysautonomia *(197)*. All of them may result in postural hypotension, impaired HR and BP responses in cardiovascular reflex tests as well as reduced HR variability. Thus, their clinical manifestations are alike in DM. Several other diseases and conditions (i.e., hereditary neuropathies, metabolic disorders, alcoholism, malignancy, drugs and toxins, infections, and connective tissue diseases) may also cause cardiovascular autonomic neuropathy, which is usually of minor clinical importance, however *(197)*.

References

1. Bannister, R. (1988) Autonomic failure, in A Textbook of Clinical Disorders of the Autonomic Nervous System (Bannister, R., ed.), Oxford Medical Publications, Oxford, UK.
2. Ewing, D. J., Campbell, I. W., Burt, A. A., and Clarke, B. F. (1973) Vascular reflexes in diabetic autonomic neuropathy. *Lancet* **2,** 1354.
3. Persson, A. and Solders, G. (1983) R–R variations in Guillain–Barré syndrome: a test of autonomic dysfunction. *Acta Neurol. Scand.* **67,** 294–300.
4. Solders, G., Persson, A., and Gutierrez, A. (1985) Autonomic dysfunction in non-diabetic terminal uraemia. *Acta Neurol. Scand.* **71,** 321–327.

5. Ewing, D. J., Campbell, I. W., and Clarke, B. F. (1980) Assessment of cardiovascular effects in diabetic autonomic neuropathy and prognostic implications. *Ann. Intern. Med.* **92**, 308–311.
6. Ewing, D. J., Campbell, I. W., and Clarke, B. F. (1980) The natural history of diabetic autonomic neuropathy. *Quart. J. Med.* **49**, 95–108.
7. Ewing, D. J., Campbell, I. W., and Clarke, B. F. (1976) Mortality in diabetic autonomic neuropathy. *Lancet* **1**, 601–603.
8. Page, M. and Watkins, P. (1978) Cardio-respiratory arrest and diabetic autonomic neuropathy. *Lancet* **1**, 14–16.
9. Lloyd-Mostyn, R. H. and Watkins, P. J. (1976) Total cardiac denervation diabetic autonomic neuropathy. *Diabetes* **25**, 748.
10. Faerman, J., Faccio, E., Milei, J., Nunez, R., Jadzinsky, M., Fox, D., et al. (1977) Autonomic neuropathy and painless myocardial infarction in diabetic patients. Histolocic evidence of their relationship. *Diabetes* **26**, 1147–1158.
11. Johnsson, R. H. and Robinson, B. J. (1988) Mortality in alcoholics with autonomic neuropathy. *J. Neurosurg.* **51**, 476.
12. Malik, M., Farrel, T., and Camm, A. J. (1990) Circadian rhythm of heart rate variability after acute myocardial infarction and its influence on the prognostic value of heart rate variability. *Am. J. Cardiol.* **66**, 1049–1054.
13. Huikuri, H. V., Niemelä, M. J., Ojala, S., Rantala, A., Ikäheimo, M. J., and Airaksinen, K. E. J. (1994) Circadian rhythms of frequency domain measures of heart rate variability in healthy subjects and patients with coronary artery disease. *Circulation* **90**, 121–126.
14. Vanoli, E., Adamson, P. B., Ba-Lin, M. P. H., Pinna, G. D., Lazzara, R., and Orr, W. C. (1995) Heart rate variability during specific sleep stages: a comparison of health subjects with patients after myocardial infarction. *Circulation* **91**, 1918–1922.
15. Frank, J. I., Ropper, A. H., and Zuñica, G. (1992) Acute intracranial lesions and respiratory sinus arrhythmia. *Arch. Neurol.* **49**, 1200–1203.
16. Barron, S. A., Rogovski, Z., and Hemli, J. (1994) Autonomic consequences of cerebral hemisphere infarction. *Stroke* **25**, 113–116.
17. Korpelainen, J. T., Sotaniemi, K. A., Suominen, K., Tolonen, U., and Myllylä, V. V. (1994) Cardiovascular autonomic reflexes in brain infarction. *Stroke* **25**, 787–792.
18. Korpelainen, J. T., Sotaniemi, K. A., Huikuri, H. V., and Myllylä, V. V. (1996) Abnormal heart rate variability as a manifestation of autonomic dysfunction in hemispheric brain infarction. *Stroke* **27**, 2059–2063.
19. Korpelainen, J. T., Huikuri, H. V., Sotaniemi, K. A., and Myllylä, V. V. (1996) Abnormal heart rate variability reflecting autonomic dysfunction in brainstem infarction. *Acta Neurol. Scand.* **94**, 337–342.
20. Naver, H. K., Blomstrand, C., and Wallin, B. G. (1996) Reduced heart rate variability after right-sided stroke. *Stroke* **27**, 247–251.

21. Nogues, M. A., Newman, P. K., Male, V. J., and Foster, J. B. (1982) Cardiovascular reflexes in syringomyelia. *Brain* **105**, 835.

22. Turkka, J. (1986) Autonomic dysfunction in Parkinson's disease. Doctoral thesis. *Acta Universitatis Ouluensis*, Series D, Medica No 142, University of Oulu, Oulu, Finland.

23. Ravits, J. M. (1997) AAEM minimonograph #48: autonomic nervous system testing. *Muscle Nerve* **20**, 919–937.

24. Omboni, S., Parati, G., DiRienzo, Wieling W., and Mancia, G. (1996) Blood pressure and heart rate variability in autonomic disorders: a critical review. *Clin. Auton. Res.* **6**, 171–182.

25. Wallin, G. B. and Elam, M. (1997) Microneurography and autonomic dysfunction, in *Clinical Autonomic Disorders* (Low, P. A., ed.), Lippincott–Raven, Philadelphia, pp. 233–243.

26. The Consensus Committee of the American Autonomic Society and the American Academy of Neurology. Consensus statement of the definition of orthostatic hypotension, pure autonomic failure, and multiple system atrophy. *Neurology* **46**, (1996) 1470.

27. Van Lieshout, J. J., Wieling, W., Karemaker, J. M., and Eckberg, D. L. (1991) The vasovagal response (Review). *Clin. Sci.* **81**, 575–586.

28. Braune, S., Auer, A., Schulte-Mönting, J., Schwerbrock, S., and Luking, C. H. (1996) Cardiovascular parameters: sensitivity to detect autonomic dysfunction and influence of age and sex in normal subjects. *Clin. Auton. Res.* **6**, 3–15.

29. Task Force of the European Society of Cardiology and the North American Society of Pacing and Electrophysiology. Heart rate variability: standards of measurements, physiological interpretation and clinical use. *Circulation* **93**, (1996) 1043–1065.

30. Diehl, R. R., Linden, D., and Berlit, P. (1997) Determinants of heart rate variability during deep breathing: basic findings and clinical applications. *Clin. Auton. Res.* **7**, 131–135.

31. Khurana, R. K. and Nicholas, E. M. (1996) Head-up tilt table test: how far and how long? *Clin. Auton. Res.* **6**, 335–341.

32. Sundkvist, G., Lilja, B., and Almer, L. O. (1980) Abnormal diastolic blood pressure and heart rate reactions to tilting in diabetes mellitus. *Diabetologia* **19**, 433–438.

33. Novak, V., Novak, P., and Low, P. A. (1997) Time-frequency analysis of cardiovascular function and its clinical applications, in *Clinical Autonomic Disorders* (Low, P. A., ed.), Lippincott–Raven, Philadelphia, pp. 323–348.

34. Khurana, R. K. and Setty, A. (1996) The value of the isometric handgrip test—studies in various autonomic disorders. *Clin. Auton. Res.* **6**, 211–218.

35. Ewing, D. J. (1988) Recent advances in the non-invasive investigation of diabetic autonomic neuropathy, in *Autonomic Failure. A Text-*

book of *Clinical Disorders of the Autonomic Nervous System* (Bannister, R., ed.), Oxford University Press, Oxford, pp. 667–689.
36. Piha, S. J. (1991) Cardiovascular autonomic reflex tests: normal responses and age-related reference values. *Clin. Physiol.* **11,** 277–290.
37. Turkka, J., Suominen, K., Tolonen, U., Sotaniemi, K., and Myllylä, V. V. (1997) Selegeline diminishes cardiovascular autonomic responses in Parkinsons disease. *Neurology* **48,** 662–667.
38. Freeman, R., Weiss, S. T., Roberts, M., Zbikowski, S. M, and Sparrow, D. (1995) The relationship between heart rate variability and measures of body habitus. *Clin. Auton. Res.* **5,** 261–266.
39. Genovely, H. and Pfeifer, M. A. (1988) RR-variation: the autonomic test of choice in diabetes. *Diabetes Metab. Rev.* **4,** 255–271.
40. Low, P. A., Opfer-Gehrking, T. L, McPhee, B. R., Fealey, R. D., Benarroch, E. E, Willner, C. L., et al. (1995) Prospective evaluation of clinical characteristics of orthostatic hypotension. *Mayo Clin. Proc.* **70,** 617–622.
41. Huikuri, H. V. (1995) Heart rate variability in coronary artery disease. *J. Intern. Med.* **237,** 349–357.
42. Karemaker, J. M. (1997) Analysis of blood pressure and heart rate variability–theoretical considerations, in *Clinical Autonomic Disorders* (Low, P. A., ed.), Lippincott–Raven, Philadelphia, pp. 309–322.
43. Peleg, S., Naor, J., Hartley, R., and Avnir, D. (1984) Multiple resolution texture and classification. *IEEE Trans. Pattern Anal. Machine. Intell.* **6,** 518–523.
44. Korpelainen, J. T., Sotaniemi, K. A., Huikuri, H. V., and Myllylä, V. V. (1997) Circadian rhythm of heart rate variability is reversibly abolished in ischemic stroke. *Stroke* **28,** 2150–2154.
45. Talman, W. T. (1985) Cardiovascular regulation and the lesions of the central nervous system. *Ann. Neurol.* **18,** 1–12.
46. Cruickshank, J. M., Neil-Dwyer, G., and Scott, A. (1974) The possible role of catecholamines, corticosteroids and potassium in the production of ECG changes associated with subarachnoid hemorrhage. *Br. Heart J.* **36,** 697–706.
47. Cechetto, D. F. (1993) Experimental cerebral ischemic lesions and autonomic and cardiac effects in cats and rats. *Stroke* **24(Suppl. I),** I-6–I-9.
48. Oppenheimer, S. M., Gelb, A., Girvin, J. P., and Hachinski, V. C. (1992) Cardiovascular effects of human insular cortex stimulation. *Neurology* **42,** 1727–1732.
49. Burch, G. E., Meyers, R., and Abilskov, J. A. (1954) A new electrocardiographic pattern observed in cerebrovascular accidents. *Circulation* **9,** 719–723.
50. Kono, T., Morita, H., Kuroiwa, T., Onaka, H., Takatsuka, H., and Fujiwara, A. (1994) Left ventricular wall motion abnormalities in patients with subarachnoid hemorrhage: neurogenic stunned myocardium. *J. Am. Coll. Cardiol.* **24,** 636–640.

51. Greenhoot, J. H. and Reichenbach, D. D. (1969) Cardiac injury and subarachnoid hemorrhage, a clinical, pathological, and physiological correlation. *J. Neurosurg.* **30,** 521–531.
52. Oppenheimer, S. M., Cechetto, D. F., and Hachinski, V. C. (1990) Cerebrogenic cardiac arrhythmias: cerebral electrocardiographic influences and their role in sudden death. *Arch. Neurol.* **47,** 513–519.
53. Hachinski, V. C., Oppenheimer, S. M., Wilson, J. X., Guiraudon, C., and Cechetto, D. F. (1992) Asymmetry of sympathetic consequences of experimental stroke. *Arch. Neurol.* **49,** 697–702.
54. Lane, R. D., Wallace, J. D., Petrosky, P. P., Schwartz, G. E., and Gradman, A. H. (1992) Supraventricular tachycardia in patients with right hemisphere strokes. *Stroke* **23,** 362–366.
55. Talman, W. T., Alonso, D. R., and Reis, D. J. (1980) Chronic lability of arterial pressure in the rat does not evolve hypertension. *Clin. Sci.* **59,** 405–407.
56. Hoff, J. T. and Reis, D. J. (1970) Localization of regions mediating the Cushing response in CNS of cat. *Arch. Neurol.* **23,** 228–240.
57. Dopa, N., Beresford, H. R., and Reis, D. J. (1975) Changes in regional blood flow and cardiodynamics associated with electrically and chemically induced epilepsy in rat. *Brain Res.* **90,** 115–132.
58. Ross, C. A., Ruggiero, D. A., and Park, D. H. (1984) Tonic vasomotor control by the rostral ventrolateral medulla: effect of electrical or chemical stimulations of the area containing C1 adrenaline neurons on arterial pressure, heart rate and plasma catecholamines and vasopressin. *J. Neurosci.* **4,** 474–494.
59. Lip, G. Y. H., Zarifis, J., Farooqi, I. S., Page, A., Sagar, G., and Beevers, D. G. (1997) Ambulatory blood pressure monitoring in acute stroke. *Stroke* **28,** 31–35.
60. Morfis, L., Schwarz, R. S., Poulos, R., and Howes, L. G. (1997) Blood pressure changes in acute cerebral infarction and hemorrhage. *Stroke* **28,** 1401–1405.
61. Korpelainen, J. (1993) Autonomic dysfunction in brain infarction. Doctoral thesis, *Acta Universitatis Ouluensis,* Series D, Medica No. 266, University of Oulu, Oulu, Finland.
62. Robinson, T. G. and Potter, J. F. (1995) Postprandial and orthostatic cardiovascular changes after acute stroke. *Stroke* **26,** 1811–1816.
63. Hsu, C. Y., Hogan, E. L., Wingfield, W., Webb, J. G., Perot, P. L., Privitera, P. J., et al. (1984) Orthostatic hypotension with brainstem tumors. *Neurology* **34,** 1137–1143.
64. Kita, Y., Ishise, J., Yoshita, Y., Aizawa, Y., Yoshio, H., Minagava, F., et al. (1993) Power spectral analysis of heart rate and arterial blood pressure oscillations in brain-dead patients. *J. Autonom. Nerv. Syst.* **44,** 101–107.
65. Novak, V., Novak, P., De Marchie, M., and Schondorf, R. (1995) The effect of severe brainstem injury on heart rate and blood pressure oscillations. *Clin. Autonom. Res.* **5,** 24–30.

66. Freitas, J., Puig, J., Rocha, A. P., Lago, P., Teixeira, J., Carvalho, M. J., et al. (1996) Heart rate variability in brain dead. *Clin. Autonom. Res.* **6,** 141–146.
67. Oppenheimer, S. M. and Cechetto, D. F. (1990) Cardiac chronotropic organisation of the rat insular cortex. *Brain Res.* **533,** 66–72.
68. Oppenheimer, S. M. (1993) The anatomy and physiology of cortical mechanisms of cardiac control. *Stroke* **24(Suppl. I),** I-3–I-5.
69. Cechetto, D. F. and Saper, C. B. (1990) Role of the cerebral cortex in autonomic function, in *Central Regulation of Autonomic Functions* (Loewy, A. D. and Spyer, K. M., eds.), Oxford University Press, New York, pp. 208–223.
70. Vingerhoets, F., Bogousslavsky, J., Regli, F., and van Malle, G. (1993) Atrial fibrillation after stroke. *Stroke* **24,** 20–26.
71. Aminoff, M. J. (1997) Other extrapyramidal disorders, in *Clinical Autonomic Disorders,* 2nd ed. (Low, P. A., ed.), Lippincott–Raven, Philadelphia, pp. 577–584.
72. Spiegel, E. A., Wycis, H. T,. Schor, S., Schwartz, H. A., and Fabioni, F. R. (1969) The incidence of vegetative symptoms in Parkinson patients with and without bradykinesia, in *Third Symposium on Parkinson's Disease* (Gillingham, F. J. and Donaldson, T. M. C., eds.), Livingstone, Edinburg, p. 200.
73. Marttila, R. (1974) Epidemiological, clinical, and virus-serological studies of Parkinson's disease. Doctoral thesis,. University of Turku.
74. Calne, D. B., Brennan, J., Spiers A. S. D., and Stern, G. M. (1970) Hypotension caused by L-dopa. *Br. Med. J.* **1,** 474–475.
75. McDowell, F. H. and Lee, J. E. (1970) Levodopa, Parkinson's disease, and hypotension. *Ann. Intern. Med.* **72,** 751–752.
76. Aminoff, M. J. and Wilcox, C. S. (1971) Assessment of autonomic function in patients with a parkinsonian syndrome. *Br. Med. J.* **4,** 80–84.
77. Appenzeller, O. and Goss, J. E. (1971) Autonomic deficits in Parkinson's syndrome. *Arch. Neurol.* **24,** 50–57.
78. Gross, M., Bannister, R., and Godwin-Austen, R. (1972) Orthostatic hypotension in Parkinson's disease. *Lancet* **22,** 174–176.
79. Barbeau, A., Mars, H., and Gillo-Joffroy, L. (1971) Adverse clinical side effects of levodopa therapy, in *Recent Advances in Parkinson's Disease* (McDowell, F. H. and Markham, C. H., eds.), Blackwell, Oxford, pp. 203–237.
80. Yahr, M. D. (1970) General discussion on clinical effects of L-dopa upon blood pressure, in *L-Dopa and Parkinsonism* (Barbeau, A. and McDowell, F. H., eds.), Davis, Philadelphia, pp. 266–268.
81. Struck, L. K., Rodnitzky, R. L., and Dobson, J. K. (1990) Stroke and its modification in Parkinson's disease. *Stroke* **21,** 1395–1399.
82. Aminoff, M. J., Gross, M., Laatz, B., Vakil, S. D., Petrie, A., and Calne, D. B. (1975) Arterial blood pressure in patients with Parkinson's disease. *J. Neurol. Neurosurg. Psychiatry* **38,** 73–77.

83. Turkka, J. T., Tolonen, U., and Myllylä, V. V. (1987) Cardiovascular reflexes in Parkinson's disease. *Eur. Neurol.* **26,** 104–112.
84. Kuroiwa, Y., Shimada, Y., and Toyokura, Y. (1983) Postural hypotension and low R–R interval variability in parkinsonism, spinocerebellar degeneration, and Shy–Drager syndrome. *Neurology* **33,** 463–467.
85. Goetz, C. G., Lutge, W., and Tanner, C. M. (1986) Autonomic dysfunction in Parkinson's disease. *Neurology* **36,** 73–75.
86. Churchyard, A., Mathias, C. J., Boonkongchuen, P., and Lees, A. J. (1997) Autonomic effects of selegiline: possible cardiovascular toxicity in Parkinson's disease. *J. Neurol. Neurosurg. Psychiatry* **63,** 228–234.
87. Turkka, J. T. (1987) Correlation of the severity of autonomic dysfunction to cardiovascular reflexes and to plasma noradrenaline levels in Parkinson's disease. *Eur. Neurol.* **26,** 203–210.
88. Turkka, J. T., Juujärvi, K. K., Lapinlampi, T. O., and Myllylä, V. V. (1986) Serum noradrenaline response to standing up in patients with Parkinson's disease. *Eur. Neurol.* **25,** 355–361.
89. Mesec, A., Sega, S., and Kiauta, T. (1993) The influence of the type, duration, severity and levodopa treatment of Parkinson's disease on cardiovascular autonomic responses. *Clin. Auton. Res.* **3,** 339–344.
90. Ørskov, L., Jakobsen, J., Dupont, E., Olivarius, B., and Christensen, N. J. (1987) Autonomic function in parkinsonian patients relates to duration of disease. *Neurology* **37,** 1173–1178.
91. Murata, Y., Harada, T., Ishizaki, F., Izumi, Y., and Nakamura, S. (1997) Autonomic dysfunction in Parkinson's disease and vascular parkinsonism. *Acta Neurol. Scand.* **96,** 359–365.
92. Thomaides, T., Bleasdale-Barr, K., Chaudhuri, K. R., Pavitt, D., Marsden, C. D., and Mathias, C. J. (1993) Cardiovascular and hormonal responses to liquid food challenge in idiopathic Parkinson's disease, multiple system atrophy, and pure autonomic failure. *Neurology* **43,** 900–904.
93. Micieli, G., Martignoni, E., Cavallini, A., Sandrini, G., and Nappi, G. (1987) Postprandial and orthostatic hypotension in Parkinson's disease. *Neurology* **37,** 386–393.
94. Lieberman, A. N., Horowitz, L., Redmond, P., Pachter, L., Lieberman, I., and Leibowitz, M. (1980) Dysphagia in Parkinson's disease. *Am. J. Gastroenterol.* **74.** 157–160.
95. Wakabayashi, K., Takahashi, H., Ohama, E., Takeda, S., and Ikuta, F. (1993) Lewy bodies in the visceral autonomic nervous system in Parkinson's Disease. *Adv. Neurol.* **60,** 609–612.
96. Dejerine, J. and Thomas, A. A. (1900) L'atrophie olivo-ponto-cérébelleuse. *Nouv. Iconog. Salpêtriére* **13,** 330–370.
97. Shy, G. M. and Drager, G. A. (1960) A neurological syndrome associated with orthostatic hypotension. *Arch. Neurol.* **2,** 511–527.
98. Adams, R. D., van Bogaert, L., and van der Eecken, H. (1961) Dégénérescences nigro-striées et cérébello-nigro-striées. *Psychiat. Neurol.* **142,** 219–259.

99. Graham, J. G. and Oppenheimer, D. R. (1969) Orhostatic hypotension and nicotine sensitivity in a case of multiple system atrophy. *J. Neurol. Neurosurg. Psychiatry* **32**, 28–34.
100. Wenning, G. K., Shlomo, Y. B., Magalhães, M., Daniel, S. E., and Quinn, N. P. (1994) Clinical features and natural history of multiple system atrophy an analysis of 100 cases. *Brain* **117**, 835–845.
101. Low, P. A. and Bannister, S. R. (1997) Multiple system atrophy and pure autonomic failure, in *Clinical Autonomic Disorders* (Low, P. A., ed.), pp. 555–575
102. Low, P. A., Walsh, J. C., Huang, C.-Y., and McLeod, J. G. (1975) The sympathetic nervous system in diabetic neuropathy—a clinical and pathological study. *Brain* **98**, 341–356.
103. Mathias, C. J., Fosbraey, P., da Costa, D. F., Thornley, A., and Bannister, R. (1986) The effect of desmopressin on nocturnal polyuria, overnight weight loss, and morning postural hypotension in patients with autonomic failure. *Br. Med. J. Clin. Res. Ed.* **293**, 353–354.
104. Smith, G. D., Watson, L. P., Pavitt, D. V., and Mathias, C. J. (1995) Abnormal cardiovascular and catecholamine responses to supine exercise in human subjects with sympathetic dysfunction. *J. Physiol.* **484**, 255–265.
105. Wilcox, C. S. and Aminoff, M. J. (1976) Blood pressure responses to noradrenaline and dopamine infusions in Parkinson's disease and the Shy–Drager syndrome. *Br. J. Clin. Pharmacol.* **3**, 207–214.
106. Cohen, J., Low, P., Fealey, R., Sheps, S., and Jiang, N. S. (1987) Somatic and autonomic function in progressive autonomic failure and multiple system atrophy. *Ann. Neurol.* **22**, 692–699.
107. Wenning, G. K., Tison, F., Shlomo, B., Daniel, S. E., and Quinn, N. P. (1997) Multiple system atrophy: a review of 203 pathologically proven cases. *Movement Disorders* **12**, 133–147.
108. Schultze, V. (1887) Über einen fall von kleinhirnschwund mit degenerationen im verlängerten marke und im rückenmarke (wahrscheinlich in folge von alkoholismus). *Virchows Arch. Pathol. Anat.* **108**, 331–343.
109. Bannister, R. and Oppenheimer, D. R. (1972) Degenerative diseases of the nervous system associated with autonomic failure. *Brain* **95**, 457–474.
110. Benarroch, E. E., Smithson, I. L., Low, P. A., and Parisi, J. E. (1998) Depletion of catecholaminergic neurons of the rostral ventrolateral medulla in multiple systems atrophy with autonomic failure. *Ann. Neurol.* **43**, 156–163.
111. Puritz, R., Lightman, S. L., Wilcox, C. S., Forsling, M., and Bannister, R. (1983) Blood pressure and vasopressin in progressive autonomic failure. Response to postural stimulation, L-dopa and nalaxone. *Brain* **106**, 503–511.
112. Kaufman, H., Oribe, E., Miller, M., Knott, P., Wiltshire-Clement, M., and Yahr, M. D. (1992) Hypotension-induced vasopressin release

distinguishes between pure autonomic failure and multiple system atrophy with autonomic failure. *Neurology* **42**, 590–593.

113. Polinsky, R. J. (1990) Clinical autonomic neuropharmacology. *Neurol. Clin.* **8**, 77–92.

114. Chokroverty, S. (1988) Sleep apnoea and respiratory disturbances in multiple system atrophy with autonomic failure, in *Autonomic Failure* (Bannister, R., ed.), Oxford Medical Publications, Oxford, pp. 432–450.

115. Paty, D. W., Oger, J. J. F., Kastrukoff, L. F., Hashimoto, S. A., Hooge, J. P. Eisen, A. A., et al. (1988) MRI in the diagnosis in MS: a prospective study in comparison of clinical evaluation evoked potentials, oligoclonal banding and CT. *Neurology* **38**, 180–185.

116. Bradley, W. E. (1978) Urinary bladder dysfunction in multiple sclerosis. *Neurology* **28**, 52–58.

117. Jensen, D., Jr. (1987) The urinary bladder in multiple sclerosis, *J. Oslo City Hosp.* **37**, 123–128.

118. Vas, C. J. (1969) Sexual impotence and some autonomic disturbances in men with multiple sclerosis. *Acta Neurol. Scand.* **45**, 166–182.

119. Cartlidge, N. (1972) Autonomic function in multiple sclerosis. *Brain* **95**, 661–64.

120. Noronha, M. J., Vas, C. J., and Aziz, H. (1968) Autonomic dysfunction (sweating responses) in multiple sclerosis. *J. Neurol. Neurosurg. Psychiatry* **31**, 19–22.

121. Elie, B. and Louboutin, J. P. (1995) Sympathetic skin response (SSR) is abnormal in multiple sclerosis. *Muscle Nerve* **18**, 185–189.

122. Caminero, A. B., Pérez-Jiménez, A., Barreiro, P., Ferrer, T. (1995) Sympathetic skin response: correlation with autonomic and somatic involvement in multiple sclerosis, *Electromyogr. Clin. Neurophysiol.* **35**, 457–462.

123. Senaratne, M. P., Carroll, D., Warren, K. G., and Kappagoda, T. (1984) Evidence for cardiovascular autonomic nerve dysfunction in multiple sclerosis. *J. Neurol. Neurosurg. Psychiatry* **47**, 947–952.

124. Sterman, A. B., Coyle, P. K., Panasci, D. J., and Grimson, R. (1985) Disseminated abnormalities of cardiovascular autonomic functions in multiple sclerosis. *Neurology* **35**, 1665–1668.

125. Pentland, B. and Ewing, D. J. (1987) Cardiovascular reflexes in multiple sclerosis. *Eur. Neurol.* **26**, 46–50.

126. Nordenbo, A. M., Boesen, F., and Andersen, E. B. (1989) Cardiovascular autonomic function in multiple sclerosis. *J. Auton. Nerv. Syst.* **26**, 77–84.

127. Anema, J. R., Heijenbrok, M. W., Faes, T. J., Heimans, J. J., Lanting, P., and Polman, C. H. (1991) Cardiovascular autonomic function in multiple sclerosis. *J. Neurol. Sci.* **104**, 129–134.

128. Vita, G., Fazio, M. C., Milone, S., Blandino, A., Salvi, L., and Messina, C. (1993) Cardiovascular autonomic dysfunction in multiple sclerosis is likely related to brainstem lesions. *J. Neurol. Sci.* **120**, 82–86.

129. Thomaides, T. N., Zoukos, Y., Chaudhuri, K. R., and Mathias, C. J. (1993) Physiological assessment of aspects of autonomic function in patients with secondary progressive multiple sclerosis. *J. Neurol.* **240**, 139–143.
130. Diamond, B. J., Kim, H., DeLuca, J., and Cordero, D. L. (1995) Cardiovascular regulation in multiple sclerosis. *Multiple Sclerosis* **1**, 156–162.
131. Frontoni, M., Fiorini, M., Strano, S., Cerutti, S., Giubilei, F., Urani, C., et al. (1996) Power spectrum analysis contribution to the detection of cardiovascular dysautonomia in multiple sclerosis. *Acta Neurol. Scand.* **93**, 241–245.
132. Linden, D., Diehl, R. R., Kretzschmar, A., and Berlit, P. (1997) Autonomic evaluation by means of standard tests and power spectral analysis in multiple sclerosis. *Muscle Nerve* **20**, 809–814.
133. Sakakibara, R., Mori, M., Fukutake, T., Kita, K., and Hattori, T. (1997) Orthostatic hypotension in a case of multiple sclerosis. *Clin. Auton. Res.* **7**, 163–165.
134. Giroud, M., Guard, O., and Dumas, R. (1988) Cardio-respiratory anomalies in disseminated sclerosis. *Rev. Neurol.* **144**, 284–288.
135. Buyse, B., Demedts, M., Meekers, J., Vandegaer, L., Rochette, F., and Kerkhofs, L. (1997) Respiratory dysfunction in multiple sclerosis: a prospective analysis of 60 patients. *Eur. Respir. J.* **10**, 139–145.
136. Tantucci, C., Massucci, M., Piperno, R., Betti, L., Grassi, V., and Sorbini, C. A. (1994) Control of breathing and respiratory muscle strength in patients with multiple sclerosis. *Chest* **105**, 1163–1170.
137. Howard, R. S., Wiles, C. M., Hirsch, N. P., Loh, L., Spencer, G. T., and Newsom-Davis, J. (1992) Respiratory involvement in multiple sclerosis, *Brain* **115**, 479–494.
138. Auer, R. N., Rowlands, C. G., Perry, S. F., and Remmers, J. E. (1996) Multiple sclerosis with medullary plaques and fatal sleep apnea (Ondine's curse). *Clin. Neuropathol.* **15**, 101–105.
139. Wennerholm, M. (1961) Postural vascular reactions in cases with migraine and related vascular headaches. *Acta Med. Scand.* **167**, 131–139.
140. Appenzeller, O., Davidson, K., and Marshall, J. (1963) Reflex vasomotor abnormalities in the hands of migrainous subjects. *J. Neurol. Neurosurg. Psychiatry* **26**, 447.
141. French, E. B., Lassers, P. W., and Desai, M. G. (1967) Reflex vasomotor responses in the hands of migrainous subjects. *J. Neurol. Neurosurg. Psychiatry* **30**, 276.
142. Hockaday, J. M. and McMillan, A. L. (1967)The effect of migraine and ergotamine upon reflex vasodilatation to radiant heating, in *Fourth European Congress on Microcirculation* (Harders, H., ed.), S. Basel Karger, Cambridge.
143. Steiner, T. J., Smith, F. R., and Rose, F. C. (1981) Vasomotor reactivity in migraine, in *Progress in Migraine Research* (Rose, F. C. and Zilkha, K. J., eds.), Pitman, Tunbridge Wells, UK, pp. 33–40.

207. Dyck, P. J., Lais, A. C., Ohta, M., Bastron, J. A., Okazaki, H., and Groover, R. V. (1975) Chronic inflammatory polyradiculoneuropathy. *Mayo Clin. Proc.* **50,** 621–637.
208. Prineas, J. W. and McLeod, J. G. (1976) Chronic relapsing polyneuritis. *Neurol. Sci.* **27,** 427–458.
209. Ingall, T. J. and McLeod, J. G., Tamura, N. (1990) Autonomic function and unmyelinated fibers in chronic inflammatory demyelinating polyradiculoneuropathy. *Muscle Nerve* **13,** 70–76.
210. Neil, H. A. W. (1992) The epidemiology of diabetic autonomic neuropathy, in *Autonomic Failure*, 3rd ed. (Bannister, R. and Mathias, C. J., eds.), Oxford University Press, Oxford, pp. 682–697.
211. Töyry, J. P., Partanen, J. V., Niskanen, L. K., Länsimies, E. A., and Uusitupa, M. I. (1997) Divergent development of autonomic and peripheral somatic neuropathies in NIDDM. *Diabetologia* **40,** 953–958.
212. Orchard, T. J., Lloyd, C. E., Maser, R. E., and Kuller, L. H. (1996) Why does diabetic autonomic neuropathy predict IDDM mortality? *Diabetes Res. Clin. Prac.* **34,** S165–S171.
213. Mulder, D. W. (1961) The neuropathies associated with diabetes mellitus: a clinical and electromyographic study of 103 unselected diabetic patients. *Neurology* **11,** 275–284.
214. Veglio, M. (1990) Autonomic neuropathy in non-insulin-dependent diabetic patients: correlation with age, sex, duration and metabolic control of diabetes. *Diabetes Metab.* **16,** 200–206.
215. Ewing, D. J., Neilson, J. M. M., Shapiro, C. M., and Reid, W. (1991) Twenty four hour heart rate variability: effects of posture, sleep, and time of day in healthy controls and comparison with bedside tests of autonomic function in diabetic patients. *Br. Heart J.* **65,** 239–244.
216. Ewing, D. J., Borsey, D. Q., Bellavere, F., and Clarke, B. F. (1981) Cardiac autonomic neuropathy in diabetes: comparison of measures of R-R interval variation. *Diabetologia* **21,** 18–24.
217. Lishner, M., Akselrod, S., Mor Avi, V., Oz, O., Divon, M., and Ravid, M. (1987) Spectral analysis of heart rate fluctuations. A non-invasive, sensitive method for the early diagnosis of autonomic neuropathy in diabetes mellitus. *J. Auton. Nerv. Syst.* **19,** 119–125.
218. Pagani, M., Malfatto, G., Pierini, S., Casati, R., Masu, A. M., Poli, M., et al. (1988) Spectral analysis of heart rate variability in assessment of autonomic diabetic neuropathy. *J. Auton. Nerv. Syst.* **23,** 143–153.
219. Freeman, R., Saul, P., Roberts, M. S., Berger, R. D., Broadbridge, C., and Cohen, R. J. (1991) Spectral analysis of heart rate in diabetic autonomic neuropathy. *Arch. Neurol.* **48,** 185–190.

PART II

The Hypothalamo–Pituitary–Adrenal System and the Heart

CHAPTER 6

Stress, the Hypothalamo–Pituitary–Adrenal System, and the Heart

Béla Bohus and S. Michiel Korte

1. Introduction

The cardiovascular system signals stress influences on humans and other animals. That physical demands changes the heart rate has been generally accepted. The prominent British physiologist Sherrington (1) suggested that natural emotional states also profoundly change the cardiovascular function: "yet heightened beating of the heart, blanching or flushing of the blood vessels, all these are prominent characters in the pantomime of natural emotion." Cannon (2) was the first to describe physiological responses to directly threatening environmental influences. His "fight and flight" reaction pattern was characterized by activation of the sympatho-adrenal system, via a mass discharge (3). This sympathetic mass discharge has long been considered to be responsible for the classical signs of stress such as tachycardia and an increase in blood pressure. Rather recently, the interest has also been focused on the other major stress system of the body (i.e., the hypothalamic–pituitary–adrenal system) as the messenger of stress effects to the heart.

The role of adrenal cortex in the nonspecific bodily responses has been proposed by Selye (4), who developed the concept of stress. In response to stress, corticosteroid hor-

From: *The Nervous System and the Heart*
Ed: G. J. Ter Horst © Humana Press Inc.

mones (aldosterone and corticosterone or cortisol) are released from the adrenal cortex via a cascade of humoral events in the hypothalamo–pituitary–adrenocortical (HPA) axis (5). The maximal activation of the adrenal cortex via the hypothalamo–pituitary mechanisms needs a certain time lag of approximately 15 min to develop. Depending on the strength of the stressor, this activation is sustained, and it takes a few hours to return to baseline activity. It is, therefore, not surprising that one of the major functions of glucocorticoids is to turn off the stress reactions, thus preventing the stress reaction from overshooting to themselves, threatening alterations of homeostasis (6). Immune, cardiovascular, and central responses to noxious stimuli would themselves become damaging if left uncontrolled by glucocorticoids. Although the sympatho-adrenal system seemed to be a more logical candidate of controlling the cardiovascular system, early experiments, particularly in adrenalectomized and corticosteroid-supplemented animals suggested the involvement of the HPA axis in heart rate regulation, using corticosteroids as the ultimate messengers. In addition, we reported that as early as 1970, the administration of the glucocorticoid cortisol results in sustained tachycardia during a conditioned fear response in the rat (7). Because it was already known that adrenal hormones profoundly affect adaptive behavior (8), it was not clear whether the corticoid influences on heart rate were directed toward central or peripheral cardiovascular regulation or were the consequences of behavioral actions such as altered emotion or motivation.

The HPA axis has long been considered a unitary system of stress reaction with corticosteroids as the only messengers. The discovery that the pituitary adrenocorticotrophic hormone (ACTH) is derived from a large precursor protein changed this view entirely. The pro-opiomelanocortin precursor is the origin of not only the ACTH, but also of the endogenous opioid β-endorphin, the family of melanocyte stimulating hormones (MSH) such as α- and β-MSH, and the structurally similar γ-MSH (9). All these peptides carry

axis and, consequently, the release of corticosteroid hormones *(56,57)*. Three daily sessions of both stressors increase the chronotropic function of pacemaker beta adrenoceptors as measured by an increased sensitivity to isoprenaline. The GR antagonist RU 38486 blocks this effect, whereas the GR agonist RU 28362 induces an increase in the beta-adrenoceptor population in nonstressed animals. Pretreatment of rats with diazepam, which blocks the stress-induced increase in the plasma level of corticosterone, prevents the development of pacemaker supersensitivity to isoprenaline *(58,59)*. Previously, it was shown that the stress of inescapable foot shock caused an increment of the chronotropic function of the pacemaker beta-2-adrenoceptors, as measured by supersensitivity to isoproterenol, epinephrine, and salbutamol *(60)*. However, a decline of the chronotropic function of pacemaker beta-1-adrenoceptors, as measured by a decrease of the maximum response to soterenol, was demonstrated *(61)*. Glucocorticoids upregulate beta-2-adrenergic receptors, but downregulate beta-1-adrenergic receptors in glioma cells, suggesting that glucocorticoids may have an opposite effect on beta-1- and beta-2-adrenergic receptors *(62)*. The ability to control the shock prevents the downregulation of the pacemaker beta-1- adrenoreceptors but not the increased participation of beta-2-adrenoreceptors in the response of the rat sinoatrial node to catecholamines after repeated inescapable stress *(61)*. Accordingly, glucocorticoids play a critical role in the modulation of the sensitivity to catecholamines of the pacemaker beta-adrenoceptors after repeated inescapable stress. This modulation of stress-induced heart function involves glucocorticoid (type II) receptors.

Dexamethasone, a potent GR agonist, stimulates the expression of atrial natriuretic peptide (ANP) mRNA in cultured rat ventricular myocytes. The GR antagonist RU38486 *(63)* abolishes this glucocortioid action. ANP mRNA is also regulated by glucocorticoids in vivo *(64,65)*. ANP can be considered as an endogenous antagonist of the renin–angiotensin–aldosterone system and the antidiuretic hormone *(66)*. Glucocorticoids also play an important role in the maintenance of Ca^{2+} transport function and myocardial contractile protein ATPases and, therefore, normal myocardial contractility *(67,68)*. These observations also demonstrate the involvement of GR-mediated processes in the local regulation of heart function.

Although all components for a specific aldosterone effect are present in the human heart (i.e., atrial and ventricular MRs) *(52)*, and the presence of 11-beta-hydroxysteroid dehydrogenase *(55)*, which converts glucocorticosteroids to inactive 11-keto congeners *(69)*, the physiological function(s) of cardiac MR sites, and their in vivo mineralocorticoid or glucocorticoid selectivity, remain to be explored.

A recent article suggests a novel aspect of the corticosteroid action on heart function *(70)*. Increasing evidence suggests that mineralocorticoid and glucocorticoid hormones affect organ functions through local synthesis. The terminal enzymes of aldosterone and corticosterone synthesis (i.e., aldosterone synthase and 11β-hydroxylase, respectively) were detected in the rat heart. The physiological activity of these enzymes is reinforced by the production of aldosterone and corticosterone in isolated rat hearts. Acute regulation of the hormone synthesis is shown by the increased production of these two hormones following angiotensin II or ACTH perfusion. Chronic regulation in the rat heart was demonstrated by increased expression of mRNA levels of 11β-hydroxylase angiotensin II and ACTH and of aldosterone synthase by angiotensin II and low sodium and high potassium diet treatments for a week. In summary, this study shows the existence of an endocrine cardiac steroidogenic system and its potential relevance for heart physiology and pathology.

3.3. The Brain as Target for Corticosteroid Actions

In the brain, the two receptor types differ in their localization, regulation, and function *(47)*. The MRs can be found in the anteroventral part of the third ventricle (AV3V area) and in the limbic brain regions such as the hippocampus, septum, and amygdala. The MRs in the AV3V area, a wellknown region in cardiovascular and volume regulation, are aldosterone sensitive. The GRs are widely distributed in the brain with highest concentration in regions involved in feedback regulation of the stress response (e.g., paraventricular hypothalamic nucleus [PVN] and hippocampus). Both MRs and GRs have been found in neurons located in the nucleus tractus solitarius (NTS) and the PVN *(49)*. These latter nuclei, together with the amygdaloid central nucleus, are intimately involved in central cardiovascular regulation *(71)*.

The limbic MRs binds both cortisol and corticosterone and aldosterone with high affinity, whereas the GRs bind corticosterone with a 10-fold lower affinity than the MRs does *(47,49)*. Therefore, at low levels of circulating corticosterone, the MR receptors are predominantly occupied, whereas after stress and during the circadian peak, both GRs and MRs are activated *(49,72,73)*. There is a growing body of evidence from De Kloet and his associates that in the course of normal diurnal variation, when the permissive (tonic) corticosteroid effects are predominant, corticosterone via MRs "prime" the stress responses, bringing them to the peak of readiness for the activities of the day. At the same time, through their suppressive actions via GRs, corticosteroids control the stress reactions, preventing them from overshooting and damaging the organism *(6,45)*. There is evidence that similar mechanisms may be active in cardiovascular control processes. For instance, experiments with intracerebroventricular administration of the selective corticosteroid receptor ligands suggest that the MR-related processes mediate pressor responses, whereas the GR exerts an inhibitory corticosteroid action on blood pressure *(74)*. Administration of the MR antagonist RU 28318 decreased, whereas aldosterone increased blood pressure. Oppositely, the GR antagonist RU 38486 caused an increase in blood pressure with a slow onset and a rather long (24–48 h) duration. The selective GR agonist RU 28362 decreased blood pressure. Adrenalectomized rats maintained on physiological saline showed a decrease in blood pressure, which could be restored by a low dose of corticosterone replacement. Chronically elevated levels of circulating corticosterone by a high dose of corticosterone replacement increased blood pressure. These changes could be blocked by intracerebroventricular administration of MR or GR antagonists, respectively. These latter findings reinforce the notion that corticosteroid influences on blood pressure regulation involve central receptor mechanisms. It should be emphasized that these experiments were carried out on conscious male rats using the indirect tail-cuff technique to measure systolic blood pressure. This method does not easily allow heart rate measurement and it requires keeping the rats in high ambient temperature. Accordingly, one can consider that the measures are taken under heat stress conditions to which the rats are repeatedly exposed. The importance of heat stress as a variable was suggested by further experiments by the same authors *(75).* They used a direct method (i.e., intra-arterial catheter implantation) for the measurement of cardiovascular parameters, including the heart rate. Intracerebroventricular administration of the MR antagonist RU 28318 reduced blood pressure, heart rate, and plasma corticosterone response to a brief restrain stress provided that the rats were previously subjected to a daily heat exposure of 32°C for 2 wk. In a subsequent study, it was shown that the antihypertensive action of centrally acting MR antagonist also depended on the circadian rhythm. In deoxycorticosterone acetate (DOCA)–salt hypertensive rats, RU 28318 decreased blood pressure in the dark (i.e., activity phase of the rats) but not during the light phase *(76).* Lesion studies in rats with mineralocorticoid hypertension suggest the involvement of MRs located in the circumventricular regions and the anterior hypothalamus *(77).* Accordingly, these studies all together favor the intimate involvement of central mineralocorticoid receptors in the control of cardiovascular regulation. Although these studies did not specify the role of GRs in these processes, other experiments provided us with ample evidence about the role of glucocorticoid-receptor-mediated processes in cardiovascular regulation.

Evidence indicates the involvement of GRs in the opioid peptide induced regulation of cardiovascular function during hemorrhagic shock. Whereas intracerebroventricular

References

1. Sherrington, C. S. (1952) Reflexes as adapted reactions: bodily resonance of emotion, in *The Integrative Action of the Nervous System, Lecture VII,* Cambridge University Press, London, p. 257.
2. Cannon, W. B. (1929) *Bodily Changes in Pain, Hunger, Fear and Rage,* Branford, Boston.
3. Cannon, W. B. (1929) Organization for physiological homeostasis. *Physiol. Rev.* **9,** 399–331.
4. Selye, H. (1976) *The Stress of Life,* McGraw-Hill, New York.
5. McEwen, B. S., De Kloet, E. R., and Rostene, W. (1986) Adrenal steroid receptors and actions in the nervous system. *Physiol. Rev.* **66,** 1121–1188.
6. Munck, A., Guyre P. M., and Holbrook N. J. (1984) Physiological functions of glucocorticoids in stress and their relationship to pharmacological actions. *Endocr. Rev.* **5,** 25–44.
7. Bohus, B., Grubits, J., and Lissák, K. (1970) Influence of cortisone on heart rate during fear extinction in the rat. *Acta Physiol. Acad. Sci. Hung.* **37,** 265–272.
8. Bohus, B. (1970) Central nervous structures and the effect of ACTH and corticosteroids on avoidance behavior: a study with intracerebral implantation of corticosteroids in the rat. *Prog. Brain Res.* **32,** 171–184.
9. Eipper, B. A. and Mains, R. E. (1980) Structure and biosynthesis of pro-adrenocorticotropin/endorphin and related peptides. *Endocr. Rev.* **1,** 1–27.
10. Lindner, E. and Scholkens, B. (1974) ACTH and α-MSH: cardiovascular and antiarrhythmic properties. *Arch. Int. Pharmacodyn. Ther.* **208,** 19–23.
11. Vale W., Rivier, C., Brown, M. R., Spiess, J., Koob, G., Swanson, L., et al. (1983) Chemical and biological characterization of corticotropin releasing factor. *Rec. Prog. Horm. Res.* **39,** 245–270.
12. Swanson, L. W. and Sawchenko, P. E. (1983) Hypothalamic integration: organization of the paraventricular and supraoptic nuclei. *Annu. Rev. Neurosci.* **6,** 269–324.
13. Dunn, A. J. and Berridge, C. W. (1990) Physiological and behavioral responses to corticotropin-releasing factor administration: is CRF a mediator of anxiety and stress responses? *Brain Res. Rev.* **15,** 71–100.
14. Akil, H., Watson, S. J., Young, E., Lewis, M. E., Khachaturian, H., and Walker J. M. (1984) Endogenous opioids: biology and function. *Annu. Rev. Neurosci.* **7,** 223–255.
15. De Souza, E. B. (1996) Corticotropin-releasing factor receptors: physiology, pharmacology, biochemistry and role in central nervous system and immune disorders. *Psychoneuroendocrinology* **20,** 789–819.

16. Steptoe, A. (1993) Stress and the cardiovascular system: a psychosocial perspective, in *Stress, From Synapse to Syndrome* (Stanford, S. C. and Salmon, P., eds.), Academic, London, pp. 119–141.

17. Bohus B. and Koolhaas, J. M. (1993) Stress and the cardiovascular system: central and peripheral physiological mechanisms, in *Stress, From Synapse to Syndrome* (Stanford, S. C. and Salmon, P., eds.), Academic, London, pp. 75–117.

18. Blanchard, R. J., Nikulina, J. N., Sakai, R. R., McKittrich, C., McEwen, B. S., and Blanchard, D. C. (1998) Behavioral and endocrine change following chronic predatory stress. *Physiol. Behav.* **63,** 561–569.

19. Sgoifo, A., Stilli, D., Aimi, B., Parmiggiani, S., Manghi, M., and Musso, E. (1994) Behavioral and electrocardiographic responses to social stress in male rats. *Physiol. Behav.* **55,** 209–216.

20. Harlow, H. J., Thorne, E. T., and Williams, E. S. (1987) Adrenal responsiveness in domestic sheep (*Ovis aries*) to acute and chronic stressors as predicted by remote monitoring of cardiac frequency. *Can. J. Zool.* **65,** 2021–2027.

21. Baldock, N. M. and Sibley, R. M. (1990) Effects of handling and transportation on the heart rate and behaviour of sheep. *Appl. Anim. Behav. Sci.* **28,** 15–39.

22. Liang, B., Verrier, R. L., Melman, J., and Lown, B. (1979) Correlation between circulating catecholamine levels and ventricular vulnerability during psychological stress in conscious dogs. *Proc. Soc. Exp. Biol. Med.* **161,** 266–269.

23. Gomez, R. E., Büttner, D. and Cannata, M. A. (1989) Open field behaviour and cardiovascular responses to stress in normal rats. *Physiol. Behav.* **45,** 767–769.

24. Obrist, P. A. (1981) *Cardiovascular Psychophysiology: A Perspective,* Plenum, New York.

25. Gärtner, K., Büttner, D., and Döhler, K. (1980) Stress response to handling and experimental procedures. *Lab. Anim.* **14,** 267–274.

26. Roozendaal, B., Koolhaas, J. M., and Bohus, B. (1991) Attenuated cardiovascular, neuroendocrine, and behavioral responses after a single footshock in central amygdaloid lesioned male rats. *Physiol. Behav.* **50,** 771–775.

27. Sgoifo, A., De Boer, S. F., Westenbroek, C., Maes, F. W., Beldhuis, H., Suzuki, T., et al. (1997) Incidence of arrhythmias and heart rate variability in wild-type rats exposed to social stress. *Am. J. Physiol.* **273,** H1754–1760.

28. Hofer, M. A. (1970) Cardiac and respiratory function during sudden prolonged immobility in wild rodents. *Psychosom. Med.* **32,** 533–547.

29. Steenbergen, Koolhaas, J. M., Strubbe, J. H., and Bohus, B. (1989) Behavioural and cardiac responses to a sudden change in environmental stimuli: effect of forced shift in food intake. *Physiol. Behav.* **45,** 729–733.

30. Buwalda, B., Koolhaas, J. M., and Bohus, B. (1992) Behavioral and cardiac responses to mild stress in young and aged rats: effects of amphetamine and vasopressine. *Physiol. Behav.* **51**, 211–216.

31. Bohus, B. (1974) Telemetred heart rate responses of the rat during free and learned behaviour. *Biotelemetry* **1**, 193–201.

32. Korte, S. M., Koolhaas, J. M., Schuurman, T., Traber, J., and Bohus, B. (1990) Anxiolytics and stress-induced behavioural and cardiac responses: a study of diazepam and ipsapirone (TVX Q 7821). *Eur. J. Pharmacol.* **179**, 393–401.

33. Sgoifo, A., De Boer, S. F., Buwalda, B., Korte-Bouws, G., Tuma, J., Bohus, B., et al. (1998) Vulnerability to arrhythmias during social stress in rats with different sympathovagal balance. *Am. J. Physiol.* **275**, H460–H466.

34. Bohus, B. (1973) Pituitary–adrenal influences on avoidance and approach behavior of the rat. *Prog. Brain Res.* **39**, 407–420.

35. Kapp, B. S., Frysinger, R. C., Gallagher, M., and Haselton, J. R. (1979) Amygdala central nucleus lesions: effect on heart rate conditioning in the rabbit. *Physiol. Behav.* **23**, 1109–1117.

36. Von Holst, D., Fuchs, E., and Stohr, W. (1983) Physiological changes in male *Tupaia belangeri* under different types of social stress, in *Biobehavioral Bases of Coronary Heart Diseases* (Dembroski, T. H., Schmidt, T. H., and Blümchen, G. eds.), Karger, Basel, pp. 382–390.

37. Korte, S. M., Smit, J., Bouws, G. A., Koolhaas, J. M., and Bohus, B. (1990) Behavioral and neuroendocrine response to psychosocial stress in male rats: the effects of the 5-HT 1A agonist ipsapirone. *Horm. Behav.* **24**, 554–567.

38. Roozendaal, B., Koolhaas, J. M., and Bohus, B. (1990) Differential effect of lesioning of the central amygdala on the bradycardiac and behavioral response of the rat in relation to conditioned social and solitary stress. *Behav. Brain Res.* **41**, 39–48.

39. Kamarck, T. and Jennings, J. R. (1991) Biobehavioral factors of sudden cardiac death. *Psychol. Bull.* **109**, 42–75.

40. Hughes, C. W. and Lynch, J. J. (1978) A reconsideration of psychological precursors of sudden death in infrahuman animals. *Am. Psychol.* **33**, 419–429.

41. Lown, B., Verrier, R., and Corbalan, R. (1973) Psychological stress and threshold for repetitive ventricular responses. *Science* **182**, 834–836.

42. Corley, K. C., Schiel, F. O. M., Mauck, H. J. P., and Greenhoot, J. (1973) Electrocardiographic and cardiac morphological changes associated with environmental stress in squirrel monkeys. *Psychosom. Med.* **35**, 361–364.

43. Nyakas, C., Prins, A. J. A., and Bohus, B. (1990) Age related alterations in cardiac response to emotional stress: relation behavioural reactivity in the rat. *Physiol. Behav.* **47**, 273–280.

44. Bohus, B. G. J. (1998) Neuroendocrinology of stress: behavioral and neurobiological considerations, in *Methods in Neuroendocrinology* (Van de Kar, L. D., ed.), CRC, Boca Raton, FL, pp. 163–180.

45. De Kloet, E. R. (1991) Brain corticosteroid receptor balance and homeostatic control. *Front. Neuroendocrinol.* **12,** 95–164.

46. Funder, J. W. (1997) Glucocorticoid and mineralocorticoid receptors: biology and clinical relevance. *Annu. Rev. Med.* **48,** 231–240.

47. De Kloet, E. R., Vreugdenhil, E., Oitzl, M. S., and Joëls, M. (1998) Brain corticosteroid balance in health and disease. *Endocr. Rev.* **19,** 269–301.

48. Handa, R. J., Price, R. H., Jr., and Wilson, M. E. (1998) Steroid hormone receptors and the assessment of feedback sensitivity, in *Methods in Neuroendocrinology* (Van de Kar, L. D., ed.), CRC, Boca Raton, FL, pp. 49–68.

49. Reul, J. M. H. M. and De Kloet, E. R. (1985) Two receptor systems for corticosterone in rat brain: microdistribution and differential occupation. *Endocrinology* **117,** 117–123.

50. Fuxe, K., Wikström, A. C., Okret, S., Agnati, L. F., Härfstrand, A., Yu, Z. Y., et al. (1985) Mapping of glucocorticoid receptor immunoreactive neurons in the rat tel- and diencephalon using a monoclonal antibody against rat liver glucocorticoid receptor. *Endocrinology* **117,** 1803–1812.

51. Van Eekelen, J. A. M., Kiss, J. Z., Westphalm, H. M., and De Kloet, E. R. (1987) Immunocytochemical study on the intracellular localization of the type 2 glucocorticoid receptor in the rat brain. *Brain Res.* **436,** 120–128.

52. Pearce, P. and Funder, J. W. (1987) High affinity aldosterone binding sites (type I receptors) in rat heart. *Clin. Exp. Pharmacol. Physiol.* **14,** 859–866.

53. Van Eekelen J. A. M., Jiang, W., De Kloet, E. R., and Bohn M. C. (1988) Distribution of the mineralocorticoid and the glucocorticoid receptor mRNAs in the rat hippocampus. *J. Neurosci. Res.* **21,** 88–94.

54. Chao, H. M., Choo, P. H., and McEwen, B. S. (1989) Glucocorticoid and mineralocorticoid receptor mRNA expression in rat brain. *Neuroendocrinology* **50,** 65–371.

55. Bonvalet J. P., Alfaidy, N., Farman, N., and Lombes, M. (1995) Aldosterone: intracellular receptors in human heart. *Eur. Heart J.* **16(Suppl. N),** 92–97.

56. De Kloet, E. R., De Kock, S., Schild, V., and Veldhuis, H. D. (1988) Antiglucocorticoid RU 38486 attenuates retention of a behaviour and disinhibits the hypothalamic–pituitary adrenal axis at different brain sites. *Neuroendocrinology* **47,** 109–115.

57. Korte, S. M., Buwalda, B., Bouws, G. A. H., Koolhaas, J. M., Maes, F. W., and Bohus, B. (1992) Conditioned neuroendocrine and cardiovas-

cular stress responsiveness accompanying behavioral passivity and activity in aged and in young rats. *Physiol. Behav.* **51,** 815–822.

58. Moura, M. J. and De Moraes, S. (1994) Forced swim stress: supersensitivity of the isolated rat pacemaker to the chronotropic effect of isoprenaline and the role of corticosterone. *Gen. Pharmacol.* **25,** 1341–1347.

59. Rahnemaye, F., Nourani, R., Spadari, R. C., and De Moraes, S. (1992) Footshock stress-induced supersensitivity to isoprenaline in the isolated pacemaker of the rat: effects of the compounds RU-38486 and RU-28362. *Gen. Pharmacol.* **23,** 787–791.

60. Bassani, R. A. and De Moraes, S. (1988) Effects of repeated footshock stress on the chronotropic responsiveness of the isolated pacemaker of the rat: role of beta-2 adrenoceptors. *J. Pharmacol. Exp. Ther.* **246,** 316–321.

61. Bassani, R. A. and Bassani, J. W. (1993) Effects of escapable and inescapable foot-shock on rat atrial beta-adrenoceptors. *Pharmacol. Biochem. Behav.* **44,** 869–875.

62. Kiely, J., Hadcock, J. R., Bahouth, S. W., and Malbon, C. C. (1994) Glucocorticoids down-regulate beta 1-adrenergic-receptor expression by suppressing transcription of the receptor gene. *Biochem. J.* **302,** 97–403.

63. Nishimori. T., Tsujino, M., Sato, K., Imai, T., Marumo, F., and Hirata, Y. (1997) Dexamethasone-induced up-regulation of adrenomedullin and atrial natriuretic peptide genes in cultured rat ventricular myocytes. *J. Mol. Cell. Cardiol.* **29,** 2125–2130.

64. Gardner, D. G., Gertz, B. J., Deschepper, C. F., and Kim, D. Y. (1988) Gene for the rat atrial natriuretic peptide is regulated by glucocorticoids in vitro. *J. Clin. Invest.* **82,** 1275–1281.

65. Gardner, D. G., Hane, S., Trachewsky, D., Schenk, D., and Baxter, J. D. (1986) Atrial natriuretic peptide mRNA is regulated by glucocorticoids in vivo. *Biochem. Biophys. Res. Commun.* **139,** 1047–1054.

66. Tan, A. C., Russel, F. G., Thien, T., and Benraad T. J. (1993) Atrial natriuretic peptide. An overview of clinical pharmacology and pharmacokinetics. *Clin. Pharmacokinet.* **24,** 28–45.

67. Narayanan, N. (1983) Effects of adrenalectomy and in vivo administration of dexamethasone on ATP-dependent calcium accumulation by sarcoplasmic reticulum from rat heart. *J. Mol. Cell. Cardiol.* **15,** 7–15.

68. Bhaskar, M., Stith, R. D., Brackett, D. J., Wilson, M. F., Lerner, M. R., and Reddy Y. S. (1989) Changes in myocardial contractile protein ATPases in chronically adrenalectomized rats with and without glucocorticoid replacement. *Biochem. Med. Metab. Biol.* **42,** 118–124.

69. Funder J. W. (1995) Steroids, hypertension and cardiac fibrosis. *Blood Press.* 2(*Suppl.*), 39–42.

70. Silvestre, J. S., Robert, V., Heymes, C., Aupetit-Faisant, B., Mouas, C., Moalic, J. M., et al. (1998) Myocardial production of aldosterone and corticosterone in the rat. Physiological regulation. *J. Biol. Chem.* **27**, 4883–4891.

71. Loewy, A. D. (1990) Central autonomic pathways, in *Central Regulation of Autonomic Function* (Loewy, A. D. and Spyer, K. D., eds.), Oxford University Press, New York, pp. 108–133.

72. Reul, J. M., van den Bosch, F. R., and De Kloet E. R. (1987) Differential response of type I and type II corticosteroid receptors to changes in plasma steroid level and circadian rhythmicity. *Neuroendocrinology* **45**, 407–412.

73. Ratka, A., Sutanto, W., Bloemers, M., and De Kloet, E. R. (1989) On the role of brain mineralocorticoid (type I) and glucocorticoid (type II) receptors in neuroendocrine regulation. *Neuroendocrinology* **50**, 117–123.

74. Van den Berg, D. T., De Kloet, E. R., Van Dijken, H. H., and De Jong, W. (1990) Differential central effects of mineralocorticoid and glucocorticoid agonists and antagonists on blood pressure. *Endocrinology* **126**, 118–124.

75. Van den Berg, D. T., De Kloet, E. R., and De Jong, W. (1994) Central effects of mineralocorticoid antagonist RU-28318 on blood pressure of DOCA–salt hypertensive rats. *Am. J. Physiol.* **267**, E927–E933.

76. Van den Berg, D. T., De Jong, W., and De Kloet, E. R. (1994) Mineralocortriocid antagonist inhibits stress-induced blood pressure response after repeated daily warming. *Am. J. Physiol.* **267**, E921–E926.

77. Goto, A., Ganguli, M., Tobian, L., Johnson, M. A., and Iwai, J. (1982) Effect of an anteroventral third ventricle lesion on NaCl hypertension in Dahl salt-sensitive rats. *Am. J. Physiol.* **243**, H614–H618.

78. Eijgelshoven, M. H., De Kloet, E. R., Van den Berg, D. T., and Van Giersbergen, P. L. (1991) Activation of glucocorticoid receptors and the effect of naloxone during hemorrhagic hypotension. *Eur. J. Pharmacol.* **205**, 183–189.

79. Sawchenko, P. E. and Bohn, M. C. (1989) Glucocorticoid receptor-immunoreactivity in C1, C2, and C3 adrenergic neurons that project to the hypothalamus or to the spinal cord in the rat. *J. Comp. Neurol.* **285**, 107–116.

80. Minson, J., Llewellyn-Smith, I., Neville, A., Somogyi, P., and Chalmers, J. (1990) Quantitative analysis of spinally projecting adrenaline-synthetising neurons of C1, C2 and C3 groups in rat medulla oblongata. *J. Auton. Nerv. Syst.* **30**, 209–220.

81. Zhu, D. N., Xue, L. M., and Li, P. (1995) Cardiovascular effects of microinjection of corticoids and antagonists into the rostral ventrolateral medulla in rats. *Blood Press.* **4**, 55–62.

82. Zhu, D. N., Xue, L. M., and Li, P. (1996) Effect of central muscarine receptor blockade with DKJ-21 on the blood pressure and heart rate in stress-induced hypertensive rats. *Blood Press.* **5**, 170–177.

83. Zhu, D. N., Xue, L. M., and Li, P. (1997) The cardiovascular response to medullary cholinergic and corticoid stimulation is calcium channel dependent in rats. *Blood Press.* **6,** 171–179.

84. De Kloet E. R., Rots, N. Y., Van den Berg, D. T., and Oitzl, M. S. (1994) Brain mineralocorticoid receptor function. *Ann. NY Acad. Sci.* **746,** 8–20.

85. Korte, S. M., De Boer, S. F., De Kloet, E. R., and Bohus, B. (1995) Anxiolytic-like effects of selective mineralocorticoid and glucocorticoid antagonists on fear-enhanced behavior in the elevated plus-maze. *Psychoneuroendocrinology* **20,** 385–394.

86. Koob, G. F., Heinrichs, S. C., Pich, E. M., Menzaghi, F., Baldwin, H., Miczek, K., et al. (1993) The role of corticotropin-releasing factor in behavioural responses to stress. *Ciba Found. Symp.* **172,** 277–289.

87. Korte, S. M., Bouws, G. A. H., and Bohus, B. (1993) Central actions of corticotropin-releasing hormone (CRH) on behavioral, neuroendocrine, and cardiovascular regulation: brain corticoid receptor involvement. *Horm. Behav.* **27,** 167–183.

88. Korte, S. M., Eisinga, W., Timmerman, W., Nyakas, C., and Bohus, B. (1992) Behavioral and cardiac responses after intracerebroventricular corticotropin-releasing hormone (CRH) administration: role of adrenal cortical hormones. *Horm. Behav.* **26,** 375–384.

89. Gardiner, S. M. and Bennett, T. (1983) Post-adrenalectomy hypotension in rats; absence of baroreflex resetting or effect of naloxone. *Clin. Sci.* **64,** 371–376.

90. Fisher, L. A., Jessen, G., and Brown, M. R. (1983) Corticotropin-releasing factor (CRF): mechanisms to elevate mean arterial pressure and heart rate. *Regul. Pept.* **5,** 153–161.

91. Fisher, L. A. (1991) Corticotropin-releasing factor and autonomic responses to stress, in *Stress, Neuropeptides, and Systems Disease* (McCubbin, J. A., Kaufmann, P. G., and Nemeroff, C. B., eds.), Academic, New York, pp. 95–118.

92. Li, S. J., Varga, K., Archer, P., Hruby, V. J., Sharma. S. D., Kesterson, R. A., et al. (1996) Melanocortin antagonists define two distinct pathways of cardiovascular control by alpha- and gamma-melanocyte-stimulating hormones. *J. Neurosci.* **16,** 5182–5188.

93. Perrin, M., Donaldson, C., Chen, R., Blount, A., Berggren, T., Bilezikjian, L., et al. (1995) Identification of a second corticotropin-releasing factor receptor gene and characterization of a cDNA expressed in the heart. *Proc. Natl. Acad. Sci. USA* **92,** 2969–2973.

94. Stenzel, P., Kesterson, R., Yeung, W., Cone, R. D., Rittenberg, M. B., and Stenzel-Poore, M. P. (1995) Identification of a novel murine receptor for corticotropin-releasing hormone expressed in the heart. *Mol. Endocrinol.* **9,** 637–645.

95. Lovenberg, T. W., Chalmers, D. T., Liu, C., and De Souza, E. B. (1995) CRF2-α and CRF2-β receptor mRNAs are differentially dis-

tributed between the rat central nervous system and peripheral tissues. *Endocrinology* **136**, 4139–4142.

96. Heldwein, K. A., Redick, D. L., Rittenberg, M. B., Calycomb, W. C., and Stenzel-Poore, M. P. (1996) Corticotropin-releasing hormone receptor expression and functional coupling in neonatal cardiac myocytes and AT-1 cells. *Endocrinology* **137**, 3631–3639.

97. Makino, S., Asaba, K., Takaok, T., and Hashimoto, K. (1998) Type 2 corticotropin-releasing hormone receptor mRNA expression in the heart in hypertensive rats. *Life Sci.* **62**, 515–523.

98. Ikeda, K., Tojo, K., Sato, S., Ebisawa, T., Tokudome, G., Hosoya, T., et al. (1998) Urocortin, a newly identified corticotropin-releasing factor-related mammalian peptide, stimulates atrial natriuretic peptide and brain natriuretic peptide secretions from neonatal cardiomyocytes. *Biochem. Biophys. Res. Commun.* **250**, 298–304.

99. Grunt, M., Glaser, J., Schmidhuber, H., Pauschinger, P., and Born, J. (1993) Effect of corticotropin-releasing factor on isolated heart activity. *Am. J. Physiol.* **264**, H1124–H1129.

100. Overton, J. M. and Fisher, L. A. (1991) Differentiated hemodynamic responses to central versus peripheral administration of corticotropin-releasing factor in conscious rats. *J. Auton. Nerv. Syst.* **35**, 43–51.

101. Parkes, D. G., Vaughan, J., Rivier, J., Vale, W., and May, C. N. (1997) Cardiac inotropic actions of urocortin in conscious sheep. *Am. J. Physiol.* **272**, H2115–H2122.

102. Adan, R. A. and Gispen, W. H. (1997) Brain melanocortin receptors: from cloning to function. *Peptides* **18**, 1279–1287.

103. Millington, W. R., Evans, V. R., Forman, L. J., and Battie, C. N. (1993) Characterization of β-endorphin- and α-MSH-related peptides in rat heart. *Peptides* **14**, 1141–114.

104. Fodor, M., Sluiter, A., Frankhuijzen-Sierevogel, A., Wiegant, V. M., Hoogerhout, P., De Wieldt, D. J., et al. (1996) Distribution of Lys-γ²-melanocyte-stimulating hormone (Lys-γ²-MSH)-like immunoreactivity in neuronal elements in the brain and peripheral tissues of the rat. *Brain Res.* **731**, 182–189.

105. Mehrabani, P. A. and Bassett, J. R. (1990) Adrenocorticotropin binding sites in rat cardiac tissue. *Pharm. Biochem. Behav.* **35**, 99–103.

106. Fathi, Z., Iben, L. G., and Parker, E. M. (1995) Cloning, expression, and tissue distribution of a fifth melanocortin receptor subtype. *Neurochem. Res.* **20**, 107–113.

107. Chhajlani, V. (1996) Distribution of CDNA for melanocortin receptor subtypes in human tissues. *Biochem. Mol. Biol. Int.* **38**, 73–80.

108. Bohus, B. (1975) Pituitary peptides and adaptive autonomic responses. *Prog. Brain Res.* **42**, 275–283.

109. Versteeg, D. H. G., Van Bergen, P., Adan, R. A., and De Wieldt, D. J. (1998) Melanocortins and cardiovascular re gulation. *Eur. J. Pharmacol.* **360**, 1–14.

PART III

Heart Pain

CHAPTER 7

Cardiac Nociceptive Systems

Björn E. Eriksson and Christer Sylvén

1. Background

Angina pectoris, described as a radiating pain or discomfort central in the chest, is the major symptom of ischemic heart disease. The term "angina pectoris" is derived from anger (compress, strangle) and pectus (breast). Classically, the term is used for an imbalance between myocardial oxygen supply and demand resulting from atheromatous coronary disease. A puzzling fact is a poor correlation between underlying pathophysiology and symptoms. In patients with known coronary stenoses, about 60–80% of the ischemic attacks are symptomless (1,2), so-called "silent ischemia;" on the other hand, a great number of patients suffer from disabling angina pectoris without signs of ischemia.

Heberden (3) introduced the concept of angina pectoris in 1772 and is unsurpassed for the distinction of his description of the symptomatology. However, he had no possibility of differentiating between reversible myocardial ischemia and irreversible, as in myocardial infarction. The symptoms are described by most patients as a discomfort with a sensation of tightness, pressure, or pain starting in the middle of the chest and often radiating to other anatomical structures in the upper part of the body. The nature of the symptoms is dull and complex, showing an interindividual variation with regard of localization, quality, and intensity, like visceral pain

From: *The Nervous System and the Heart*
Ed: G. J. Ter Horst © Humana Press Inc.

from other structures. The complexities of the pathophysiological mechanisms in terms of nociception, neural transmission, and experience is an area given considerable attention.

Visceral pain with its character of diffuse localization, moderate intensity, and several qualities often including autonomic reflexes should be distinguished from the phenomenon of referred pain. Referral of a pain from a visceral organ to a cutaneous area of the body develops when the pain afferents radiate to the same afferent nerves in the spinal cord. Ischemic pain originating in the heart is, classically, described as referred to the left shoulder and arm.

2. Nociceptive Pain

"Pain is an unpleasant sensory and emotional experience associated with actual or potential tissue damage (nociceptive event), or described in terms of such damage." This is the definition of pain adopted by the International Association for the Study of Pain (IASP) *(4).*

There is experimental and clinical evidence that acute and chronic pains are subserved by partially different pain-generating mechanisms. It is obvious that pain associated with ischemia and also inflammation, ulcers, tumor growth, and so forth is often the result of to ongoing "nociceptive events." On the contrary, in pain caused by an altered or damaged nervous processing of pain (neuropathic pain) deafferentation, central, idiopathic, or psychogenic, it is generally not possible to identify noxious stimuli as the cause of pain *(5).*

The presence or absence of ongoing "nociceptive events," ischemia in atheromatous coronary disease, is of crucial importance for the diagnosis and treatment of angina pectoris. According to the distinction between ischemia or not, a strategy has to be tailored for the treatment of these two principally different conditions, ischemia-induced angina pectoris and Syndrome X (i.e., angina pectoris-like pains in the absence of any disease in major coronary arteries).

Nociception in somatic pain is thought to act through specific receptors, nociceptors, resulting in excitation of afferent nerves. The nociceptors are specialized low-threshold receptors in the afferent neural cell membrane sensitive to thermal, mechanical, or chemical stimuli. A moderately intensive but specific stimulus can produce pain.

In angina pectoris, a visceral pain, primary sympathetic afferents are thought to be excited by mechanical or chemical stimuli. However, so far, no specific nociceptor has been found in the heart. Excitation of afferent nerves is, therefore, believed to act by modulation and spatio-temporal summation of unspecific physiological stimuli (6).

Generally, nociception is mediated by myelinated rapid conducting Aδ–fibers giving a rapid and distinct character of pain (like in somatic pain) and C-fibers, which are unmyelinated and slow, resulting in a dull and indistinct pain (like visceral pain).

The pain afferents in somatic pain and partially in cardiac pain project to the dorsal horn of the spinal cord. The filtered or enhanced activity in spinal neurons radiates further in axons crossing over the median toward the midbrain and thalamus through several pathways (Chapter 8). Modulation of the nerve activity is a common phenomenon in these pathways and also in the thalamus. An important split of the flow of impulses is seen in the thalamic level. One part is relayed to the limbic system, where emotional and affective reactions are created (Chapter 2). Another part relayed to cortical structures for discrimination, localization, and evaluation of the quality of the pain perception (7) (Chapter 8). Both of these projections are end stations generating the information that the patient expresses and the clinician has to consider. The afferent nerve activity involved in nociception may also reach the hypothalamus, which generates neuroendocrinological effects and autonomic reflexes (Chapters 2 and 3). Pain is therefore creating a general impact on the attention and well-being of the individual (Chapter 13).

3. Neuropathic Pain

Neuropathic pain is caused by changes in a peripheral nerve, a nervous circuit, or the central handling of afferent stimuli. This pain has mainly been studied in the field of somatic pain. If the origin is peripheral in the nervous system (e.g., an injured nerve), a spontaneous (ectopic) activity in the nerve itself or in a neurinoma could be the stimuli causing the pain. Cell membranes on injured axons can change through an increased expression of sodium channels, which results in an abnormal excitability and sensitivity (8).

An upregulation of α_2-receptors on the cell membrane of the injured nerve could give rise to excitation by transmitted norepinephrine and contribute to sympathetic-maintained pain (reflex sympathetic dystrophy or causalgia). Furthermore, a growth of sympathetic nerve terminals are seen close to the injured nerve, which further contributes to sympathetic-induced excitation of the nerve (9,10).

Central neuropathic pain can be generated by changes in the balance between afferent transmission and inhibitory activity from the midbrain and spinal cord. This may result in an intermittent and low nerve activity that normally does not pass through the gates in the ganglia and dorsal horn, which in such conditions passes without effective modulation.

Nociceptive pain in the intact nervous system is modified by endogenous pain-controlling systems (inhibition), the efficacy of which determines the final pain perception (Chapter 8 and 9). From the sensory cortex and hypothalamic region radiates descending pathways that pass through many synapses in several regions before reaching the dorsal horn of the spinal cord (Chapter 2). In the periaqueductal gray (PAG) region (Chapter 8) are many local neurons and mediators responsible for gating of the descending activity, which finally modulate the inhibition in the dorsal horn and medulla oblongata (7). Normally, descending (inhibitory) pathways are inhibited by a tonic release of the neurotransmitter GABA via GABA$_A$ receptors. This continuous inhibition acts as a brake for at least a part of the descending system. An increased activity in local glutamate-, β-endorphin-, and substance P-containing neurons has the ability to decrease the GABA-ergic tone through stimulation of enkephaline-containing neurons (7). These mechanisms may increase the descending pain inhibitory activity. Morphine and electric stimulation in the dorsal horn enhances descending pain inhibition through counteracting the effect of GABA.

Pain not evoked from the wounded area but from surrounding tissues is called secondary pain. This additive nociceptor activation in the periphery may be evoked by reflex activity elicited during myocardial ischemia, for example. The resulting perception is further modified by individual tolerance and endurance.

4. Anginal Chest Pain

Myocardial ischemia is the major stimulus for anginal chest pain, although this unfavorable oxygen supply does not always result in chest pain. The majority of ischemic attacks and acute myocardial infarction (AMIs) are symptomless. When angina pectoris is present in a person, stable or unstable, the majority of the ischemic attacks will be asymptomatic.

Angina pectoris is a late phenomenon in the ischemic cascade *(12)*. This latency differs distinctly from the rapid appearance of somatic pain. Following the onset of myocardial ischemia, wall-motion abnormalities and electrocardiogram (ECG) changes precede the onset of angina. When experimental ischemia has been induced by coronary occlusion or during percutaneous transluminal coronary angioplasty (PTCA), the systolic and diastolic function of the heart is impaired before ECG changes develop after about 20 s. Angina pectoris develops after 30 s or even later if it occurs at all. During spontaneous attacks, the onset of angina pectoris can be delayed for several minutes. This suggests that a sufficient duration of ischemia and a sufficient severity are necessary for the development of angina pectoris *(13)*. As can be expected for a complex, multicausal process, there is not a known mechanistic link; rather, there is a probabilistic or chaotic association between the severity and duration of myocardial ischemia and pain generation *(14)*. Heberdeen did not differentiate between chest pain caused by AMI and

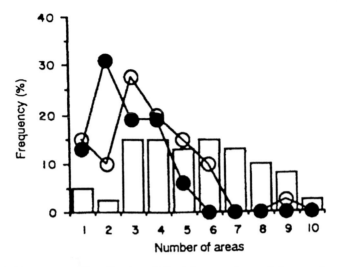

Fig. 1. Frequency distribution (%) of the number of chest-related body surface areas with pain in acute myocardial infarction (AMI), non-AMI, and nonischemic chest pain. □: AMI; ○: non-AMI; ●: nonischemic.

reversible ischemia. Based on the use of the ECG, this differentiation of underlying pathophysiology was not conceptualized until Keefer did so in 1928 *(15)*.

In an attempt to evaluate the diagnostic power of pain presentation in a coronary care unit, we studied the pain localization, extension, character, and intensity in 80 consecutive patients *(16)*. Major and unexpected findings were that the anginal chest pain was moderate in intensity, the mean number of reported qualities were between 3 and 4, and the description was aching, burning, pressing/throbbing, dyspnoea/suffocating, or anxiogenic. Moreover, the extension of chest pain in patients with AMI was wider, but the intensity was similarly moderate. No differences in quality and intensity distributions of the major chest pain have been reported in angina pectoris because of reversible myocardial ischemia or acute myocardial infarction *(17,18)* (Fig. 1).

Patients with angina pectoris, whether it is the result of reversible or irreversible ischemia, report their pain quality as being either aching, burning, pressing/throbbing, dyspnoea/suffocating, and/or feeling anxious. This is typical for

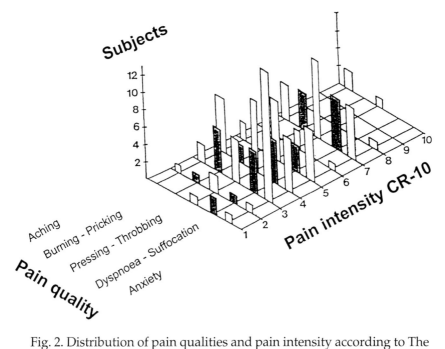

Fig. 2. Distribution of pain qualities and pain intensity according to The Borg CR-10 scale in patients suffering from acute myocardial infarction.

visceral pain and suggests that it is caused by activation of the limbic and hypothalamic systems (see above) (Fig. 2) (Chapters 2, 3, 6, 8, and 9). In terms of location of pain, there is a great overlap between patients with anterior and inferior localizations of their myocardial infarction (Fig. 3) and this is in keeping with studies in patients with isolated coronary stenosis in the right and left coronary arteries. When these were compared, no specific localization of the chest pain was found *(19)*. A patient with isolated right coronary artery stenosis could report pain from the left chest wall and the left arm, and a patient with isolated left coronary artery stenosis could report pain from the right chest wall and the right arm. Thus, when the pain is localized, it is roughly localized to the chest, but within this wide body area further localization appears not to be related to the local myocardial area where the nociceptive event takes place. Hypothetically, the localization central in the chest could be the result of the vis-

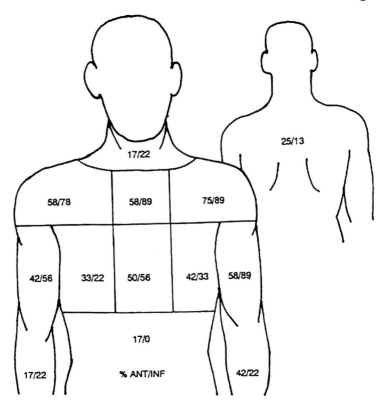

Fig. 3. Frequency (%) of pain in 13 chest-related areas in anterior (ANT) and inferior (INF) acute myocardial infarction.

ceral nociceptive component and the radiating pain could be the result of referred pain. These characteristics of ischemic cardiac pain may be compared to the rapid appearance and distinctness of somatic pain both in terms of localization, high intensities, and specific quality *(20)*.

No specific nerve endings are present to mediate pain in the heart. Rather, mediation of pain has been supposed to be dependent on an alarm reaction in which neural sensitization dramatically increases the intensity of the overall myocardial nerve traffic that otherwise is controlling or integrating myocardial function on a beat-to-beat basis *(21)*. Such reflex activation may be viewed as a visceral autonomic response to a nocious event, in distinction to the somatic pain response of nerves specialized for mediating pain. In comparison to somatic pain, this visceral pain is of a primitive character.

The nonspecific structure and function, the complexity, and a reported individual variation *(21,22)* of the morphology of the cardiac autonomic nervous system may explain the absence of pain or the presence of unspecific symptoms in the majority of patients suffering from myocardial ischemia. Also, when angina pectoris is manifest, its slow onset, its diffuse character, and its moderate pain intensity may depend on its neurological substrate.

5. Cardiac Nervous System

Theoretically, anginal pain is thought to be generated by mechanical or chemical stimuli. No specific nociceptor has been found in the myocardium. Excitation of neurons is generated by two different principal processes *(23)*. One is a rapid and spatially exact response acting via ion-channel-linked receptors. The other is a slow process, several hundreds of milliseconds longer than the channel-linked process, acting via a non-channel-linked receptor causing synaptic modulation. Modulatory processes are spatially diffuse and involve changed metabolism of the neuron mediated by G-proteins and enzymatic reactions. A nociceptive event could cause increased production of neuropeptides such as substance P, calcitonin-gene-related peptide (CGRP), neurokinin A (NKA), and glutamate *(7)* in the affected neuron. These substances will increase the sensitivity for nociceptive events.

Spatial and temporal summation of evoked neural activity is another important process. With increasing intensity of stimulus, the afferent neuronal response becomes enhanced with time to a level that a simple stimulus could not affect. In diseased states, a painful sensation could develop as a result of a high-intensity activation of tonic low-threshold receptors.

During occlusion of a coronary artery, there is also an increased impulse activity from mechanoreceptors *(24)* and it has been hypothesized that dilatation of large vessels and the heart could cause the appearance of pain *(25)*. Davies et al. *(13)* showed that neither the rate nor the magnitude of left ventricular dilation influences the presence or absence of anginal pain. This is consistent with the observation that myocardial biopsies can be taken without any sensation of pain. On the contrary, increased cardiac pain was reported during stretching of coronary arteries at balloon inflation even though the severity of myocardial ischemia decreased *(26)*. However, different stimuli may cause an unspecific increase in neuronal activity and this, according to the intensity hypothesis, together with other stimuli (e.g., chemical), could cause anginal pain. Afferent and efferent sympathetic nerves as studied in the canine heart project to about 260 ganglia (Chapters 1 and 2). These ganglia contain about 20,000 neurons, of which about 80% may be local circuit neurons *(27)*. It has been proposed that a first regulation and gating of the afferent signals takes place in these intrinsic cardiac ganglia *(26)* and that the intrinsic cardiac nervous system acts as a little brain within the heart *(27)*. Apparently, during normal states, the intrinsic cardiac nervous system develops beat-to-beat regulatory functions of cardiac vascular tone, contractility, and electricity. The intrinsic cardiac nervous system utilizes excitatory and inhibitory synapses. Administration of neurochemicals to such intrinsic neurons modify their activity. Such responses could be evoked by substances such as bradykinin, substance P, oxytocin, acetylcholine, nicotine, adenosine, and ATP *(29)*. As a result of such neuronal responses cardiovascular variables such as heart rate, frequency of ectopy and inotropy can be modulated *(30)*.

Interestingly, the oxygen consumption in the cardiac intrinsic neurons is about one-third of that in the myocardium. Proximal coronary arteries supply the intrinsic cardiac neurons and the acute coronary thrombosis or spasm could directly affect the integrity and function and be responsible for the genesis of pain.

Only a minority of the cardiac afferent axons project to cell bodies in the dorsal root ganglia. About 90% of the cell

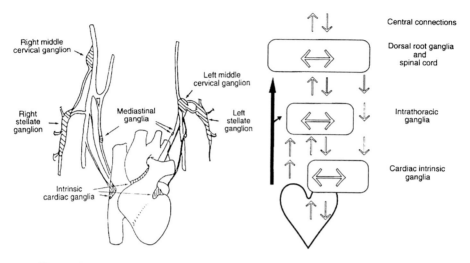

Fig. 4. Anatomical and schematic functional representation of intrathoracic ganglia where neurons regulating the heart are located.

bodies from axons originating from the heart are situated in the intrinsic cardiac nervous system, mediastinal, and other intrathoracic ganglia *(31)*. The majority of nerves in intrathoracic ganglia may be local circuit neurons *(22)*. The extrinsic cardiac nervous system in the intrathoracic ganglia integrates information and generates cardio-cardiac reflexes (Fig. 4). No spatial representation and no left/right localization of afferent and efferent nerves innervating different cardiac regions have been found. The mediastinal ganglia are connected not only to the heart but also to other thoracic organs such as the esophagus, the skin of the cranial abdomen, the thorax, and arms. This could contribute to referral of the cardiac pain and the complexity of anginal pain perception.

Primary Aδ- and C-fibers project with cell bodies in the dorsal root ganglia C6-Th5 of the spinal cord *(32)* (Chapters 8 and 9). However, secondary afferents, with already filtered signals, from intracardiac and intrathoracic ganglia also project into the spinal cord *(33)*. In the spinal cord, the signal crosses over the median and the main ascending nociceptive signal is projected within the spinothalamic and spinoreticular tracts to centers in the brain and brainstem. A small number of fibers are also ascending ipsilaterally (Chapters 8 and 9).

Convergence of visceral afferents with somatic afferents at spinothalamic neurons can be one explanation for the phenomenon of referred pain to a body surface in the same dermatome from which the heart is innervated. At the spinal level, a modulation of the signal from descending inhibitory neurons and somatic input will occur via several interneurons responsible for regulating input and output in the spinal cord (Chapters 8 and 9).

Aδ-Fibers from somatic pain (e.g., localized cutaneous pain sensations) project to the lateral part of the thalamus (neothalamus) for connection to the primary and secondary cortical sensory areas (SI and SII), which are somatotopically organized. Visceral pain such as heart pain is mainly conducted via C-fibers and project to the medial part of the thalamus (paleothalamus) and is not topically organized. Axonal branching takes place to the reticular system and the hypothalamus. The hypothalamus also receives input from the reticular formation in the brainstem, including the PAG. Activation of the hypothalamus and the limbic system via the middle cingulate cortex and the prefrontal cortex is responsible for the aggressive/defensive behavior and emotions and motivational interactions associated with pain experience (Chapter 2).

From positron emission tomography (PET) studies (Chapter 10) during angina pectoris, an increased activity in the thalamus, hypothalamus, and the reticular tissue has been reported as opposed to pains of neuropathic and cancerous origins, where the activity is decreased (34). Cortical activation during angina pectoris is located bilateral in the prefrontal corticis. No activities in the sensory cortex, the Brodman areas 1 and 2, as in somatic pain, could be seen.

The neural activation pattern related to anginal pain clearly explains the complexity and diffuse symptomatology. A slow appearance in relation to the noxious event, its diffuse character and interindividual variations, its activation of autonomic reflexes, and the emotional correlate as a part of the pain experience are the most important features of anginal chest pain. The organization of the nervous system of the heart is one probable basis for the complex characteristics of anginal chest pain.

6. Myocardial Ischemia

A major underlying cause of the anginal chest pain is myocardial ischemia, described as an imbalance between myocardial oxygen supply and demand, generally caused by insufficient blood perfusion as a manifestation of atheromatous coronary artery disease. A shortage of oxygen results in anaerobic metabolism and the low blood flow results in accumulation of metabolites. An "ischemic cascade" (presented earlier) starts and could generate anginal pain late during the ischemic event.

In 1932, Lewis postulated that a pain messenger must be present between the ischemic cardiomyocyte and the central nervous system to evoke a pain response (35). The Lewis criteria for a pain messenger substance are substantial release during ischemia, excitation of cardiac nerves, and provocation of pain. There have been many putative candidate substances for being the pain messenger in the heart. Lactate, potassium, serotonin, bradykinin, adenosine triphosphate, and adenosine have been implicated. Of candidate substances, so far only adenosine fulfills the Lewis criteria.

Malliani concluded in 1986 that there is no evidence of any specific high-threshold-pain receptor in the myocardium. Neither the specificity nor the intensity hypothesis could explain the appearance of angina pectoris. He suggested that activation has to occur according to a specific code based on a specific spatio-temporal activation sequence where a discrete limited amount of the myocardium is activated (36).

7. Lactate

The blood lactate concentration is an index of anaerobic metabolism. Increased lactate levels in muscle and blood indicates an anaerobic supplement to the aerobic production of ATP. Some glycolysis seems to be lactate producing also in muscles, which are active in fully aerobic conditions (37). Even at rest, the blood lactate concentration is about 1 mM. The elimination of lactate from the blood has a half-life of 15 min. During aerobic circumstances hydrolysis of one ATP molecule produces about one proton at the muscle cell pH. However, during the oxidative phosphorylation, all the products of ATP hydrolysis are reutilized. This means no net accumulation of H^+ in aerobic metabolism. In anaerobic glycolysis, hydrogen ions are only partially reutilized when glycogen is converted to lactate. In humans, there could be a drop in muscle ATP concentrations to about half of the initial concentration. This drop represents a potential increase in the proton concentration of about 25 times (38). This could be of importance for the genesis of ischemic pain.

A decreased pH could activate polymodal nerves at a pH of 4.6 or less (39) and, therefore, could be a pain-producing substance. Experimentally, during forearm and leg ischemia, the time course of pain is not equal to the time course for the lactate increase. The appearance and disappearance of pain occur more rapidly than changes in lactate concentration (14). Myocardial ischemia develops when the rate of myocardial oxygen consumption (MVO_2) exceeds the coronary capacity to deliver oxygen. Induced myocardial ischemia leads to anaerobic glycolysis in the tissue, resulting in a release of lactate, contrary to the normally perfused heart, which extracts lactate.

Patients with McArdle's syndrome, a deficiency of phosphofructokinase, are reported to have exertional muscular pains in spite of low lactate levels (40). Patients with claudication have, at symptom, limited exercise in the quadriceps femoris muscle of the diseased leg lactate levels that are not higher but similar to the lactate levels in healthy controls (41). Therefore, lactate and proton concentrations do not seem to play a major role as a pain messenger in the ischemic heart.

8. Bradykinin

The kinins are small polypeptides that are split away from α_2-globulins in the plasma or tissue fluids. The kinins

are potent vasodilator substances. Different types of pro-
teolytic enzymes can split the kinins from the globulin, the
most important is kallikrein. As kallikrein becomes activated,
it creates bradykininogen that is converted by tissue enzymes
to bradykinin. Bradykininogen is formed during the inflammatory process in the vasculature (Chapter 12). The half-life
of bradykinin in plasma is about a few minutes and is then
digested by the enzyme carboxypeptidase or by angiotensin-
converting enzyme (Chapter 11). Bradykinin has the powerful effects of arteriolar dilatation and also increased capillary
permeability. Experimentally, an injection of 1 µg of bradykinin into the brachial artery increases the blood flow six-
fold *(42)*. Even smaller amounts injected locally into the
tissues can cause marked edema because of an increase in
capillary pore size.

   Bradykinin is one of the most powerful excitatory substances on afferent nerves known. However, during PTCA
occlusion of a coronary artery with signs of myocardial
ischemia, no bradykinin was released into the coronary sinus
(43). Intracoronarily injected bradykinin did not cause typical angina pectoris-like pain, but the patient experienced an
unspecific discomfort or pain located over the whole body
(44). The pain is counteracted by cyclooxygenase inhibitors
(Crea, personal communication).

9. Potassium

   An increase in potassium ion (K^+) concentration causes
vasodilatation. This results from the ability of potassium ions
to inhibit smooth-muscle contraction. Potassium is essential
for the membrane potential regulated by the sodium–potassium ion pump in the cellular membrane.

   Potassium in high intravenous concentrations acts as a
local irritant with a capacity to depolarize nerves. During
normal conditions, the ratio intracellular to extracellular concentrations is 4 : 150 mmol. In experimental preparations,
10–30 mmol concentrations are needed for unspecific depolarization of nerves *(45)*.

During myocardial ischemia in man, the coronary sinus potassium concentration increased only about 0.4 mmol *(46)*. One major concern is that anions also have to be transferred over the cellular membrane, which could be one explanation for the comparatively low extracellular potassium concentrations obtained during coronary occlusion.

Furthermore, magnesium has the ability to counteract the algogenic actions of potassium, a potentially antialgogenic mechanism that could be active during ischemic release of magnesium.

10. Substance P

Substance P is found in the basal ganglia, hypothalamus, and primary pain fibers radiating to the dorsal horn of the spinal cord. It is generally believed to cause excitation. During an inflammation (e.g., in the vasculature), substance P is released from the nerve endings. Substance P (and CGRP) increase the blood flow and the endothelial permeability and activate inflammatory and immune cells (Chapter 12).

During a nociceptive event, an increased synthesis in ganglion cells of neuropeptides such as substance P and CGRP is induced. They are then transported to and accumulated in the peripheral nerve endings and can become released when the nerve is excited. The transport increases also to the central parts of the primary afferent nerve in the spinal cord where substance P participates in pain transmission *(7)*.

Substance P infusion into the coronary artery or into the femoral artery does not in itself provoke pain from the corresponding vascular bed. Substance P added to adenosine enhances the adenosine-provoked pain, suggesting a further enhancement of adenosine-provoked neural sensitization emphasizing the polymodal character of cardiac afferent nerve stimulation *(43)*.

11. Serotonin

Serotonin (5-hydroxitryptamine [5-HT]) is present in large concentrations in the gastrointestinal tract and also in

inverse relationship between the dose needed for the provocation of pain and the amount of tissue exposed to adenosine was found. More adenosine is needed for the provocation of pain in the lower arm than in the leg. When administration of adenosine was done in the distal two-thirds of the left anterior descending coronary artery *(66)*, less pain was reported than when adenosine was given at the ostium of the left coronary artery *(64)*. This is an indication of adenosine acting as an enhancer of spatial and temporal summation of autonomic afferent nerve traffic resulting in pain. These observations are in line with reports that there is a dose-response relationship between the dose of adenosine given and sympathetic nerve traffic in humans *(67)*.

In animal studies, epicardial application of adenosine in physiological concentrations excites cardiac neurons in dorsal root ganglia *(68)*. No-dose ganglion activity was noted in a canine model, either excited or inhibited *(69)*. Therefore, it is obvious that adenosine, as the only substance currently known, fulfills the Lewis criteria with substantial release during myocardial ischemia, ability of excitation of cardiac nerves, and provocation of anginal chest pain. Theophylline reduces the ischemic pain following lower arm ischemic work *(14)*. This indicates the pain-provoking properties of endogenous release of adenosine (Fig. 6).

12.3. Analgesic Effects of Adenosine

Adenosine has been shown to have neuromodulatory effects. The effect of adenosine, depending on activation of the receptors and their differing effects on different targets, can be either activation or inhibition of heart rate, blood pressure, vascular tone, and neural activity *(69)* (Fig. 7). Adenosine has prominent pain-provoking properties, as demonstrated earlier, but in addition to its algesic effects, adenosine has also been reported to have analgesic effects.

A number of groups have shown antinociceptive effects by endogenously administered adenosine, suggesting a central mechanism of action *(55)*. Enogenous adenosine administered into the vascular bed has, because of the short half-life

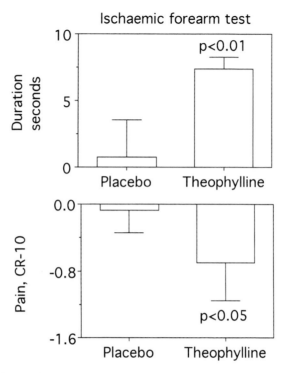

Fig. 6. Effects of theophylline on the duration and intensity of pain in the ischemic forearm test in healthy volunteers.

of adenosine, no ability to pass the blood-brain barrier. There are, however, different opinions regarding the site of action and adenosine receptor activation. Adenosine may act via A1 and A2 receptors, both of which have been shown to exist in the dorsal horn of the spinal cord *(6)*. Modulatory effects of adenosine can involve presynaptic decrease of Ca^{2+} currents or A1-receptor-mediated inhibition of currents in the dorsal horn *(70)*. Adenosine has also been demonstrated to induce hyperpolarization on striatal neurons, as a result of an increased potassium conductance *(71)*. This could be a mechanism in the spinal cord too. Antinociceptive effects of adenosine have been noted after intrathecal, intra-arterial, and intravenous administration of adenosine *(72,73)*.

Experimental studies in man have shown analgesic effects of adenosine on forearm ischemia, on heat pain

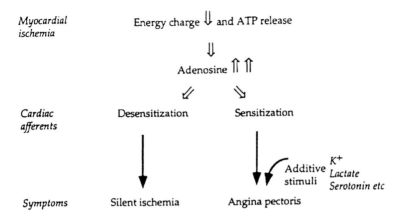

Fig. 7. Current view on the peripheral algenic/analgenic neuro-modulator effects of adenosine in myocardial ischemia.

threshold, and on mustard-oil-provoked allodynia *(72)*. During ischemia, these adenosine effects are similar in magnitude to those of morphine, which emphasizes the tentative importance of adenosine for the manifestation of silent or painful myocardial ischemia.

Administration of adenosine, at approximately 100 μg/kg/min may exert an antinociceptive effect in patients during anesthesia and surgery, expressed as a lower need for end-tidal isoflunane (ET-ISO) than expected *(74)*.

The analgesic potential of adenosine during myocardial ischemia was studied in patients with coronary artery disease and exercise-limiting angina pectoris *(75)*. Patients were given a low dose of adenosine or placebo in a double-blind, crossover fashion by continuous iv infusion before and during two exercise tests. Adenosine decreased the experience of chest pain, whereas hemodynamic and electrocardiographic signs of myocardial ischemia did not change (Fig. 8). Recently, adenosine in a continuous intravenous administration has been shown to have analgesic effects during the ischemic forearm test and the adenosine receptor theophylline counteracted this effect *(73)*.

The antinociceptive effect of adenosine has been suggested to be operative mainly in dorsal horn neurons at the spinal

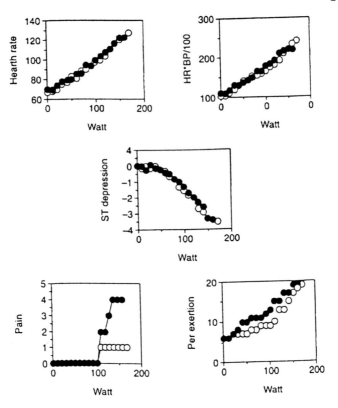

Fig. 8. Representative results from exercise stress test from one patient. The figure shows change in heart rate (beats per minute, upper left), change in double product (beats per minute × mm Hg/100, upper right), ST-depression (mV, middle), chest pain quantited with the Borg CR-10 scale (lower left), and perceived general exertion quantited with Borg RPE scale, 6-20 (lower right). Adenosine (○) was infused at a rate of 35 μg/kg/min. The study was performed in a double-blind, crossover fashion with placebo (●).

level, where adenosine may inhibit small-diameter sensory fibers by both presynaptic and postsynaptic mechanisms. However, in a formalin test in mice, peripheral coadministration of formalin and receptor-phenylisopropyladenosine (R-PIA) (a high-affinity A1 adenosine receptor agonist) resulted in more pronounced antinociceptive effects than when formalin and R-PIA were administered simultaneously but at different cutaneous sites. These observations

Circulation (Zucker, I. H. and Gilmore, J. P., eds.), CRC, Boca Raton, FL, pp. 1–37.

23. Alberts, B., Bray, D., Lewis, J., Raff, M., Roberts, K., and Watson, J. D. (1989) *Molecular Biology of the Cell.* Garland, New York.

24. Thorén, P. (1979) Role of cardiac vagal C-fibers in cardiovascular control. *Rev. Physiol. Biochem. Pharmacol.* **86**, 1–94.

25. MacAlpin, R. N. (1980) Coronary arterial spasm. *J. Hist. Med.* **35**, 288–311.

26. Sylvén, C. and Crea, F. (1994) Mechanism of the anginal pain: the key role of adenosine, in *From Molecular Biology to Integrative Physiology, Adenosine and Adenosine Nucleotides* (Belardinelli, L. and Pelleg, A., eds.), Kluwer, Boston, pp. 315–325.

27. Huang, M. H., Sylvén, C., Horackova, M., and Armour, J. A. (1995) Ventricular sensory neurons in canine dorsal root ganglia: effects of adenosine and substance. *Am. J. Physiol.* **269**, R318–R324.

28. Armour, J. A., Yuan, B. X., and Butler, C. K. (1990) Cardiac responses elicited by peptides administered to canine intrinsic cardiac neurons. *Peptides* **11**, 753–761.

29. Huang, M. H., Sylvén, C., Smith, F. M., Pelleg, A., and Armour, J. A. (1995) Cardiac sensory neurons tonically activated by endogenous adenosine and substance. *Am. J. Physiol.* **269**, R318–R329.

30. Murphy, D. A. and Armour, J. A. (1992) Human cardiac nerve stimulation. *Ann. Thorac. Surg.* **54**, 502–506.

31. Hopkins, D. A. and Armour J. A. (1989) Ganglionic distribution of afferent neurons innervating the canine heart and cardiopulmonary nerves. *J. Auton. Nerv. Syst.* **26**, 213–222.

32. Hillarp, N. Å. (1970) Peripheral autonomic mechanisms, in *Handbook of Physiology, Sect. 1, Neurophysiology* (Field, J., ed.), American Physiological Society, Washington, DC, pp. 979–1006.

33. Quigg, M. (1991) Distribution of vagal afferent fibers of the Guinea Pig heart labeled by anterograde transport of conjugated horseradish peroxidase. *J. Auton. Nerv. Syst.* **36**, 13–24.

34. Rosen, S. D., Paulesu, E., Frith, C. D., Frackoviak, R. S. J., Davies, G. J., Jones, T., et al. (1994) Central nervous pathways mediating angina pectoris. *Lancet* **344**, 147–150.

35. Lewis, T. (1932) Pain in muscular ischemia—its relation to anginal pain. *Arch. Intern. Med.* **49**, 713–727.

36. Malliani, A. (1986) The elusive link between transient myocardial ischemia and pain. *Circulation* **73**, 201–204.

37. Connett, R. J., Gayeski, T. E. J., and Honig, C. R. (1984) Lactate accumulation in fully aerobic working dog gracilis muscle. *Am. J. Physiol.* **246**, H120.

38. Hochacka, P. N. and Mommsen, T. P. (1983) Protons and anaerobiosis. *Science* **219**, 1391.

39. Ushida, Y. and Murao, S. (1975) Acid induced excitation of afferent cardiac sympathetic nerve fibers. *Am. J. Physiol.* **228**, 33–37.

40. Sahlin, K., Areskog, N. H., Hallen, R. C., Henriksson, K. G., Infeldt, C., and Lewis, S. F. (1990) Impaired oxidative metabolism increases adenine nucleotide breakdown in McArdle's disease. *J. Appl. Physiol.* **69,** 1231–1235.
41. Pernow, B., Sahlin, B., Waahrren, J., Cronestrand, R., and Ekeström, S. (1975) Leg blood flow and muscle metabolism in occlusive arterial disease of the leg before and after reconstructive surgery. *Clin. Sci. Mol. Med.* **49,** 265–275.
42. Guyton, A. C. (1986) *Textbook of Medical Physiology,* W. B. Saunders, Philadelphia, p. 242.
43. Eldar, M., Schulhoff, N., Ohlstein, E., Hollander, G., Greengart, A., and Lichstein, E. (1992) The pain of myocardial ischemia: is it mediated by Bradykinin? *Eur. Heart J.* **13(Suppl.),** 363 (abstract).
44. Rafflebeul, W., Bassenge, E., and Lichtlen, P. (1989) Competition between endothelium-dependent and nitroglycerin induced coronary vasodilatation. *Z. Kardiol.* **78(Suppl. 3),** 45–47.
45. Keele, C. A. and Armstrong, D. (1964) Substances producing pain and itch, in *Monographs of the Physiological Society, No. 12* (Barcroft, H., Dawson, H., and Paton, W. D. M., eds.), Arnold, London, pp. 89–106.
46. Webb, S. C. and Poole-Wilson, P. A. (1986) Potassium exchange in the human heart during atrial pacing and myocardial ischemia. *Br. Heart J.* **55,** 554–559.
47. Fossel, E. T., Morgan, H. E., and Ingvall J. S. (1980) Measurement of changes in high energy phosphates in the cardiac cycle by using gated 31-P nuclear magnetic resonance. *Proc. Natl. Acad. Sci. USA* **77,** 3654–3658.
48. Arch, J. R. S. and Newsholme, E. A. (1978) The control of the metabolism and the hormonal role of adenosine assays, in *Biochemistry* (Campell, P. and Aldridge, W., eds.), Academic, London, pp. 88–123.
49. Biaggioni, I., Onrot, J., Hollister, A. S., and Robertsson, D. (1986) Cardiovascular effects of adenosine infusion in man and their modulation by dipyridamole. *Life Sci.* **39,** 2229–2236.
50. Sollevi, A. (1986) Cardiovascular effects in man; possible implications. *Prog. Neurobiol.* **27,** 319–349.
51. Edlund, A., Fredholm, B. B., Patriani, P., Patrono, C., Wennmalm, Å., and Wennmalm, M. (1983) Release of two vasodilators—adenosine and prostacycline—from isolated rabbit hearts during controlled hypoxemia. *J. Physiol.* **340,** 487–501.
52. Bardenheuer, H., Hofling, B., Fabry, A., and Peter, K. (1987) Increased adenosine production by the heart during acute coronary occlusion in man. *Anesthesiology* **67,** A31.
53. Pelleg, A. and Porter, R. S. (1990) The pharmacology of adenosine. *Pharmacotherapy* **10(3),** 157–174.

84. Kemp, H., Vokonas, P., Cohn, P., and Gorlin, R. (1973) The anginal syndrome associated with normal coronary angiograms: report of a six year experience. *Am. J. Med.* **54,** 735–742.
85. Opherk, D., Schuler, G., Wettaur, K., Manthey, J., Schwarz, F., and Kubler, W. (1989) Four year follow up in patients with angina pectoris and normal coronary angiograms (Syndrome X). *Circulation* **80,** 1610–1616.
86. Rosen, S. D., Uren, N. G., Kaski, J. C., Tousoulis, D., Davies, G. J., and Camici, P. G. (1994) Coronary vasodilator reserve, pain perception and sex in patients with Syndrome X. *Circulation* **90,** 50–60.
87. Cannon, R. O., Quyyumi, A., Schenke, W. H., Fananazapir, L., Tucker, E. E., Gaughan, A. Q. M., et al. Epstein, S. E. (1990) Abnormal cardiac sensitivity in patients with chest pain and normal coronary arteries. *J. Am. Coll. Cardiol.* **16,** 1359–1366.
88. Eriksson, B., Svedenhag, J., Martinsson, A., and Sylvén, C. (1995) Effect of epinephrine infusion on chest pain in Syndrome X in the absence of signs of myocardial ischemia. *Am. J. Cardiol.* **75,** 241–245.
89. Rosen, S. D., Paulesu, E., Frackowiak, R. S. J., and Camici, P. G. (1995) Regional brain activation compared in angina pectoris and Syndrome X. *Circulation* **92(Suppl. I),** 651.

CHAPTER 8

The Neuroanatomy
of Cardiac Nociceptive Pathways
Differential Representations

of "Deep" and "Superficial" Pain

Kevin A. Keay, Colin I. Clement,
and Richard Bandler

1. Definitions of Pain and Its Central Representation

Cardiac pain is usually associated with behavioral and physiological changes that often include behavioral quiescence, hyporeactivity, bradycardia, hypotension, nausea, and sometimes vomiting. Pain of cardiac origin is also commonly associated with patterns of referral to deep structures of the head, neck, and chest *(1–6)*. The clinical symptoms of angina are typical to those of other pains of visceral origin insofar as they include quiescence, nausea, vomiting, "deep" referred pain, and sometimes even "a feeling of impending death" *(7)*. This pattern of response was described elegantly more than 50 years ago by Sir Thomas Lewis *(8)*, who called attention to the remarkable similarity of the behavioral and physiological responses to pain arising from the viscera and those associated with pain arising from deep somatic structures (muscles, joints, periosteum). In a series of experiments conducted by Lewis and Kellgren *(9)*, it was shown that after injection of hypertonic saline into the interspinous ligaments at C6 to T1, the subjects (many of them angina sufferers)

From: *The Nervous System and the Heart*
Ed: G. J. Ter Horst © Humana Press Inc.

experienced pain that was remarkably similar to previously experienced cardiac pain. The perceptual experience and reactions evoked by visceral and deep somatic pain were so distinct from those evoked by pain of cutaneous origin that Lewis further suggested that there must be a *fundamental separation of the central neural circuits* involved in processing deep versus cutaneous pain.

> The difference in the qualities of skin pain and of deep pain is so clear and each belongs so exclusively to the corresponding structures that it would perhaps seem unsafe to class both together under the one unqualified term pain. It has been the usage; but these two sensations have not been shown to possess the common properties which the use of a single term would imply. If we are right in believing that the system of fibres subserving cutaneous pain passes to an appropriate and exclusive part of the sensorium which determines this particular sensation, we are brought to consider whether or not fibres subserving pain derived more deeply connect to a distinct part of the sensorium. Although both follow the path of the anterolateral tract, as has been shown by the abolition in both cases in which this tract has been divided surgically, we should bear in mind the possible serious fallacy of regarding both types as represented in a common centre.

A survey of the basic pain research literature, however, leads one to the conclusion that Lewis' suggestion of different central mechanisms mediating deep versus cutaneous pain has been ignored for the most part. Disappointingly, his detailed and extensive observations appear to have contributed little to shaping the questions addressed by research into the central representation of pain. Likely explanations for this lie in a combination of technical limitations and specific biases.

For the main part, studies of the central representation of pain have relied largely on single-unit electrophysiological techniques within the spinal cord and, to a lesser extent, the thalamus. The very nature of this technique and its attendant methodologies have largely restricted our view to the representation of *acute, cutaneous noxious stimuli*. Such stimuli are easily quantifiable and reproducible and can be used repeatedly in a single experiment. Investigations using noxious deep somatic or noxious visceral stimuli are more difficult, as the stimuli have less reproducibility and are often limited by the number of times a stimulus can be presented. Thus, studies of deep somatic or visceral pain using these techniques are relatively few (although *see* refs. *10–15*).

A second bias is a focus on the phenomenon of the central convergence of deep and cutaneous nociceptive inputs, which has its origins in the clinical observations of "referred pain." Many studies utilizing noxious deep somatic or noxious visceral stimuli use them primarily to identify spinal neurons with convergent (cutaneous and deep) inputs. Thus, although there exist numerous maps of the distribution and extent of spinal neurons with noxious cutaneous receptive fields, there are many fewer comparable maps available for noxious visceral responses alone. Our knowledge of noxious visceral representations in the spinal cord is probably quite conservative, as the information has been deduced largely from studies of deep and cutaneous convergence. To our knowledge, no systematic attempt has been made to evaluate Lewis' proposition of distinct central substrates for pain of deep versus cutaneous origin.

1.1. A Definition of Pain

Contemporary definitions of pain, as, for example, the one agreed upon by the International Association for the Study of Pain (IASP) *(16)*,

> Pain is an unpleasant sensory and emotional experience associated with actual or potential tissue damage, or described in terms of such damage.

stress the fact that pain has, in addition to its obvious sensory component, significant *emotional, affective,* and *motivational* dimensions. It has been suggested that such dimensions are a primary purpose of pain. For example, Wall *(17)* has written that

Pain is better classified as an awareness of a need state than
as a sensation. It serves more to promote healing than to avoid
injury. It has more in common with the phenomena of hunger and thirst than it has with seeing or hearing.

It follows that an understanding of the central neural
circuits that mediate pain-related emotional, affective, or
motivational state changes offers a method to define the central nervous system (CNS) regions critical for the different
pain states defined by Lewis (8). Given the distinct and different behavioral and physiological changes that accompany
deep versus superficial pain, this framework may help to
define regions involved in processing pain of cardiac origin.

2. Representation of Cardiac Pain in the Spinal Cord

2.1. Anatomical Studies

Primary afferent fibers from the abdominal and thoracic
viscera are often called sympathetic afferents. The term arises
from their trajectory in association with the sympathetic
efferent innervation of the viscera. However, primary afferent fibers innervating pelvic viscera follow a trajectory associated with the parasympathetic efferent innervation of this
region. To avoid confusion, perhaps a better term for primary afferents innervating pelvic, abdominal, and thoracic
viscera is *visceral afferents* (*see* refs. *18* and *19*).

In general, visceral afferents of the thoracic, abdominal,
and pelvic viscera terminate in laminae I, V, and X of the
dorsal horn refs. *20–49* (*see* Fig. 1). In the case of the heart,
visceral afferents travel in the inferior cardiac nerve, the
middle cardiac nerve, and then as discrete fibers traversing
the upper and middle thoracic sympathetic ganglia. Cardiac
(visceral) afferents project into the lower cervical and upper
thoracic spinal cord segments where, similar to other primary
afferents, they may ascend or descend one to three spinal
cord segments before synapsing. For example, anatomical
tracing studies using anterograde transport of horseradish-
peroxidase in cat have shown that the inferior cardiac nerve
terminates most densely in segments T2–T6, specifically in

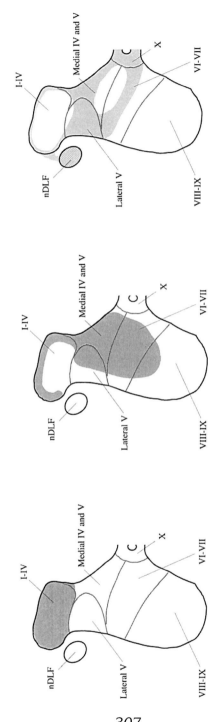

Fig. 1. Schematic coronal cross sections of spinal cord, comparing the laminar distributions of cutaneous, deep somatic (muscle), and visceral primary afferent fibers. I–IV: Laminae I to IV of the dorsal horn; medial IV and V: medial part of laminas IV and V; lateral V: lateral part of lamina V; VI–VII: laminae VI and VII of the intermediate horn; VIII–IX: laminae VIII and IX of the ventral horn; LSN: lateral spinal nucleus X: lamina X; nDLF: nucleus of the

307

laminae I, V, and X and in the dorsal portion of lamina VII. No labeling was detected in laminae II–IV *(20,50)*. A seemingly identical laminar pattern of visceral afferent terminations is also seen following injection of anterograde tracer into the pelvic nerves *(21–23,51)*, kidney *(24,25)*, the greater splanchnic nerve *(26–28,52)*, the hypogastric nerve *(29,30)*, and the lumbar colonic nerves *(53)*. Thus, visceral afferent fibers, irrespective of segmental levels of termination, share strikingly similar laminar distributions.

Similarities exist also in the patterns of laminar termination of afferents arising from deep somatic structures (i.e., muscles and joints). These afferents have selective patterns of termination in laminae I/IIo, IV and V, with additional terminations in laminae VI, VII, and VIII, and, to a lesser extent, lamina X (*see* Fig. 1 and refs. *26,31–37,54*). Thus, visceral and deep somatic afferents terminate, in common, in laminae I and V, but visceral afferents alone terminate profusely in lamina X. This pattern of termination of afferents arising from deep structures contrasts greatly with patterns of termination of cutaneous afferents, which selectively target laminae I, II, and III *(38–40)*. Furthermore, cutaneous afferents usually terminate in a spatially restricted manner within these laminae, in contrast to the generally more widespread distribution within laminae of visceral and deep somatic afferents *(15)*. It is evident, then, that afferents arising from deep somatic and visceral structures have similar laminar distributions and patterns of termination, which, furthermore, are distinct from those shown by cutaneous afferent fibers. However, the question remains as to precisely how these termination patterns relate to "nociceptive" afferents?

2.2. Functional Studies

Experimental manipulations for noxious stimulation of the heart have utilized, for the most part, epicardial, intracardiac, or intravenous administration of algesic compounds (e.g., bradykinin, 5-hydroxytryptamine [5-HT]). These techniques have been reviewed extensively; (see, for example, ref. *50*). Single-unit recording studies have shown that such noxious stimulation of the heart activates neurons in laminae I and V of the thoracic and lower cervical spinal cord, consistent with the findings of the anatomical experiments described above. Furthermore, neurons within these laminae often receive convergent inputs from other superficial and deep somatic structures *(1–4,55)*.

The immunohistochemical detection of the protein product of the *c-fos* immediate-early gene *(Fos)* can also be used as a marker for defining neuronal activation in the CNS, following a peripheral stimulus *(56–60)*. The use of immediate-early gene expression has the advantage of identifying, with single-cell resolution, populations of neurons that respond to specific manipulations. The identification of such extensive populations is not possible with single-unit electrophysiological recording techniques.

During the past decade, this technique has been used widely to identify populations of neurons involved in processing different classes of pain. Such data have made it possible to begin to define pathways which are activated specifically by models of "cardiac pain." More fundamentally, these data suggest that cardiac pain shares common neuronal substrates with other deep painful stimuli, all of which produce similar emotional state changes.

Intravenous i.v. injections of the algesic substance 5-HT (1) depolarizes C-fibers in the cervical vagus *(61)*; (2) depolarizes primary afferent neurons in the nodose ganglion *(62,64)* and (3) evokes angina-like sensations of chest tightening and nausea in man *(64)*. Studies in our laboratory (in the freely moving and halothane-anesthetized rat) using iv injection of 5-HT and the *c-fos* methodology have shown that significant Fos expression is evoked in neurons in laminae I, IIo, IV, V, and X, the ventral horn, and the nucleus of the dorsolateral fasciculus (DLF) within spinal segments T1–L2 (*see* Fig. 2) *(65)*.

A comparison of the segmental and laminar correspondence of iv 5-HT evoked Fos expression, with the patterns of termination of the cardiac afferent fibers defined using anatomical tracing techniques, reveals a remarkable agreement. Compare the visceral schematic in Fig. 1, with the iv 5-HT-evoked

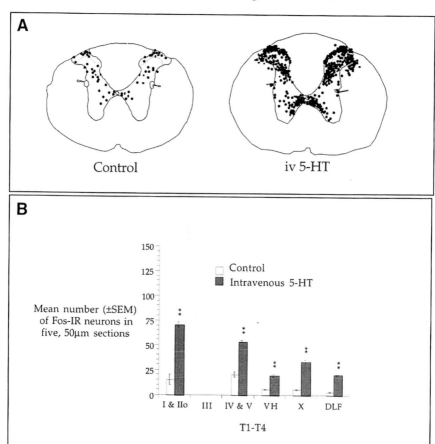

Fig. 2. Panel **A** shows camera-lucida reconstructions of coronal sections through the upper thoracic spinal cord of the rat. The section on the left shows the location of neurons expressing the immediate-early gene *c-fos* in the control condition (anaesthesia only); the section on the right shows *c-fos* expression (i.e., neuronal activation) evoked by cardiac pain induced by intravenous injections of 5-hydroxytryptamine. Panel **B** shows a histogram illustrating data from Clement et al. *(65)* showing the laminar distribution of *c-fos* expression following iv, 5-HT. It shows clearly that this model of cardiac pain evokes increased neuronal activity in laminae I/II, IV, and V, the ventral horn (VH), lamina X, and the dorsolateral fasciculus (DLF).

Fos expression in Fig. 2A (right panel). The Fos findings also fit well with the spinal cord segments and laminae from which neurons responsive to noxious stimulation of the heart have been recorded using single-unit electrophysiological techniques in rat and primate *(1,2,4,6,41)*.

The patterns of Fos expression following noxious stimulation of deep somatic structures show a similar laminar distribution to that evoked by iv 5-HT, although at different segmental levels. For example, as illustrated in Fig. 3, injections of algesic substances into hindlimb muscles (triceps surae) or the knee joint evoked increased Fos expression restricted to neurons in laminae I, IIo, IV, and V, ventral horn, and the nucleus of the DLF (*see also* ref. *66–68*) (Fig. 3). These observations fit well with Lewis' suggestion of common spinal representations of pain of visceral and deep somatic origin. In further support of the idea of "deep pain" neurons in the spinal cord is the common observation that visceral pain is most often referred to deep somatic structures and that neurons that respond to noxious visceral stimuli respond also to noxious stimulation of deep somatic structures *(1–6)*.

In contrast to the above (*see* Fig. 4), cutaneous noxious stimulation (20-s immersion of hindpaw in 53°C water) elevates Fos expression mainly in neurons in laminae I, II, and III *(69)*. This further highlights the clear laminar differences in the spinal representation of cutaneous pain versus deep pain. Noxious manipulations that affect both superficial and deep tissues, as, for example, the "formalin test," in which a subcutaneous formalin injection is made into the plantar surface of the hindpaw, evoke Fos expression in laminae of the superficial and deep dorsal horn and the ventral horn (*see* Fig. 4). The pattern reflects a combination of the patterns seen as a result of noxious deep somatic and noxious cutaneous stimuli *(48,56,59,66,68–70)*.

3. Cardiac Pain and the Upper Cervical Spinal Cord

A somewhat unexpected finding following iv 5-HT was a significant increase in Fos-expressing neurons within the upper cervical spinal cord (UCC:C1–2); specifically in laminae I, IV, V, and X and the nucleus of the DLF (*see* Fig. 5). In fact, the actual numbers of UCC Fos-positive neurons

L4 Spinal Segments

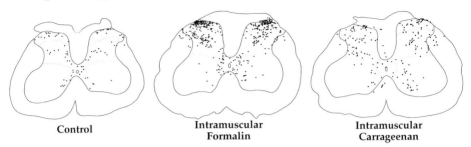

Control   Intramuscular Formalin   Intramuscular Carrageenan

Fig. 3. Camera-lucida drawings of coronal spinal cord segments at the L4 level in the rat, showing the expression of the immediate early gene *c-fos* (a marker of neuronal activation) following either (1) anesthesia alone (left), (2) bilateral injection (0.05 mL) of formalin (5%) into the triceps surae muscle (middle), (3) bilateral injection (0.05 mL) of carrageenan (type IV, 2%) into the triceps surae muscle (right). Note the labeling in both the superficial and deep dorsal horns (laminae I/IIo, IV, and V) as well as label in the ventral horn and in the dorsolateral fasciculus (DLF).

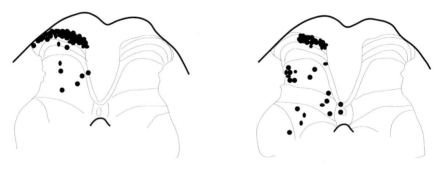

Cutaneous Thermal Stimulus   Subcutaneous Formalin

Fig. 4. Schematic showing the location of spinal cord neurons expressing Fos protein immunoreactivity 2 h after either (left) a cutaneous thermal stimulus (20-s immersion of hindpaw in 53°C water) to the hindpaw, or (right) a subcutaneous injection of formalin into the hindpaw. Note that a "pure" cutaneous stimulus such as noxious heat applied to the skin evokes increased neuronal activity primarily in laminae I and IIo, whereas a mixed noxious cutaneous and noxious deep somatic stimulus as occurs with subcutaneous formalin evokes Fos expression in laminae I–V and in the ventral horn. (Modified from ref. **69**.)

exceeded the numbers at the segmental level. Clement and colleagues have described also a similar UCC pattern of activation following ip injection of acetic acid and injection of algesic substances into muscle (triceps surae) *(65)*.

Clearly then, UCC neurons receive visceral and deep somatic nociceptive signals that ascend from lower spinal segments. Significant activation of UCC neurons also has been reported following noxious stimulation of trigeminally innervated structures; for example, deep neck muscles (personal observations), the superior sagittal sinus *(71)*, dura, tongue, temporomandibular joint, and cornea *(72–74)*.

It is important to note the significant overlap in the patterns of UCC activation following noxious stimulation of trigeminally innervated regions and following noxious visceral or noxious deep somatic stimulation. These stimuli all evoke activation of UCC neurons in laminae I/IIo, IV, and V and the nucleus of the dorsolateral fasciculus. The partial overlap within the UCC of noxious trigeminal and noxious cardiac representations likely underlies the incidence of ischemic pain of cardiac origin being referred to the head and neck region (i.e., clinical presentation of cardiac ischemia such as toothache, jaw ache, or ear ache *(1–6,75)*. As there are no direct primary cardiac afferent projections to the C1–2 segments, an indirect pathway is required. Most likely this is the result of ascending propriospinal connections, although supraspinal projections that then descend to the UCC may also contribute *(76–78)*.

4. Cardiac Pain, the Vagus, and the Nucleus of the Solitary Tract

In addition to cardiac afferents to the spinal cord, there is clinical evidence that the vagus may play also a role in relaying noxious information of cardiac origin specifically from the inferior–posterior surface of the heart *(50)*. Visceral afferent vagal fibres terminate exclusively in the nucleus of the solitary tract. Interestingly, electrophysiological studies have revealed the existence of a population of NTS "deep

UCC

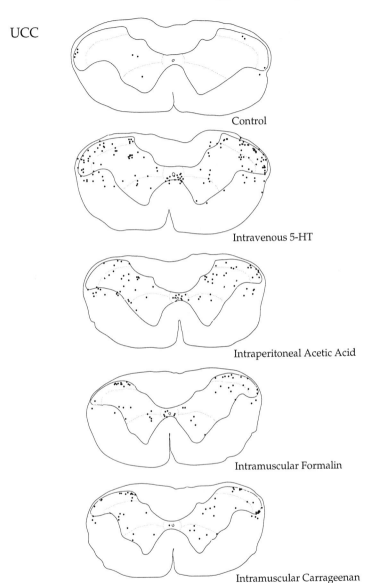

Control

Intravenous 5-HT

Intraperitoneal Acetic Acid

Intramuscular Formalin

Intramuscular Carrageenan

Fig. 5. *(opposite page)* Camera-lucida drawings of coronal sections of the first cervical spinal cord segment in the rat. Each section illustrates the location of activated neurons (in five 50-µm sections) as determined by the expression of the immediate early gene *c-fos* following noxious visceral (iv, 5HT or ip, acetic acid) or noxious deep somatic stimuli (bilateral injection [0.05 mL] of either formalin (5%) or carrageenan [type IV, 2%] [5%] into the triceps surae muscles). Modified from ref. *65*.

from the SI cortex (areas 3b and 1). In humans, painful esophageal distension produces cerebral-evoked potentials, which correspond to massed neuronal responses in SI *(136)*. Thus, SI contains representations of both deep and cutaneous pain. Whether these representations are topographically separable has yet to be examined.

Similar to SI, single-unit recording studies in primate and rat have revealed nociceptive-specific neurons in SII *(137–139)*. In humans, Greenspan and Winfield *(140)*, have reported unilaterally increased mechanical and thermal (heat and cold) thresholds with unaltered affective responses in a patient in whom a tumor was localized by magnetic resonance imaging, in the posterior parietal operculum (the region that corresponds to SII) *(141)*. Neurosurgical removal of the tumor resulted in reinstatement of "normal" sensation. This case is claimed by the authors to support a role for SII in sensory-discriminative aspects of pain processing. Human studies have revealed also that electrical stimulation of SII cortex evokes "pain" *(142)*; and specific lesions of SII have been reported to produce asymbolia for pain *(143)*; that is, although able to distinguish different types of painful stimuli from each other, a patient does not produce the usual affective, motor, or verbal responses to pain. There are also clinical reports of constant burning pain over the contralateral body, following damage to SII *(144)*. In addition to the burning pain, a specific thermal and cutaneous analgesia was reported, an observation consistent with a role for SII in the sensory discriminative aspects of pain processing.

Thus, a body of data supports a role for both SI and SII in pain processing. Both regions receive inputs from the ventroposterior nucleus of the thalamus, which contains "nociceptive neurons." In addition, SII receives projections from the nociresponsive intralaminar thalamic nuclei. The response properties of SII neurones are, however, quite different from those of the SI cortex. SII neurons have large receptive fields, which are often bilateral, which contrasts with the spatially restricted fields of SI neurons. These observations led to the suggestion that SII is important for a "conscious perception" of pain *(138)*. There are, however, no studies to date that have investigated the processing of visceral pain in SII, although the thalamic regions (ventroposterior and posterior nuclei) projecting to SII contain neurons responsive to noxious visceral events *(43,77,145,146)*.

8. "Pain" Networks in Other Thalamo-Cortical Areas?

8.1. Parafascicular/Centromedian Thalamus and the Anterior Cingulate Cortex

The intralaminar nuclei of the thalamus include the centromedian (Cm) and parafascicular (Pf) nuclei. These nuclei are spino-recipient, with more than 50% of the neurons projecting to this region being located within the upper cervical spinal cord *(91,92)*. The centromedian and parafascicular nuclei are also projected upon by the vlPAG *(147,* see Fig. 8)*. That projections to Cm and Pf arise from regions of major convergence of noxious visceral and noxious deep somatic inputs places these nuclei within a potential "deep pain network." Neurons in the Cm and Pf nuclei have been shown to respond to deep noxious inputs *(148–153)*.

Both the Cm and Pf nuclei project to the anterior cingulate cortex (area 24). Inactivation of the anterior cingulate cortex in the rat by local anesthetic injection, significantly reduced the behavioral responses to subcutaneous injections of formalin into the paw *(154)*, suggesting that it plays a critical role in the mediation of the "chronic" behavioral responses to deep painful stimuli. Furthermore, the anterior cingulate cortex has been shown to play a critical role in the establishment of learned avoidance of both noxious cutaneous (foot shock) *(155)* and noxious "visceral" stimuli (eye shock) *(156)*. On balance, these data suggest a role for the anterior cingulate in learned pain avoidance and "chronic" pain behaviors. Single-unit recording studies have shown that anterior cingulate neurons respond to acute, cutaneous noxious stimuli *(157)*. In human positron emission tomography (PET) studies, the anterior cingulate area shows large blood flow

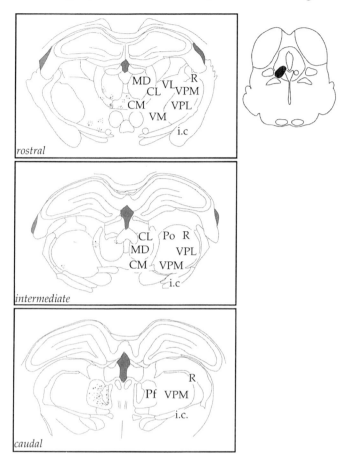

Fig. 8. Panel illustrating projections from the ventrolateral column of the PAG to the centromedian and parafascicular nuclei of the thalamus. At the top right of the figure is a schematic reconstruction of a site of injection of the anterograde tracer, biotinylated dextran amine into the depressor region of the ventrolateral PAG. The left portion of the figure shows three coronal sections through the thalamus of the rat, illustrating the location of anterogradely labeled varicosities and terminals following the injection shown. The sections are arranged from rostral (top) to caudal (bottom). Note that the vlPAG projects strongly to the centromedian, centrolateral, and parafascicular nuclei of the thalamus. CM: Central medial nucleus; CL: centrolateral nucleus; MD: mediodorsal nucleus; VM: ventromedial nucleus; VL: ventrolateral nucleus; VPL: ventral posterolateral nucleus; VPM: ventral posteromedial nucleus; G: gelatinosus nucleus; R: reticular nucleus; Po: posterior nucleus; fr: fasciculus retroflexus; PF: parafascicular nucleus; ic: internal capsule.

changes *(158,159)*. Both the single-unit recording studies and the PET studies have, for the most part, focused on easily replicable noxious cutaneous stimuli; thus, the question as to whether deep noxious stimuli activate this region has not been addressed.

The anterior cingulate region projects predominantly (although not exclusively) to the lateral column of the PAG in the rat and the primate *(160–163)*. In the rat, but apparently not in the primate, it projects also to the nucleus of the solitary tract, the dorsal motor nucleus of the vagus, and directly to the intermediolateral cell column of the spinal cord *(160,164)*. Such pathways allow for cortical modulation of the different behavioral and autonomic changes that characterize the response to pain of superficial or deep origin *(165,166)*. Projections from the anterior cingulate cortex back to the Pf nucleus of the thalamus, as well as the PAG, provide routes via which responsiveness to a noxious stimulus might be modulated *(167)*.

8.2. Submedius Thalamic Nucleus and Orbito-Medial Frontal Cortex

The nucleus submedius is a strong candidate within the intralaminar thalamic group of nuclei to form part of a central "deep pain network." The nucleus submedius receives substantial spinal input arising exclusively from neurons in laminae V, VI, VII, and X and the nucleus of the dorsolateral fasciculus. These are precisely the spinal cord laminae that receive the bulk of visceral and deep somatic afferents and are activated by noxious visceral and noxious deep somatic stimuli *(20,22,23,25,26,29,30,44–49,53,59,65,66,68,168,169)*. The nucleus submedius provides a major source of afferent drive onto the orbital, as well as the anterior cingulate cortices. Single-unit recording studies have shown that intense noxious stimuli (including noxious visceral stimuli) activate neurones in nucleus submedius. The cells, however, showed no modality specificity; that is, irrespective of the tissue stimulated, the salient feature for evoking alterations in neuronal activity appeared to be the persistence and intensity of the noxious stimulus. These observations led Snow and colleagues *(170)* to suggest that this region is involved in producing affective changes ("suffering") in response to severe pain.

Orbito-medial prefrontal cortical regions are thought to influence the affective "tone" of behavior. After lobotomy or prefrontal leukotomy (i.e., surgical removal or disconnection of the orbito-medial prefrontal region), individuals suffering from "unbearable chronic pain" report an end to their "suffering," although they are still able to perceive the presentation of a noxious stimulus *(171)*. Grantham *(172)* reported that lesions of a discrete region of prefrontal cortex, the infero-medial orbital cortex, produced an "indifference" to, but not an end to, chronic pain. Tranel et al. reported that following orbital-prefrontal cortical lesions in people, persistent aversive stimuli cease to have a negative reinforcing quality (173). Similarly, in rats, orbital-prefrontal cortical lesions or application of local anesthetic to the ventrolateral orbital cortex abolish attempts to "switch-off" an aversive foot-shock stimulus (174). More recently, PET studies in humans have also shown that the orbital cortex is activated in chronic, "ongoing" pain states resulting from peripheral nerve damage (175). It is interesting to note that Hsieh and colleagues (176) similar to both Talbot et al. (159) and Jones et al. (158) report no significant blood flow changes in the orbital cortex following acute, cutaneous painful stimuli. This difference may, therefore, reflect that orbital-cortical regions are activated only by chronic or intense pain states.

Select orbital-cortical regions project selectively onto the ventrolateral column of the PAG in both rat and primate *(160)*. These projections provide a route via which the orbital-prefrontal cortex might mediate and/or modulate the behavioral and physiological responses to deep or persistent pain. In support of this suggestion are the observations that orbital-cortex stimulation evokes an opioid-mediated analgesia *(177,178)*. One component of the passive emotional coping style response mediated by the vlPAG is an opioid-mediated analgesia (101–104). The orbital cortex also has extensive connections with specific hypothalamic and amygdaloid regions, which places this region in a pivotal position in the circuits which could contribute to emotional learning associated with pain (e.g., refs. *160* and *179*).

9. Conclusions: A Neuroanatomy of Cardiac Pain ?

Lewis' view that there exists a fundamental separation within the central nervous system of the processing of superficial (cutaneous) and deep (deep somatic and visceral) pain has begun to be addressed. In particular, the use of immediate-early gene expression as a marker of neuronal activation has made it possible to begin to define populations of neurons responsive to deep painful stimuli (*see* Fig. 9). With respect to cardiac pain, the following conclusions are proposed as a statement of our current knowledge.

- At the level of the spinal cord a clear separation between superficial and deep pain has emerged. Cardiac pain activates neurons in the same spinal laminae as other types of visceral and deep somatic pain.
- The role of the UCC in ascending pain pathways has, for the main part, been ignored. This is a curious oversight given that approximately 50% of the neurons that contribute to ascending spinothalamic, spinohypothalamic, and spinomesencephalic pathways are found within the UCC. Further, the extensive spinal and trigeminal convergence that occurs within the UCC likely underlies the referral of cardiac pain to regions of the shoulder, head, and neck.
- The precise location(s) of spinal neurons that are activated by cardiac pain and give rise to supraspinal projection are not known. This represent an important next step in defining a central neuroanatomy of cardiac pain
- The role of the NTS in central "pain" circuitry remains controversial. Spinal and vagal projections to the NTS likely contribute significantly to the autonomic, behavioral, and antinociceptive changes associated with acute or chronic pain of cardiac origin.
- Above the level of the NTS, little is known of the repre-

sentations of any pain of visceral origin, including cardiac pain. Although anatomical outlines have been established (*see* Fig. 9), much remains to be done.

Acknowledgments

The experimental work described in this chapter was performed with the financial support of the National Health Medical Research Council ([NHMRC], Australia). The authors thank Prof. Michael J. Cousins for his comments on an earlier draft of the manuscript. They also thank Jason R. Potas for assistance with the figurework in this chapter.

Fig. 9. *(continued on opposite page)* Panel **A** illustrates schematically the major sources of visceral and deep somatic nociceptive signals to the thalamus, midbrain (PAG), and rostral pons (PB). It shows that ascending information arising from deep noxious stimulation is relayed rostrally by either "segmental" spinal cord, the upper cervical spinal cord, and/or the nucleus of the solitary tract. Different midbrain and thalamic regions receive distinct combinations of spinal or NTS inputs. Not illustrated are the projections from the PAG and PB to the thalamus. Panel **B** illustrates schematically the input/output connections of the (vlPAG) (the only brain region known to both receive convergent noxious visceral and noxious deep somatic inputs, and to integrate the behavioral and physiological responses characteristic of deep pain) with the thalamus and cortex. The panel includes those cortical regions for which a role in pain processing has been established. These two panels indicate those regions that current evidence suggests likely comprise a "deep pain " (including cardiac pain) central network. SM: Nucleus submedius of the thalamus; VMpo: posterior ventromedial nucleus of the thalamus; CM: centromedian nucleus of the thalamus; Pf: parafascicular nucleus of the thalamus; VPm: ventroposterior nucleus of the thalamus medial portion; VPl: ventroposterior nucleus of the thalamus lateral portion; lPAG: lateral PAG region; vlPAG: ventrolateral PAG region; lcPB: lateral crescent region of the parabrachial nucleus; dlPB: dorsolateral region of the parabrachial nucleus; clPB: central lateral region of the parabrachial nucleus; AntC: anterior cingulate cortex; SI: primary somatosensory cortex; MPO: median preoptic area; BNST: bed nucleus of the stria terminalis.

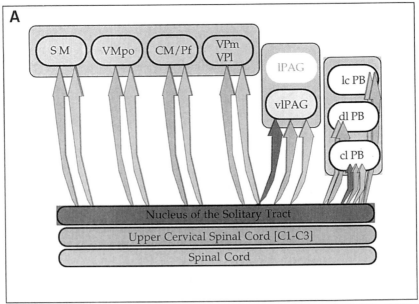

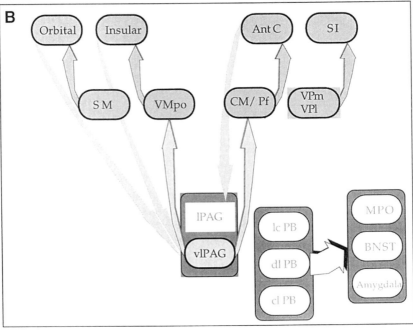

References

1. Ammons, W., Blair, R., and Foreman, R. (1984) Greater splanchnic excitation of primate T1-T5 spinothalamic neurons. *J. Neurophysiol.* **51,** 592–603.
2. Ammons, W., Girardot, M., and Foreman, R. (1985) T2–T5 spinothalamic neurons projecting to medial thalamus with viscerosomatic input. *J. Neurophysiol.* **54,** 73–89.
3. Blair, R., Weber, R., and Foreman, R. (1981) Characteristics of primate spinothalamic tract neurons receiving viscerosomatic convergent inputs in T3–T5 segments. *J. Neurophysiol.* **46,** 797–811.
4. Bolser, D., Hobbs, S., Chandler, M., Ammons, W., Brennan, T., and Foreman, R. (1991) Convergence of phrenic and cardiopulmonary spinal afferent information on cervical and thoracic spinothalamic tract neurons in the monkey: Implications for referred pain from diaphragm and heart. *J. Neurophysiol.* **65,** 1042–1054.
5. Bonica, J. (1990) *Management of Pain.* Lea and Febiger, London.
6. Foreman, R. (1989) Organization of the spinothalamic tract as a relay for cardiopulmonary sympathetic afferent fibre activity, in *Progress in Sensory Physiology* Springer-Verlag, Heidelberg, pp. 1–51.
7. Proccacci, P., Zoppi, M., and Maresca, M. (1994) Heart and vascular pain, in *Textbook of Pain* (Wall, P. D. and Melzack, R., eds.), Churchill-Livingstone, Edinburgh, pp. 541–544.
8. Lewis, T. (1942) *Pain.* McMillan, London.
9. Lewis, T. and Kellgren, R. D. (1939) Observations related to referred pain, viscerosomatic reflexes and other associated phenomena. *Clin. Sci.* **4,** 47.
10. Bernard, J. F. and Besson, J. M. (1990) The spino (trigemino) pontoamygdaloid pathway: electrophysiological evidence for an involvement in pain processes. *J. Neurophysiol.* **63,** 473–490.
11. Bernard, J. F., Huang, G. F., and Besson, J. M. (1994) The parabrachial area: electrophysiological evidence for an involvement in visceral nociceptive processes. *J. Neurophysiol.* **71,** 551–569.
12. Cervero, F. (1983) *Mechanisms of Visceral Pain.* Academic, London.
13. Cervero, F. (1991) Mechanisms of acute visceral pain. *Br. Med. Bull.* **47,** 549–560.
14. Foreman, R. and Blair, R. (1988) Central organization of sympathetic cardiovascular response to pain. *Annu. Rev. Physiol.* **50,** 607–622.
15. Ness, T. and G. Gebhart (1990) Visceral pain: a review of experimental studies. *Pain* **41,** 167–234.
16. Merskey, H. and Bogduk, N. (1994) *Classification of Chronic Pain: IASP Task Force on Taxonomy.* IASP, Seattle, WA.
17. Wall, P. D. (1979) On the relation of injury to pain. *Pain* **6,** 253–264.
18. Janig, W. (1995) The sympathetic nervous system in pain. *Eur. J. Anaesthesiol.* **12,** 53–60.

19. Janig, W. and Habler, H. (1995) Visceral-autonomic integration, in *Visceral Pain: Progress in Pain Research and Management* (Gebhart, G., eds.), IASP, Seattle, WA, pp. 311–348.
20. Kuo, D., Oravitz, J., and De Groat, W. (1984) Tracing of afferent and efferent pathways in the left inferior cardiac nerve of the cat using retrograde and transganglionic transport of horseradish peroxidase. *Brain Res.* **321,** 111–118.
21. De Groat, W. C. (1986) Spinal cord projections and neuropeptides in visceral afferent neurones. *Prog. Brain Res.* **67,** 165–187.
22. Nadelhaft, I. and Booth, A. (1984) The location and morphology of preganglionic neurons and the distribution of visceral afferents from the rat pelvic nerve: a horseradish peroxidase study. *J. Comp. Neurol.* **226,** 238–245.
23. Nadelhaft, I., Roppolo, J., Morgan, C., and DeGroat, W. (1983) Parasympathetic preganglionic neurons and visceral primary afferents in monkey sacral spinal cord revealed following application of horseradish peroxidase to pelvic nerve. *J. Comp. Neurol.* **216,** 36–52.
24. Ciriello, J. and Calaresu, F. (1983) Central projections of afferent renal fibres in the rat: an anterograde transport study of horseradish peroxidase. *J. Auton. Nerv. Syst.* **8,** 273–285.
25. Kuo, D., Nadelhaft, I., Hisamitsu, T., and De Groat, W. (1983) Segmental distribution and central projection of renal afferent fibres in the cat studied by transganglionic transport of horseradish peroxidase. *J. Comp. Neurol.* **216,** 162–174.
26. Cervero, F. and Connell, L. A. (1984) Distribution of somatic and visceral primary afferent fibres within the thoracic spinal cord. *J. Comp. Neurol.* **230,** 88–98.
27. Cervero, F. and Tattersall, J. E. (1987) Somatic and visceral inputs to the thoracic spinal cord of the cat: marginal zone (lamina I) of the dorsal horn. *J. Physiol.* **388,** 383–395.
28. Kuo, D. C. and De Groat, W. C. (1985) Primary afferent projections of the major splanchnic nerve to the spinal cord and gracile nucleus of the cat—an anatomical study using transganglionic transport of horseradish peroxidase. *J. Comp. Neurol.* **231,** 421–434.
29. Morgan, C., De Groat, W., and Nadelhaft, I. (1986) The spinal distribution of visceral primary afferent neurons which send axons into the hypogastric nerves of the cat. *J. Comp. Neurol.* **243,** 23–40.
30. Neuhuber, W. (1982) The central projections of visceral primary afferent neurons of the inferior mesenteric plexus and hypogastric nerve and the location of the related sensory and preganglionic sympathetic cell bodies in the rat. *Anat. Embryol.* **164,** 413–425.
31. Craig, A. D. and Mense, S. (1983) The distribution of afferent fibres from the gastrocnemius-soleus muscle in the dorsal horn of the cat, as revealed by the transport of horseradish peroxidase. *Neurosci. Lett.* **41,** 233–238.

32. Mense, S. and Prabharkar, N. R. (1986) Spinal termination of nociceptive afferent fibres from deep tissues in the cat. *Neurosci. Lett.* **66**, 169–174.
33. Mysicka, A. and Zenker, W. (1981) Central projections of muscle afferents from the sternomastoid nerve in the rat. *Brain Res.* **211**, 257–265.
34. Nyberg, G. and Blomqvist, A. (1984) The central projections of muscle afferent fibres to the lower medulla and upper spinal cord: an anatomical study in the cat with the transganglionic transport method. *J. Comp. Neurol.* **230**, 99–109.
35. Pfaller, K. and Arvidsson, J. (1988) Central distribution of trigeminal and upper cervical afferents in the rat studied by anterograde transport of horseradish peroxidase conjugated to wheat germ agglutinin. *J. Comp. Neurol.* **268**, 91–108.
36. Prihoda, M., Hiller, M.-S., and Mayr, R. (1991) Central projections of cervical primary afferent fibres in the guinea pig: an HRP and WGA-HRP tracer study. *J. Comp. Neurol.* **308**, 418–431.
37. Swett, J. E. (1983) Few C-fibres from muscle terminate in lamina II of the spinal cord of the cat. *J. Physiol.* **345**, 157P.
38. Florence, S., Wall, J., and Kaas, J. (1991) Central projections from the skin of the hand in squirrel monkeys. *J. Comp. Neurol.* **311**, 563–578.
39. Molander, C. and Grant, G. (1985) Cutaneous projections from the rat hindlimb foot to the substantia gelatinosa of the spinal cord studied by transganglionic transport of WGA-HRP conjugate. *J. Comp. Neurol.* **237**, 476–484.
40. Nyberg, G. and Blomqvist, A. (1985) The somatotopic organization of forelimb cutaneous nerves in the brachial dorsal horn: An anatomical study in the cat. *J. Comp. Neurol.* **242**, 28–39.
41. Hobbs, S. F., Chandler, M. J., Bolser, D. C., and Foreman, R. D. (1992) Segmental organization of visceral and somatic input onto C3–T6 spinothalamic tract cells of the monkey. *J. Neurophysiol.* **68**, 1575–1588.
42. McKitrick, D. and Calaresu, F. (1993) Expression of Fos in central nervous system elicited by afferent stimulation in femoral nerve. *Brain Res.* **632**, 127–135.
43. Chandler, M. J., Hobbs, S. F., Bolser, D. C., and Foreman, R. D. (1991) Effects of vagal afferent stimulation on cervical spinothalamic tract neurons in monkeys. *Pain* **44**, 81–87.
44. Cervero, F. (1983) Somatic and visceral inputs to the thoracic spinal cord of the cat: effects of noxious stimulation of the biliary system. *J. Physiol.* **337**, 51–67.
45. Cervero, F. and Tattersall, J. (1985) Cutaneous receptive fields of somatic and viscero-somatic neurons in the thoracic spinal cord of the cat. *J. Comp. Neurol.* **237**, 325–332.
46. Cervero, F. and Tattersall, J. (1985) Somatotopic organisation in the thoracic spinal cord of the cat. *J. Physiol. (Lond.)* **361**, 45P.

47. Cervero, F. and Tattersall, J. (1986) Somatic and visceral sensory integration in the thoracic spinal cord. *Prog. Brain Res.* **67,** 189–205.

48. Morgan, C., Nadelhaft, I., and DeGroat, W. (1981) The distribution of visceral primary afferents from the pelvic nerve to Lissauer's tract and the spinal grey matter and its relationship to the sacral parasympathetic nucleus. *J. Comp. Neurol.* **201,** 415–440.

49. Traub, R., Pechman, P., Iadarola, M., and Gebhart, G. (1992) Fos-like proteins in the lumbosacral spinal cord following noxious and non-noxious colorectal distention in the rat. *Pain* **49,** 393–403.

50. Meller, S. T. and Gebhart, G. F. (1992) A critical review of the afferent pathways and the potential chemical mediators involved in cardiac pain. *Neurosci.* **48,** 501–524.

51. Morgan, M. M. (1991) Differences in antinociception evoked from dorsal and ventral regions of the caudal and periaqueductal gray matter, in *The Midbrain Periaqueductal Gray: Functional, Anatomical, and Neurochemical Organization* (Depaulis, A. and Bandler, R., eds.), Plenum, New York, pp. 139–150.

52. Kuo, D. C., Yang, G. C. H., Yamasaki, D. S., and Krauthamer, G. M. (1982) A wide field electron-microscopic analysis of the fibre constituents of the major splanchnic nerve in the cat. *J. Comp. Neurol.* **210,** 49–58.

53. Morgan, C., Nadelhaft, I., and De Groat, W. (1986) The spinal distribution of visceral primary afferent neurons which send axons into the lumbar colonic nerves of the cat. *Soc. Neurosci. Abs.*

54. Schaible, H. G., Schmidt, R. F., and Willis, W. D. (1986) Responses of spinal cord neurones to stimulation of articular afferent fibres in the cat. *J. Physiol.* **372,** 575–593.

55. Gebhart, G. and Ness, T. (1991) Central mechanisms of visceral pain. *Can. J. Physiol. Pharmacol.* **69,** 627–634.

56. Bullit, E. (1990) Expression of c-fos-like protein as a marker for neuronal activity following noxious stimulation in the rat. *J. Comp. Neurol.* **296,** 517–530.

57. Curran, T. (1984) Viral and cellular fos proteins. *Cell* **36,** 259–268.

58. Dragunow, M. and Faull, R. (1989) The use of c-fos as a metabolic marker in neuronal pathway tracing. *J. Neurosci. Methods* **29,** 261–265.

59. Hunt, S. P., Pini, A., and Evans, G. (1987) Induction of c-fos-like protein in spinal cord neurons following sensory stimulation. *Nature* **328,** 632–634.

60. Lanteri-Minet, M., dePommery, J., Herdegen, T., and Weil-Fugaza, J. (1993) Differential time course and spatial expression of Fos, Jun and Krox24 proteins in spinal cord of rats undergoing subacute or chronic somatic inflammation. *J. Comp. Neurol.* **333,** 223–235.

61. Neto, F. R. (1978) The depolarising action of 5-HT on mammalian non-myelinated nerve fibers. *Eur. J. Pharmacol.* **49,** 351–356.

62. Stansfield, C. E. and Wallis, D. I. (1985) Properties of visceral primary afferent neurons in the nodose ganglion of the rabbit. *J. Neurophysiol.* **54,** 245–260.

63. Wallis, D. I., Stansfield, C. E., and Nash, H. L. (1982) Depolarising responses recorded from nodose ganglion cells of the rabbit evoked by 5-hydroxytryptamine and other substances. *Neuropharmacology* **21**, 31–40.

64. Page, I. H. and McCubbin, J. W. (1953) The variable arterial pressure response to serotonin in laboratory animals and man. *Circ. Res.* **1**, 354–362

65. Clement, C., Keay, K., Podzebenko, K., Gordon, B., and Bandler, R. (1999) Spinal sources of noxious visceral and noxious deep somatic afferent drive onto the ventrolateral periaqueductal gray of the rat. *J. Comp. Neurol.*, submitted.

66. Lanteri-Minet, M., Isnardon, P., De Pommery, J., and Menetrey, D. (1993) Spinal and hindbrain structures involved in visceroception and visceronociception as revealed by the expression of Fos, Jun and, Krox-24 proteins. *Neurosci.* **55**, 737–753.

67. Menetrey, D. and dePommery, J. (1991) Origins of spinal ascending pathways that reach central areas involved in visceroception and visceronociception in the rat. *Eur. J. Neurosci.* **3**, 249–259.

68. Menetrey, D., Gannon, A., Levine, J. D., and Basbaum, A. I. (1989) Expression of c-fos protein in interneurons and projection neurons of the rat spinal cord in response to noxious somatic, articular and visceral stimulation. *J. Comp. Neurol.* **285**, 177–195.

69. Williams, S., Evans, G., and Hunt, S. (1990) Changing patterns of c-fos induction in spinal neurons following thermal cutaneous stimulation in the rat. *Neurosci.* **36**, 73–81.

70. Owler, B., Clement, C., Keay, K., and Bandler, R. (1994) Deep somatic and visceral noxious stimuli evoke Fos expression in different spinal cord laminae and a common region of the nucleus of the solitary tract. *Proc. Aust. Neurosci. Soc.* **5**, 200.

71. Kaube, H., Keay, K. A., Hoskin, K. L., Bandler, R., and Goadsby, P. J. (1993) Expression of c-Fos-like immunoreactivity in the caudal medulla and upper cervical spinal cord following stimulation of the superior sagittal sinus in the cat. *Brain Res.* **629**, 95–102.

72. Hathaway, C., Hu, J., and Bereiter, D. (1995) Distribution of Fos-like immunoreactivity in the caudal brainstem of the rat following noxious chemical stimulation of the temporomandibular joint. *J. Comp. Neurol.* **356**, 444–456.

73. Kemper, R., Meijler, W., and TerHorst, G. (1997) Trigeminovascular stimulation in conscious rats. *NeuroReport* **8**, 1123–1126.

74. Strassman, A. M. and Voss, B. P. (1993) Somatotopic and laminar organization of Fos-like immunoreactivity in the medullary and upper cervical dorsal horn induced by noxious facial stimulation. *J. Comp. Neurol.* **331**, 495–516.

75. White, J. (1957) Cardiac pain. *Circulation* **16**, 644–655.

76. Fu, Q., Chandler, M., McNeill, D., and Foreman, R. (1992) Vagal afferent fibres excite upper cervical neurons and inhibit activity of lumbar spinal cord neurons in the rat. *Pain* **51**, 91–100.

77. Hobbs, S. F, Oh, U., Chandler, M. J., Fu, Q., Bolser, D., and Foreman, R. (1992) Evidence that C1 and C2 proprispinal neurons mediate the inhibitory effects of viscerosomatic spinal afferent input on primate spinothalamic tract neurons. *J. Neurophysiol.* **67,** 852–860.

78. Zhang, J., Chandler, M., and Foreman, R. (1996) Thoracic visceral inputs use upper cervical segments to inhibit lumbar spinal neurons in rats. *Brain Res.* **709,** 337–342.

79. Person, R. J. (1989) Somatic and vagal afferent convergence on solitary tract neurons in cat: electrophysiological characteristics. *Neurosci.* **30,** 283–295.

80. Gieroba, Z. J. and Blessing, W. W. (1994) Depressor neurons in caudal medulla demonstrated by Fos expression following activation of cardiopulmonary vagal (Bezold-Jarisch) receptors. *Proc. Aust. Neurosci. Soc.* **5,** 189.

81. Bonaz, B., V. Plourde, and Y. Tache (1994) Abdominal surgery induces Fos immunoreactivity in the rat brain. *J. Comp. Neurol.* **349,** 212–222.

82. Lanteri-Minet, M., Weil-Fugazza, J., DePommery, J., and Menetrey, D. (1994) Hindbrain structures involved in pain processing as revealed by the expression of c-Fos and other immediate early gene proteins. *Neurosci.* **58,** 287–298.

83. Traub, R., Lim, F., Sengupta, J., Meller, S., and Gebhart, G. (1994) Noxious distention of viscera results in differential c-Fos expression in second order sensory neurons receiving sympathetic or parasympathetic input. *Neurosci. Lett.* **180,** 71–75.

84. Traub, R., Sengupta, J., and Gebhart, G. (1996) Differential c-Fos expression in the nucleus of the solitary tract and spinal cord following noxious gastric distension in the rat. *Neurosci.* **74,** 873–884.

85. Zittel, T., DeGiorgio, R., Brecha, N., Sternini, C., and Raybould, H. (1993) Abdominal surgey induces c-fos expression in the nucleus of the solitary tract in the rat. *Neurosci. Lett.* **159,** 79–82.

86. Dean, C. and Seagard, J. (1995) Expression of c-fos protein in the nucleus tractus solitarius in response to physiological activation of carotid baroreceptors. *Neurosci.* **69,** 249–257.

87. Erickson, J. and Millhorn, D. (1991) Fos-like protein is induced in neurons of the medulla oblogata after stimulation of the carotid sins nerve in awake and anesthetised rats. *Brain Res.* **567,** 11–24.

88. McKitrick, D., Krukoff, T., and Calaresu, F. (1992) Expression of c-fos protein in rat brain after electrical stimulation of the aortic depressor nerve. *Brain Res.* **599,** 215–222.

89. Rutherford, S., Widdop, R., Sannajust, F., Loius, W., and Gundlach, A. (1992) Expression of c-fos and NGFI-A messenger RNA in the medulla oblongata of the anesthetised rat following stimulation of vagal and cardiovascular afferents. *Mol. Brain Res.* **13,** 301–312.

90. Mehler, W. R. (1969) Some neurological species differences—a posteriori. *Ann. NY Acad. Sci.* **167,** 424–468.

91. Carstens, E. and Trevino, D. (1978) Anatomical and physiological properties of ipsilaterally projecting spinothalamic neurons in the second cervical segment of the cat's spinal cord. *J. Comp. Neurol.* **182**, 167–184.

92. Carstens, E. and Trevino, D. (1978) Laminar origins of spinothalamic projections in the cat as determined by the retrograde transport of horseradish peroxidase. *J. Comp. Neurol.* **182**, 161–165.

93. Bandler, R. and Keay, K. A. (1996) Columnar organization in the midbrain periaqueductal gray and the integration of emotional expression, in *The Emotional Motor System, Progress in Brain Research*, vol. 107 (Holstege, G., Bandler, R., and Saper, C., eds.), Elsevier, Amsterdam, pp. 285–300.

94. Bandler, R. and Shipley, M. (1994) Columnar organization in midbrain periaqueductal gray: modules for emotional expression? *Trends Neurosci.* **17**, 379–389.

95. Beitz, A. J. (1995) Periaqueductal gray, in *The Rat Nervous System* (Paxinos, G., eds.), Academic, San Diego, pp. 173–182.

96. Carrive, P. (1991) Functional organization of PAG neurons controlling regional vascular beds, in *The Midbrain Periaqueductal Gray Matter: Functional, Anatomical and Neurochemical Organization* (Depaulis, A. and Bandler, R., eds.), Plenum, New York, pp. 67–100.

97. Depaulis, A., Keay, K. A., and Bandler, R. (1994) Quiescence and hyporeactivity evoked by activation of cell bodies in the ventrolateral midbrain periaqueductal gray of the rat. *Exp. Brain Res.* **99**, 75–83.

98. Keay, K. A, Crowfoot, L. J., Floyd, N. S., Henderson, L. A., Christie, M. J., and Bandler, R. (1997) Cardiovascular effects of microinjections of opioid agonists into the "depressor region" of the ventrolateral periaqueductal gray region. *Brain Res.* **762**, 61–71.

99. Lovick, T. A. (1992) Inhibitory modulation of the cardiovascular defence response by the ventrolateral periaqueductal grey matter in rats. *Exp. Brain Res.* **89**, 133–139.

100. Zhang, S. P., Bandler, R., and Carrive, P. (1990) Flight and immobility evoked by excitatory amino acid microinjection within distinct parts of the subtentorial periaqueductal grey of the cat. *Brain Res.* **520**, 73–82.

101. Behbehani, M. and Fields, H. (1979) Evidence that an excitatory connection between the periaqueductal gray and nucleus raphe magnus mediates stimulation produced analgesia. *Brain Res.* **170**, 85–93.

102. Fields, H. and Basbaum, A. (1978) Brainstem control of spinal pain-transmission neurons. *Ann. Rev. Physiol.* **40**, 217–248.

103. Jensen, T. and Yaksh, T. (1992) Brainstem excitatory amino acid receptors in nociception: microinjection mapping and pharmacological characterization of glutamate sensitive sites in the brainstem associated with algogenic behavior. *Neurosci.* **46**, 535–547.

104. Jensen, T. S. and Yaksh, T. L. (1984) Spinal monoamine and opioid systems partially mediate an analgesia produced by glutamate at brainstem sites. *Brain Res.* **363,** 114–127.
105. Duggan, A. W. (1983) Injury, pain and analgesia. *Proc. Aust. Physiol. Pharmacol. Soc.* **14,** 218–240.
106. Benus, R. F., Bohus, B., Koolhaas, J. M., and van-Oortmerssen, G. A. (1991) Heritable variation for aggression as a reflection of individual coping strategies. *Experientia* **47,** 1008–1019.
107. Engel, G. L. and Schmale, A. H. (1972) Conservation-withdrawal: a primary regulatory process for organismic homeostasis. *CIBA Found. Symp.* **8,** 57–76.
108. Henry, J. P. and Stephens, P. M. (1977) *Stress Health and the Social Environment: A Sociobiological Approach to Medicine.* Springer-Verlag, New York.
109. Depaulis, A., Keay, K. A., and Bandler, R. (1992) Longitudinal neuronal organisation of defensive reactions in the midbrain periaqueductal gray region of the rat. *Exp. Brain Res.* **90,** 307–318.
110. Keay, K. A., Feil, K., Gordon, B. D., Herbert, H., and Bandler, R. (1997) Spinal afferents to functionally distinct penaqriaqueductal grey columns in the rat: An anterograde and retrograde tracing study. *J. Comp. Neurol.* **385,** 207–229.
111. Clement, C. I., Keay, K. A., and Bandler, R. (1998) Medullary catecholaminergic projections to the ventrolateral periaqueductal gray region activated by halothane anaesthesia. *Neuroscience* **86,** 1273–1284.
112. Herbert, H. and Saper, C. B. (1992) Organization of medullary adrenergic and noradrenergic projections to the periaqueductal gray matter in the rat. *J. Comp. Neurol.* **315,** 34–52.
113. Keay, K. A., Clement, C. I., Owler, B., Depaulis, A., and Bandler, R. (1994) Convergence of deep somatic and visceral nociceptive information onto a discrete ventrolateral midbrain periaqueductal gray region. *Neurosci.* **61,** 727–732.
114. Clement, C. I., Keay, K. A., Owler, B. K., and Bandler, R. (1996) Common patterns of increased and decreased Fos expression in midbrain and pons evoked by noxious deep somatic and noxious visceral manipulations in the rat. *J. Comp. Neurol.* **366,** 495–515.
115. Keay, K. A. and Bandler, R. (1998) Vascular head pain selectively activates the ventrolateral PAG in the cat. *Neurosci. Lett.* **245,** 58–60.
116. Tassorelli, C. and Joseph, S. A. (1995) Systemic nitroglycerin induces fos immunoreactivity in brainstem and forebrain structures of the rat. *Brain Res.* **682,** 167–181.
117. Keay, K. A. and Bandler, R. (1993) Deep and superficial noxious stimulation increases Fos-like immunoreactivity in different regions of the midbrain periaqueductal grey of the rat. *Neurosci. Lett.* **154,** 23–26.
118. Bernard, J. and Bandler, R. (1998) Parallel circuits for emotional coping behaviour: New pieces in the puzzle. *J. Comp. Neurol.* **401,** 429–436.

119. Cechetto, D., Standaert, D., and Saper, C. (1985) Spinal and trigeminal dorsal horn projections to the parabrachial nucleus in the rat. *J. Comp. Neurol.* **240,** 153–160.
120. Feil, K. and Herbert, H. (1995) Topographic organization of spinal and trigeminal somatosensory pathways to the rat parabrachial and Kölliker–Fuse nuclei. *J. Comp. Neurol.* **353,** 506–528.
121. Herbert, H., Moga, M., and Saper, C. (1990) Connections of the parabrachial nucleus with the nucleus of the solitary tract and medullary reticular formation in the rat. *J. Comp. Neurol.* **293,** 540–580.
122. Bernard, J., Bester, H., and Besson, J. (1996) Involvement of the spino-parabrachio-amygdaloid and -hypothalamic pathways in the autonomic and affective-emotional aspects of pain. *Prog. Brain. Res.* **107,** 243–255.
123. Bernard J. F. and Besson, J. M. (1990) The spino(trigemino)-ponto amygdaloid pathway: electrophysiological evidence for an involvement in pain processes. *J. Neurophysiol.* **63,** 473–490.
124. Bernard J. F., Huang, G. F., and Besson, J. M. (1994) The parabrachial area: electrophysiological evidence for an involvement in visceral nociceptive processes. *J. Neurophysiol.* **71,** 1646–1660.
125. Saper, C. (1995) The spinoparabrachial pathway: shedding new light on an old path. *J. Comp. Neurol.* **353,** 477–479.
126. Krout, K., Jansen, A., and Loewy, A. (1998) Periaqueductal gray matter projection to the parabrachial nucleus in rat. *J. Comp. Neurol.* **401,** 437–454.
127. Fernandez De Molina, A. and Hunsperger, R. W. (1962) Organization of the subcortical system governing defence and flight reactions in the cat. *J. Physiol. (Lond.)* **160,** 200–213.
128. Sherrington, C. (1906) *The Integrative Action of the Nervous System.* Yale University Press, New Haven, CT.
129. Woodworth, R. S. and Sherrington, C. S. (1904) A pseudaffective reflex and its spinal path. *J. Physiol. (Lond.)* **31,** 234–243.
130. Woolf, C. (1984) Long term alterations in the excitability of the flexion reflex produced by peripheral tissue injury in the chronic decerebrate rat. *Pain* **18,** 325–343.
131. Bandler, R. (1988) Brain mechanisms of aggression as revealed by electrical and chemical stimulation: Suggestion of a central role for the midbrain periaqueductal grey region. *Prog. Psychobiol. Physiol. Psychol.* **13,** 67–154.
132. Lamour, Y., Willer, J. C., and Guillbaud, G. (1983) Rat somatosensory (SmI) cortex. I. Characteristics of neuronal responses to noxious stimulation and comparison to responses to non-noxious stimulation. *Exp. Brain Res.* **49,** 35–45.
133. Chudler, E. H., Anton, F., Dubner, R., and Kenshalo, J. D. R. (1990) Responses of nociceptive SI neurons in monkeys and pain sensation in humans elicited by noxious thermal stimulation: effect of interstimulus interval. *J. Neurophysiol.* **63,** 559–569.

134. Kenshalo, D. R., Jr. and Isensee, O. (1983) Responses of primate SI cortical neurons to noxious stimuli. *J. Neurophysiol.* **50,** 1479–1496.

135. Chandler, M. J., Hobbs, S. F., Fu, Q.-G., Kenshalo, D. R., Jr., Blair, R. W., and Foreman, R. D. (1992) Responses of neurons in ventroposterolateral nucleus of primate thalamus to urinary bladder distention. *Brain Res.* **571,** 26–34.

136. Castell, D., Wood, J., Frieling, T., Wright, F., and Vieth, R. (1990) Cerebral electrical potentials evoked by ballon distention of the human oesophagus. *Gastroenterology* **98,** 662–666.

137. Andersson, S. A. (1978) Cortical response after spinal lesions and tooth pulp stimulation. *Neurosci. Res. Prog. Bull.* **16,** 125–136.

138. Burton, H., Mitchell, G., and Brent, D. (1982) Second somatosensory area in the cerebral cortex of cats: somatotopic organisation and architecture. *J. Comp. Neurol.* **210,** 109–135.

139. Carreras, M. and Andersson, S. A. (1963) Functional properties of neurons of the anterior ectosylvian gyrus of the cat. *J. Neurophysiol.* **26,** 100–126.

140. Greenspan, J. D. and Winfield, J. A. (1992) Reversible pain and tactile deficits associated woth a cerebral tumor compressing the posterior insula and parietal operculum. *Pain* **50,** 29–39.

141. Roberts, T. S. and Akert, K. (1963) Insular and opercular cortex and its thalamic projections in *Macaca mulatta. Scheiz. Arch. Neurol. Neurochir. Psychiatry* **92,** 1–46.

142. Penfield, W. G. and Boldrey, E. (1937) Somatic motor and sensory representation in the cerebral cortex of man as studied by electrical stimulation. *Brain* **60,** 389–443.

143. Berthier, M., Starkstein, S., and Leiguarda, R. (1988) Asymbolia for pain: a sensory disconnection syndrome. *Ann. Neurol.* **24,** 41–49.

144. Schmahmann, J. D. and Leifer, D. (1992) Parietal pseudothalamic pain syndrome. Clinical features and anatomic correlates. *Arch. Neurol.* **49,** 1032–1037.

145. Al-Chaer, E. D., Feng, Y., and Willis, W. D. (1998) A role for the dorsal column in nociceptive visceral input into the thalamus of primates. *J. Neurophysiol.* **79,** 3143–3150.

146. Asato, F. and Yokota, T. (1989) Responses of neurons in nucleus ventralis posterolateralis of the cat thalamus to hypogastric inputs. *Brain Res.* **488,** 135–142.

147. Floyd, N. S., Keay, K. A., and Bandler, R. (1996) A calbindin-immunoreactive "deep pain" recipient thalamic nucleus in the rat. *NeuroReport* **7,** 622–626.

148. Bon, K., Lanteri-Minet, M., de Pommery, J., Michiels, J. F., and Menetrey, D. (1997) Cyclophosphamide cystitis as a model of visceral pain in rats: minor effects at mesodiencephalic levels as revealed by the expression of c-fos, with a note on Krox-24. *Exp. Brain Res.* **113,** 249–264.

149. Yen, C. T., Fu, T. C., and Chen, R. C. (1989) Distribution of tha-lamic nociceptive neurons activated from the tail of the rat. *Brain Res.* **498**, 118–122.

150. McClung, R. E and Dafny, N. (1980) The parafascicular nucleus of thalamus exhibits convergence input from the dorsal raphe and the spinal tract of the trigeminal nerve. *Brain Res.* **197**, 525–531.

151. Zagami, A. S. and Lambert, G. A. (1990) Stimulation of cranial ves-sels excites nociceptive neurones in several thalamic nuclei of the cat. *Exp. Brain Res.* **81**, 552–566.

152. Dostrovsky, J. O. and Guillbaud, G. (1990) Nociceptive responses in medial thalamus of the normal and arthritic rat. *Pain* **40**, 93–104.

153. Peschanski, M., Guillbaud, G., and Gautron, M. (1981) Posterior intralaminar region in rat: neuronal responses to noxious and non-noxious cutaneous stimuli. *Exp. Neurol.* **72**, 226–238.

154. Vaccarino, A. L. and Melzack, R. (1989) Analgesia produced by the injection of lidociane into the anterior cingulum bundle of the rat. *Pain* **39**, 213–219.

155. Gabriel, M., Kubota, Y., Sparenborg, S., Straube, K., and Vogt, B. A. (1991) Effects of cingulate cortex lesions on avoidance learning and training-induced unit acivity in rabbits. *Exp. Brain Res.* **86**, 585–600.

156. Gibbs, C. M. and Powell, D. A. (1991) Single unit activity in the dorsomedial prefrontal cortex during the expression of discrimi-native bradycardia in rabbits. *Behav. Brain Res.* **43**, 79–92.

157. Sikes, R. W. and Vogt, B. A. (1992) Nociceptive neurons in area 24 of the rabbit cingulate cortex. *J, Neurophysiol.* **68**, 1720–1732.

158. Jones, A. K. P., Friston, K., and Frackowiack, R. S. J. (1991) Cere-bral localisation of responses to pain in man using positron emmision tomography. *Science* **255**, 215–216.

159. Talbot, J., Marrett, S., Evans, A. C., Meyer, E., Bushnell, M. C., and Duncan, G. C. (1991) Multiple representations of pain in the human cerebral cortex. *Science* **251**, 1355–1358.

160. An, X., Bandler, R., Öngür, D., and Price, J. (1998) Prefrontal cortical projections to longitudinal columns in the midbrain periaqueductal gray in macaque monkeys. *J. Comp. Neurol.* **401**, 455–479.

161. Beitz, A. J. (1982) The organisation of afferent projections to the midbrain periaqueductal gray of the rat. *Neurosci.* **7**, 133–159.

162. Christie, M. J., James, L. B., and Beart, P. M. (1986) An excitatory amino acid projection from rat prefrontal cortex to periaqueductal gray. *Brain Res. Bull.* **16**, 127–129.

163. Morrell, J. I., Greenberger, L. M., and Pfaff, D. W. (1981) Hypotha-lamic, other diencephalic, and telencephalic neurons that project to the dorsal midbrain. *J. Comp. Neurol.* **201**, 589–620.

164. Hurley, K. M., Herbert, H., Moga, M. M., and Saper, C. B. (1991) Efferent projections of the infralimbic cortex of the rat. *J. Comp. Neurol.* **308**, 249–276.

165. Devinsky, O. and Luciano, D. (1993) The contribution of the cingulate cortex to human behaviour, in *Neurobiology of Cingulate Cortex and Limbic Thalamus* (Vogt, B. A. and Gabriel, M., eds.), Birkåuser, Boston.

166. Neafsey, E. J. (1990) Prefrontal cortical control of the autonomic nervous system: anatomical and physiological observations. *Prog. Brain Res.* **85,** 147–166.

167. Royce, G. J. (1983) Cells of origin of corticothalamic projections upon the centromedian and parafascicular nuclei in the cat. *Brain Res.* **258,** 11–21.

168. Hammond, D., Presley, R., Gogas, K., and Basbaum, A. (1992) Morphine or U-50,488 suppresses Fos protein-like immunoreactivity in the spinal cord and nucleus tractus solitarii evoked by a noxious visceral stimulus in rat. *J. Comp. Neurol.* **315,** 244–253.

169. Lu, Y., Jin, S., Xu, T., Qin, B., Li, J., Ding, Y., et al. (1995) Expression of c-fos protein in substance P receptor-like immunoreactive neurons in response to noxious stimuli on the urinary bladder: an observation in the lumbosacral cord segments of the rat. *Neurosci. Lett.* **198,** 139–142.

170. Snow, P. J., Lumb, B. M., and Cervero, F. (1991) The representation of prolonged and intense, noxious somatic and visceral stimuli in the ventrolateral orbital cortex of the cat. *Pain* **48,** 89–99.

171. Freeman, W. and Watts, J. W. (1946) Pain of organic disease relieved by prefrontal lobotomy. *Proc. Roy. Soc. Med.* **39,** 445–447.

172. Grantham, E. G. (1951) Prefrontal lobotomy for relief of pain with a report of a new operative technique. *J. Neurosurg.* **8,** 405–410.

173. Tranel, D., Damasio, A. R., and Damasio, H. (1988) Impaired autonomic reactions to emotional and social stimuli in patients with bilateral orbital damage and acquired sociopathy. *Soc. Neurosci. Abstr.* **14,** 1288.

174. Cooper, S. J. (1975) Anaesthetisation of the prefrontal cortex and response to noxious stimulation. *Nature* **254,** 439–440.

175. Hsieh, J. C., Belfrage, M., Stone-Elander, S., Hansson, P., and Ingvar, M. (1995) Central representation of chronic ongoing neuropathic pain studied by positron emission tomography. *Pain* **63,** 225–236.

176. Hsieh, J. C., Ståhle-Bäckdahl, M., Hägermark, Ö., Stone-Elander, S., Rosenquist, G., and Ingvar, M. (1995) Traumatic nociceptive pain activates the hypothalamus and the periaqueductal gray: a positron emission tomography study. *Pain* **64,** 303–314.

177. Hardy, S. (1985) Analgesia evoked by prefrontal stimulation. *Brain Res.* **339,** 281–285.

178. Oleson, T., Kirkpatrick, D., and Goodman, S. (1980) Elevation of pain threshold to tooth shock by brain stimulation in primates. *Brain Res.* **194,** 79–95.

179. Öngür, D., An, X., and Price, J. (1998) Prefrontal cortical projections to the hypothalamus in macaque monkeys. *J. Comp. Neurol.* **401,** 480–505.

CHAPTER 9

Neurophysiology of Heart Pain

Robert D. Foreman

1. Introduction

Chest pain is often a symptom that causes a person to seek treatment from a physician and, often, a cardiologist. The public has been informed that chest pain is usually the result of a "heart attack" or ischemic heart disease. It is true that the chest pain might be indicative of ischemic heart disease resulting from coronary stenosis and/or coronary spasm. However, this pain could also signal noncardiac symptoms such as esophageal disease or even inflammation of the muscle and joint of the chest. The picture of chest pain and ischemic heart disease is further complicated by the fact that severe ischemic episodes may or may not be associated with angina pectoris. All these events are dependent on how the central nervous system processes information received from thoracic visceral organs and somatic structures, the state of the peripheral and central nervous system at the time these events occur, and the psychological state of the person experiencing these sensations. Our understanding about the central mechanisms involved with these events are limited, therefore, the scope of this chapter will be limited to spinal cord processing related to angina pectoris.

The purpose of this chapter is to provide a neurophysiological basis for the pain associated with ischemic heart disease. Authors of other chapters provided information about

From: *The Nervous System and the Heart*
Ed: G. J. Ter Horst © Humana Press Inc.

the stimuli that activate cardiac receptors leading to the perception of pain and address the regions in the brain where the nociceptive information from the heart is processed. This chapter will discuss the processing of cardiac nociceptive information in the spinal cord and its transmission to the thalamus, where information is relayed to structures in the forebrain that are critical for the pain perception.

Patients describe angina pectoris as a chest pain that may radiate to the throat, neck, or ulnar aspect of the left arm, sometimes reaching the little finger. Less often, it radiates to the neck and jaw, or either the right or both arms. Intensity and pain location often varies from person to person and from time to time. Angina pectoris may also be associated with the subjective sensation of anguish and fear of impending death. Heberden (1), who experienced angina pectoris, described its most typical manifestation as retrosternal with crushing, burning or squeezing character.

2. Spinal Cord Processing of Visceral Information from the Heart

Cell bodies of the sympathetic afferent fibers from the heart and coronary arteries are concentrated in the dorsal root ganglia of the T2–T6 spinal segments, but they can spread as far as the C8–T9 segments (2,3). Axons of dorsal root ganglion cells enter the tract of Lissauer and terminate in the same segment or ascend and descend a few segments before penetrating the gray matter (2). Some of these axons arch over the dorsal rim of the gray matter and enter lamina I, whereas others travel along the lateral edge of the gray matter and terminate primarily in laminae V, VII, and X. When compared to somatic afferents, the density of innervation is much less and more diffuse for sympathetic afferent fibers. This diffuse and extensive organization of sympathetic afferent fibers most likely contributes to the poorly localized nature of angina pectoris. These fibers can either directly or indirectly activate cells with axons projecting to the supraspinal structures that are involved with pain perception.

4. Ascending Pathways Transmitting Noxious Cardiac Information

Cells of origin of ascending pathways, propriospinal neurons, and interneurons are in the gray matter of the spinal cord. Of the cells in the upper thoracic gray matter, the spinothalamic tract (STT) cells are the most studied system of the ascending pathways for transmitting visceral afferent information from the heart to the brain. Cell bodies in the STT in the upper thoracic segments are located predominantly in laminae I and V, but some cells may be sprinkled in other laminae, especially lamina VII *(4–7)*. The STT axons generally cross to the contralateral side within one or two segments and then ascend in the anterolateral quadrant, however, about 10–15% of the axons ascend on the ipsilateral side and some are in the dorsolateral quadrant *(5,8)*. These cells usually receive converging information from the upper thoracic segments and somatic structures and ascend to the lateral and medial thalamus *(6,7,9,10)*.

The lateral thalamus is composed of the ventroposterolateral, ventroposteromedial, and ventroposteroinferior nuclei. Cells of the lateral thalamus relay information to the primary somatosensory cortex and, possibly, to the secondary somatic cortex. Some evidence exists to suggest that visceral information projects to the somatosensory cortex *(11–13)*. Information processed in this cortical area appears to contribute sensory discrimination *(14,15)*.

Ascending pathways carrying visceral and somatic information also project to the medial thalamus, consisting primarily of the centralis lateralis and centrum medianum–parafascicularis nuclei *(16–18)*. These nuclei send information to the association cortex, including the insular cortex, amygdala, and cingulate gyrus *(19–22)*. These nuclei may be primarily responsible for the motivational affective components of pain, including autonomic adjustments *(14,23–25)*.

3.1. Common Pain of Angina Pectoris: Chest and Arm

Generally, three main clinical characteristics are associated with angina pectoris: (1) Nociceptive information from the heart is generally felt as pain in somatic structures innervated by the same spinal segments that innervate the heart (26); (2) This pain is referred to proximal and axial body structures but generally not to distal limbs (27); (3) The pain is generally deep and aching, not a superficial or cutaneous pain (28). This subsection will address the studies to explain the possible neurophysiological mechanisms that contribute to pain associated with myocardial ischemia.

3.1.1. Convergence

Electrical stimulation of cardiopulmonary afferent fibers strongly excites about 80% of the STT cells in the T1–T6 segments (29) and 60% of the neurons in the C5–C6 segments (Fig. 1). These same cells receive convergent input from the overlying chest and arms. Chemical stimulation of the heart with algesic chemicals, such as bradykinin, activate cardiac afferent fibers that excite STT cells in the T1–T5 spinal segments (7,10) (Fig. 2). These same cells also receive convergent input from afferent fibers innervating somatic structures. In contrast to thoracic and mid-cervical STT cells, cells in the cervical enlargement (C7 and C8) receive very little, if any, input from stimulation of cardiopulmonary afferent fibers (Fig. 1B); their somatic innervation is from the distal forelimb and hand. This lack of visceral activation of cells most likely means that pain would not be referred to the distal forelimb and head; this fits with clinical observations (30–32). Because cardiopulmonary fibers enter the spinal cord primarily in the upper thoracic segments and they do not excite C7–C8 STT cells, the afferent input must be dependent on other routes to activate the C4–C6 STT cells. For example, cardiopulmonary afferent fibers from upper thoracic segments may activate a propriospinal pathway that makes direct or indirect synaptic connections with upper cervical STT cells (33). Another route may be afferent branches of the T2 and T3 sympathetic fibers that travel in the zone of Lissauer for several segments. This suggestion is based on the observation that visceral afferents branch for long distances as they send collaterals into the gray matter (34). This

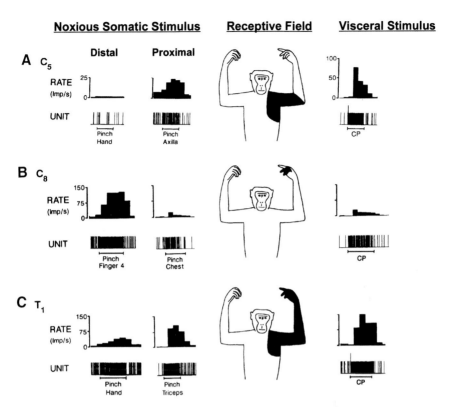

Fig. 1. Segmental organization of STT cells based on their responses to noxious somatic stimuli, somatic receptive fields, and electrical stimulation of the cardiopulmonary afferent fibers (visceral stimulus). (A), (B), and (C) represent STT cells in the C4–C6, C7–C8, and T1–T5 segments, respectively. Upper tracings in each panel are the discharge rate of the cells in impulses per second (imp/s) and the lower panels represent extracellular action potentials after passing through a window discriminator. The rate delayed unit activity by 1 s because action potentials were collected in 1-s bins. Horizontal bars in each panel are the stimulus periods. Somatic receptive fields are represented by black areas on monkey figures.

innervation is less likely because this would mean that collaterals would abruptly stop their innervation of the cervical enlargement. It is possible that neurochemical messages from these cells during development may prevent collaterals from forming in these segments, but, at present, this is speculation. In summary, convergence of visceral and

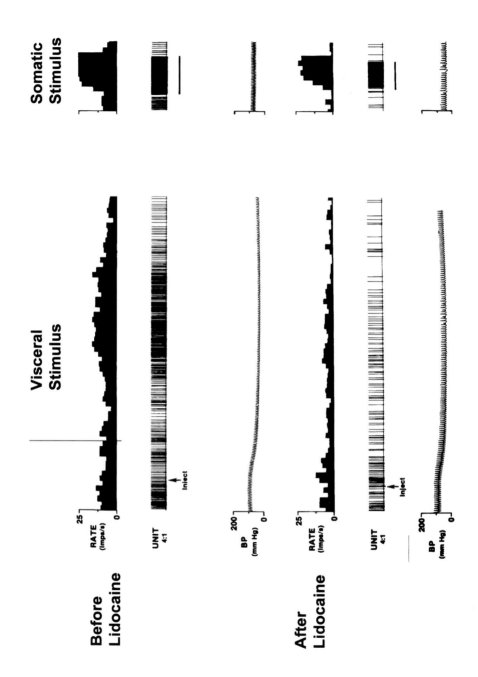

Visceral Stimulus

Somatic Stimulus

Before Lidocaine

RATE (Imps/s)

25

0

UNIT 4:1

Inject

BP (mm Hg)

200

0

After Lidocaine

RATE (Imps/s)

25

0

UNIT 4:1

Inject

BP (mm Hg)

200

0

somatic input onto a common pool of STT cells provides a substrate for explaining the referral of pain to somatic structures.

3.1.2. Proximal and Axial Referral

Neurophysiological observations support human studies that angina pectoris is most commonly felt in the proximal and axial regions of the left arm and chest. The frequency distribution of angina pectoris shows that pain radiates from the chest more than 95% of the time and radiates 30–60% of the time to the left proximal shoulder. Less frequently, pain is felt further down the arm *(31,35,36)*. Stimulation of the cardiopulmonary afferent fibers strongly excites approximately 80% of the STT cells with proximal somatic receptor fields, but only weakly excites 35% of the cells with distal somatic input *(29)* (Fig. 3). Thus, there is a highly significant relationship of cells with excitatory visceral input and proximal axial fields.

3.1.3. Muscle-like Pain

Angina pectoris is a pain that is described as deep, diffuse, dull, and suffering. These same sensations are often expressed for muscle pain. In contrast, cutaneous pain is usually sharp and well focused. Similarities between muscle

Fig. 2. *(opposite page)* Convergence of visceral and somatic input onto a T_3 STT cell. Before lidocaine, bradykinin (0.4 µg/kg) representing the visceral stimulus was injected into the heart via the left atrial appendage. The top tracing in each panel is the discharge rate of the cell in impulses per second (imp/s), the middle tracing is extracellular action potentials after passing through a window discriminator, and the bottom tracing is blood pressure (PB in mm Hg). Arrows indicate when bradykinin was injected. Activity increased after approximately a 20-s delay. The somatic stimulus was a noxious pinch to skin and muscle. The fall in blood pressure did not contribute to the response because an equivalent fall in blood pressure using nitropresside did not elicit a cell response. The lower panel shows that the cell response to bradykinin was eliminated after 2% lidocaine was perfused over the heart to anesthetize cardiac receptors. The cell was still responsive to the somatic input after lidocaine. The bar under the somatic stimulus is the duration of the pinch.

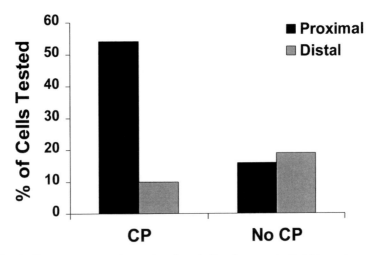

Fig. 3. Comparisons of proximal and distal somatic field locations with cardiopulmonary (CP) afferent input onto STT cells. Cells responding to CP input were much more likely to have somatic input from proximal fields ($p < 0.001$) than cells with distal inputs. All STT cells were tested to determine if they were activated by cardiopulmonary stimulation.

pain and visceral pain were shown in patients suffering from angina pectoris *(28)*. Patients were asked to compare pain provoked by a hypertonic saline solution injected into the muscles surrounding the interspinus ligament of the left eighth cervical or first thoracic spinal segment with their angina pectoris. These patients stated that the onset, continuation, segmental localization, and character very closely mimicked anginal pectoris *(28)*. Further evidence for interactions between muscle and visceral organs is the referred muscle hyperalgesia resulting from a diseased visceral organ *(37)*. Calculosis of the upper urinary tract leads to the development of muscular hyperalgesia in patients, with less involvement of overlying cutaneous structures *(38,39)*. These clinical observations are supported by experimental studies. Noxious stimulation of the ureter results in muscular hyperalgesia and central sensitization of dorsal horn cells *(40–42)*. These results are from pelvic structures, but very likely hyperalgesia also results from angina pectoris.

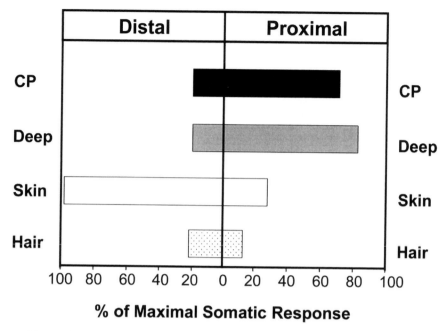

Fig. 4. Comparison of STT activity with electrical stimulation cardiopulmonary afferent fibers and manipulation of distal (left panel) and proximal (right panel) somatic receptive fields. The Percentage of maximal somatic response is the fraction of the largest response of STT cells from any of the somatic areas tested with noxious pinch and hair movement. Distal receptive fields were on the hand and lower arm. The proximal fields were on the chest and upper arm. Responses were classified as visceral from cardiopulmonary (CP) afferent input, muscle (deep), cutaneous pinch (skin) and hair movement (hair).

Our work also supports the interaction between muscle and visceral inputs. The STT cells excited by visceral stimuli are more likely to be excited with deep input (i.e., muscle input than responses to cutaneous input) *(29,43)*. To test the hypothesis, responses of STT cells were recorded from the thoracic segments of the primate during stimulation of cardiopulmonary afferent fibers. These same STT cells were also tested for somatic input by pinching the skin and muscle of somatic receptive fields in the hands and the proximal arm and chest (Fig. 4). Muscle stimulation most powerfully excited STT cells that receive input primarily from the proximal arm and chest region. Their response reaches 88% of the maximal somatic response that can be elicited from all neurons with proximal somatic input. Cutaneous stimulation alone only achieves less than 33% of the maximal somatic response for cells with proximal fields. Cells with proximal somatic fields are strongly excited during cardiopulmonary afferent stimulation, with their activity reaching approximately 70% of the maximal somatic response. In contrast, pinching the skin alone on the hand and fingers generates the greatest responses in STT cells, and these responses do not increase when skin and muscle are pinched together. The STT cells with distal cutaneous fields were minimally excited by cardiopulmonary afferent fiber stimulation. These results provided evidence that visceral input from cardiopulmonary afferents converged most commonly with muscle afferent input onto the same STT cells, whereas the visceral stimulus has little effect on STT cells with primarily cutaneous input. Because visceral afferents converge on STT cells with afferent input from deep tissue, visceral pain, such as that resulting from myocardial ischemia, mimics muscle pain. Thus, pain is felt predominantly as a deep or localized suffering pain, generally in proximal structures such as muscles, tendons, and ligaments.

3.2. Uncommon Pain of Angina Pectoris: Neck and Jaw Pain

A less common feature of angina pectoris is pain referred to the neck and jaw region (31). This pain sometimes remains or even appears after surgical sympathectomy is used to reduce the incidence of refractory angina pectoris (44–46). This pain was attributed to transmission of nociceptive information in vagal afferent fibers, which are commonly thought to transmit innocuous sensory information. Neurophysiological studies show that stimulation of vagal and sympathetic afferent fibers (Fig. 5) and chemical stimulation of the heart excite STT neurons in the C1–C3 segments (47,48). Vagal stimulation serves as a much more potent stimulus than cardiopulmonary afferent fibers (Fig. 5). Vagal stimulation mark-

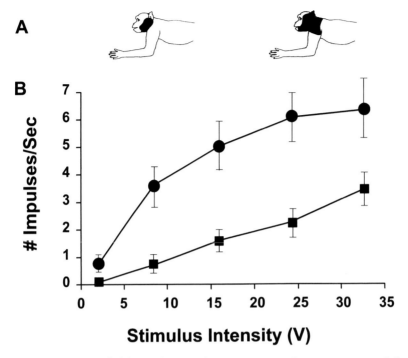

Fig. 5. Somatic fields and stimulus–response characteristics of thoracic vagal (●) and cardiopulmonary (■) afferent fibers converging on C1–C2 STT cells. Blackened areas on the monkey figures are representative of the common locations of somatic receptive fields for C1–C2 STT cells. The top curve in **(B)** shows the effects of varying stimulus intensity (2–33 V, 1 Hz, 0.1 ms, single pulse or two pulses 3 ms apart) for the vagus nerve. Data (means ±SE, $n = 14$) are numbers of impulses per second produced in the first peak of peristimulus histograms (50 sweeps). The bottom curve in (B) shows the effects of varying stimulus intensity for stimulation of cardiopulmonary afferent fibers with the same parameters and information described for the vagus except $n = 9$.

edly increases the cell activity, and the C-fiber input was more commonly observed with vagal stimulation than cardiopulmonary afferent stimulation. Somatic receptive fields for these C1–C3 STT neurons are most commonly on the neck, jaw, ear, and upper arm (Fig. 5). Overlapping terminations of primary afferent fibers from different regions could explain why the receptive fields of the head and upper body have variable locations. Although cardiopulmonary afferent input seems to play a subordinate role, this pathway nevertheless excites neurons in the C1–C3 segments. These cells are a long distance from the entry zone of the cardiac afferent fibers; that is, primarily the T2–T6 dorsal root ganglia (2,49). It is possible that the cardiac information is conducted via a propriospinal pathway. As we showed that transection of the ventrolateral quadrants in rats eliminates the cardiac input to the C1–C3 spinal neurons, most likely a propriospinal pathway is involved in the transmission of cardiac information (50). Such a pathway carrying visceral information very likely also exists in the monkey. This is based on the evidence that excitory responses of the T1–T5 STT cells are attenuated or abolished after the ventrolateral quadrant of the spinal cord near the T7 segment is cut (51). Thus, it is likely that a pool of neurons in the C1–C3 segments of the spinal cord provide a neural substrate for referred pain originating from the heart and perceived in the neck and jaw region.

4. Other Ascending Pathways for Transmitting Visceral Information

4.1. The Anterolateral Pathways

The anterolateral quadrant of the spinal cord also contains other ascending tracts that may transmit noxious information to the regions of the brain important for pain perception (52–54). One such pathway projects to the parabrachial region of the pons that may serve as an important relay for visceral nociceptive information. Cell bodies for this pathway are primarily from lamina I and terminate in the lateral parabrachial area (55–58). Cells receiving this input project to the amygdala (59), the ventromedial nucleus of the thalamus, and the retrochiasmatic area of the hypothalamus (60). This system might contribute to the emotional-affective behavioral and autonomic reactions to noxious events.

Other pathways, including the spinoreticular pathway (61), the spinomesncephalic (62,63), the spinosolitary (64), and spinohypothalamic tract (65) may all be involved with conveying information from the heart, but much less information is known about the visceral responsiveness of these pathways. Future studies will help us determine how these particular pathways contribute to the overall cardiac pain experience that is felt during myocardial ischemia.

4.2. The Dorsal Column Pathway

For years, the dorsal column pathway was characterized as a route that transmitted innocuous somatic and, to a less extent, visceral information. Recent evidence shows that dorsal column pathways play a role in transmitting nociceptive visceral information, specifically from pelvic organs (66–70). Patients are relieved of their pelvic cancer pain after a small lesion is made in the midline of the dorsal column at the T10 spinal level (71). In animal studies, gentle or noxious stimulation of reproductive organs or noxious colorectal distension excites gracile nucleus neurons that most likely reach this pathway via the postsynaptic dorsal column pathway (10,66). Colorectal responses of cells in the ventroposterolateral nucleus of the rat thalamus are reduced after a limited dorsal column lesion, showing that visceral input can be transmitted via the dorsal columns (67). Much less work has been done for the afferent input from the heart to the dorsal columns and thalamus. Recordings from neurons of the ventroposterolateral nucleus of the thalamus show that both the STT and dorsal column pathways play a role in transmitting information from the heart and thoracic region to the thalamus (72). Thus, multiple ascending pathways transmit visceral information, but the coded messages resulting from action potentials that are transmitted in each pathway must be evaluated to understand how each one contributes to the sculpting of visceral sensation in the brain (72). We have shown that activation of cardiopulmonary afferent fibers elicited significantly fewer evoked action potentials at a shorter latency in fewer cuneothalamic neurons compared to the evoked activity of STT cells. Furthermore, most cuneothalamic neurons respond primarily to non-noxious somatic stimuli, whereas STT neurons respond primarily or solely to noxious pinching of somatic fields. Thus, differences in neuronal

responses to noxious stimulation of cardiopulmonary afferent fibers show that a dorsal column pathway and the ventrolateral pathways to the ventroposterolateral thalamus may
play distinct roles in the transmission and integration of pain
associated with coronary artery disease. Much more work
needs to be done to understand how these different contributions can explain the characteristics of cardiac pain.

5. Central Sensitization of Visceral Afferent Information

Injured visceral organs have the potential to send signals that continually bombard neurons in the spinal gray
matter. This bombardment could activate mechanisms in
spinal cells that provide a functional substrate for hyperal-
gesic states resulting from visceral disease. Previous studies
have examined central sensitization for somatic components,
but the visceral studies lag behind (73). Central sensitization
has been studied in organs other than the heart, but it is
included here because this type of sensitization may occur
with ischemic heart disease. In humans, repeated noxious
balloon distensions of the colorectal region gradually increase
pain sensitivity and expand overlying somatic areas of pain
referral (74). Recordings from neurons in animal models support the findings observed in human studies. Somatic receptive fields expand for spinal neurons receiving input from
noxious stimulation of the gallbladder, but not for those cells
receiving only somatic input (75). Thus, the conditioning visceral stimulus is selective, because only those neurons
responsive to a visceral afferent input change their sensitization to somatic input. An additional important characteristic of these responsive neurons is that referred pain tends
to outlast the duration of the noxious visceral stimulus. This
observation correlates well with the clinical experience that
hyperalgesia is felt after the painful episode is passed. These
results raise the possibility that central sensitization of STT
cells and neurons in the gray matter could intensify the pain
experience resulting from cardiac pain.

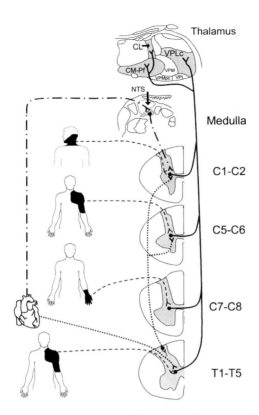

Fig. 6. *(continued on opposite page)* Schematic diagram of neural mechanisms that could explain referred pain characteristics of angina pectoris. The solid black (⎯⎯) line originating in the spinal gray matter and ending in the thalamus represents the spinothalamic tract cells from different segments of the spinal cord. Blackened areas on the figures are representative somatic receptive fields and the broken lines (. . .) are somatic nerves. The (– – –) line represents the cardiopulmonary afferent fibers that enter the T1–T5 spinal segments and the ascending pathway that bypasses C7–C8 segments and enters upper cervical segments. The (.__.__.__.) line is the vagus nerve that synapses in the nucleus tractus solitarius of the medulla, and then descends to the C1–C2 segments. CL: Nucleus, centralis lateralis; CMPf: centrum medianum parafascicular nucleus; VPI: ventral posteroinferior nucleus; VPLc: ventral posterolateral nucleus, caudal part; VPM: ventral posteromedial nucleus; VPMpc: ventral posteromedial nucleus, parvocellular part; NTS: nucleus tractus solitarius.

6. Summary

In summary, afferent input from the heart excites STT cells in the thoracic and upper cervical segments of the spinal cord (Fig. 6). These cells received convergent input from the overlying somatic structures. Thus, this information forms the basis for understanding the pain resulting from ischemic heart disease. However, the huge variations in the expression of pain of overlying somatic structures and silent ischemia raise important issues about how information is processed, modulated, and perceived. These variations could occur in the intrinsic and extrinsic ganglia, the dorsal root ganglia, neuronal mechanisms in the spinal cord, and descending pathways from supraspinal structures.

Acknowledgments

The author gratefully acknowledges Carrie Hulka for typing the manuscript and Patrick Whelan for the illustrations. The work of the author was supported by grants HL227321, HL52986, and NS35471 from the National Institutes of Health.

References

1. Heberden, W. (1772) Some account of a disorder of the breast. *Med. Trans.* **2,** 59–67.
2. Kuo, D. C., Oravitz, J. J., and de Groat, W. C. (1984) Tracing of afferent and efferent pathways in the left inferior cardiac nerve of the cat using retrograde and transport of horseradish peroxidase. *Brain Res.* **321,** 111–118.
3. Vance, W. H. and Bowker, R. C. (1983) Spinal origins of cardiac afferents from the region of the left anterior descending artery. *Brain Res.* **258,** 96–100.
4. Trevino, D. L. (1976) The origin and projections of a spinal nociceptive and thermoreceptive pathway, in *Sensory Functions of the Skin* (Zotterman, Y., ed.), Pergamon, Elmsford, NY, pp. 367–77.
5. Apkarian, A. V. and Hodge, C. J., Jr. (1989) Primate spinothalamic pathways II. The cells of origin of the dorsolateral and ventral spinothalamic pathways. *J. Comp. Neurol.* **288,** 474–492.
6. Ammons, W. S., Girardot, M.-N., and Foreman, R. D. (1985) T_2–T_5 spinothalamic neurons projecting to medial thalamus with viscerosomatic input. *J. Neurophysiol.* **54,** 73–89.
7. Ammons, W. S., Girardot, M.-N., and Foreman, R. D. (1985) Effects of intracardiac bradykinin on T_2–T_5 medial spinothalamic cells. *Am. J. Physiol.* **249,** R147–R152.
8. Willis, W. D., Kenshalo, D. R., and Leonard, R. B. (1979) The cells of origin of the primate spinothalamic tract. *J. Comp. Neurol.* **188,** 543–74.

9. Blair, R. W., Weber, R. N., and Foreman, R. D. (1981) Characteristics of primate spinothalamic tract neurons receiving viscerosomatic convergent inputs in T_3–T_5 segments. *J. Neurophysiol.* **46,** 797–811.
10. Blair, R. W., Weber, R. N., and Foreman, R. D. (1982) Responses of thoracic spinothalamic neurons to intracardiac injection of bradykinin in the monkey. *Circ. Res.* **51,** 83–94.
11. Bruggemann, J., Shi, T., and Apkarian, A. V. (1997) Viscero-somatic neurons in the primary somatosensory cortex (SI) of the squirrel monkey. *Brain Res.* **756(1–2),** 297–300.
12. Follett, K. A. and Dirks, B. (1994) Characterization of responses of primary somatosensory cerebral cortex neurons to noxious visceral stimulation in the rat. *Brain Res.* **656(1),** 27–32.
13. Chandler, M. J., Hobbs, S. F., Fu, Q.-G., Kenshalo, D. R., Blair, R. W., and Foreman, R. D. (1992) Responses of neurons in ventroposterolateral nucleus of primate thalamus to urinary bladder distention. *Brain Res.* **571,** 26–34.
14. Melzack, R. and Wall, P. D. (1982) *The Challenge of Pain.* Basic Books, New York.
15. Price, D. D. and Dubner, R. (1977) Neurons that subserve the sensory-discriminative aspects of pain. *Pain* **3,** 307–338.
16. Boivie, J. (1979) An anatomical reinvestigation of the termination of the spinothalamic tract in the monkey. *J. Comp. Neurol.* **186,** 343–370.
17. Mehler, W. R., Feferman, M. E., and Nauta, W. J. H. (1960) Ascending axon degenerating following anterolateral cordotomy. An experimental study in the monkey. *Brain* **83,** 718–751.
18. Craig, A. D. and Dostrovsky, J. O. (1997) Processing of nociceptive information at supraspinal levels, in *Anesthesia: Biologic Foundations* (Yaksh, T. L., ed.), Lippincott-Raven, Philadelphia, pp. 624–642.
19. Bentivoglio, M., Macchi, C., and Albanese, A. (1981) The cortical projections of the thalamic intralaminar nuclei as studies in cat and rat with the multiple-fluorescence retrograde tracing technique. *Neurosci. Lett.* **26,** 5–10.
20. Berendse, H. W. and Groenewengen, V. H. (1991) Restricted cortical termination fields of the midline and intralaminar thalamic nuclei in the rat. *Neuroscience* **42,** 73–102.
21. Herkenham, M. (1980) Laminar organization of thalamic projections to the rat neocortex. *Science* **207,** 532–535.
22. Sadikot, A. F., Parent, A., and Francois, C. (1990) The center median and parafascicular thalamic nuclei project respectively to the sensorimotor and associate limbic striatal territories in the squirrel monkey. *Brain Res.* **510,** 161–65.
23. Albe-Fessard, D. and Besson, J. M. (1973) Convergent thalamic and cortical projections. The nonspecific system, in *Handbook of Sensory Physiology* (Iggo, A., ed.), Springer-Verlag, Berlin, pp. 489–560.
24. Casey, K. L. and Jones, E. G. (1978) Supraspinal mechanisms: an overview of ascending pathways: brainstem and thalamus. *Neurosci. Res. Prog. Bull.* **16,** 103–118.

25. Melzack, R. and Casey, K. L. (1968) Sensory, motivational and central control determinants of pain, in *The Skin Senses* (Kenshalo, D. R. ed.), Charles C Thomas, Springfield, IL, pp. 423–443.

26. Ruch, T. C. (1961) Pathophysiology of pain, in *Neurophysiology* (Ruch, T. C., Patton, H. D., Woodbury, J. W., and Towe, A. L., eds.), W. B. Saunders, Philadelphia, pp. 350–368.

27. Bonica, J. J. (1990) *Management of Pain.* Lea & Febiger, London, pp. 133–179.

28. Lewis, T. (1942) *Pain.* Macmillan, New York.

29. Hobbs, S. F., Chandler, M. J., Bolser, D. C., and Foreman, R. D. (1992) Segmental organization of visceral and somatic input onto C_3–C_6 spinothalamic tract cells of the monkey. *J. Neurophysiol.* **68,** 1575–1588.

30. Harrison, T. R. and Reeves, T. J. (1968) Patterns and causes of chest pain, in *Principles and Problems of Ischemic Heart Disease.* YearBook Medical, Chicago, pp. 197–204.

31. Sampson, J. J. and Cheitlin, M. D. (1971) Pathophysiology and differential diagnosis of cardiac pain. *Prog. Cardiovasc. Dis.* **23,** 507–531.

32. Procacci, P. and Zoppi, M. (1989) Heart pain, in *Textbook of Pain.* Churchill Livingstone, Edinburgh, pp. 410–419.

33. Nowicki, D. and Szulczyk, P. (1986) Longitudinal distribution of negative cord dorsum potentials following stimulation of afferent fibres in the left inferior cardiac nerve. *J. Auton. Nerv. Syst.* **18,** 185–197.

34. Sugiura, Y., Terul, N., and Hosoya, Y. (1989) Difference in distribution of central terminals between visceral and somatic unmyelinated (C) primary afferent fibers. *J. Neurophysiol.* **62,** 834–840.

35. Bennet, J. R. and Atkinsson, M. (1966) The differentiation between oesophageal and cardiac pain. *Lancet* **ii,** 1123–1127.

36. Sylvén, C. (1989) Angina pectoris. Clinical characteristics, neurophysiological and molecular mechanisms. *Pain* **36,** 145–167.

37. Giamberardino, M. A., Valente, R., and Vecchiet, L. (1993) Muscular hyperalgesia of renal/ureteral origin, in *New Trends in Referred Pain and Hyperalgesia* (Giamberardino, M. S., Vecchiet, L., Albe-Fessard, D., and Lindblom, L., eds.), Elsevier, Amsterdam, pp. 149–160.

38. Giamberardino, M. A., de Bigotina, P., Martegiani, C., and Vecchiet, L. (1994) Effects of extracorporal shock-wave lithotripsy on referred hyperalgesia from renal/ureteral calculosis. *Pain* **56,** 77–83.

39. Vecchiet, L., Giamberardino, M. A., Dragani, L., and Albe-Fessard, D. (1989) Pain from renal ureteral calculosis: evaluation of sensory thresholds in the lumbar area. *Pain* **36,** 289–295.

40. Giamberardino, M. A., Dalal, A., Valente, R., and Vecchiet, L. (1996) Changes in activity of spinal cells with muscular input in rats with referred muscular hyperalgesia from ureteral calculosis. *Neurosci. Lett.* **203,** 89–92.

41. Giamberardino, M. A., Valente, R., Affaitati, G., and Vecchiet, L. (1997) Central neuronal changes in recurrent visceral pain. *Int. J. Clin. Pharm. Res.* **17(2/3),** 63–66.

42. Laird, J. M. A., Roza, C., and Cervero, F. (1996) Spinal dorsal horn neurons responding to noxious distension of the ureter in anesthetized rats. *J. Neurophysiol.* **76(5)**, 3239–3248.
43. Foreman, R. D. (1993) Spinal mechanisms of referred pain, in *New Trends in Referred Pain and Hyperalgesia* (Giamberardino, M. A., Vecchiet, L., Albe-Fessard, D., and Lindblom, U., eds.), Elsevier, Amsterdam, pp. 47–57.
44. Lindgren, I. and Olivercrona, H. (1947) Surgical treatment of angina pectoris. *J. Neurosurg.* **4**, 19–39.
45. Meller, S. T. and Gebhart, G. F. (1992) A critical review of the afferent pathways and the potential chemical mediators involved in cardiac pain. *Neuroscience* **48(3)**, 501–524.
46. White, J. C. and Bland, E. F. (1948) The surgical relief of severe angina pectoris. Methods employed and end results in 83 patients. *Medicine* **27**, 1–42.
47. Chandler, M. J., Zhang, J., and Foreman, R. D. (1996) Vagal, sympathetic and somatic sensory inputs to upper cervical (C_1–C_3) spinothalamic tract neurons in monkeys. *J. Neurophys.* **76(4)**, 2555–2567.
48. Chandler, M. J., Zhang, J., and Foreman, R. D. (1995) Pericardial injections of inflammatory chemicals excite upper cervical (C_1–C_3) spinothalamic tract (STT) cells in monkeys. *Soc. Neurosci.* **21(1)**, 260.4 (abstract).
49. Hopkins, D. A. and Armour, J. A. (1989) Ganglionic distribution of afferent neurons innervating the canine heart and cardiopulmonary nerves. *J. Auton. Nerv. Syst.* **26**, 213–222.
50. Zhang, J., Chandler, M. J., Miller, K. E., and Foreman, R. D. (1997) Cardiopulmonary sympathetic afferent input does not require dorsal column pathways to excite C_1–C_3 spinal cells in rats. *Brain Res.* **771**, 25–30.
51. Ammons, W. S., Blair, R. W., and Foreman, R. D. (1984) Greater splanchnic excitation of primate T_1–T_5 spinothalamic neurons. *J. Neurophysiol.* **51**, 592–603.
52. White, J. C. and Sweet, W. M. (1969) *Pain and the Neurosurgeon. A Forty-Year Experience.* Charles C Thomas, Springfield, IL, p. 560.
53. Vierck, C. J., Greenspan, J. D., Ritz, L. A., and Yeomans, D. C. (1986) The spinal pathways contributing to the ascending conduction and the descending modulation of pain sensations and reactions, in *Spinal Afferent Processing* (Yaksh, T. L., ed.), Plenum, New York, pp. 275-329.
54. Gybels, J. M. and Sweet, W. H. (1989) Neurosurgical treatment of persistent pain. physiological and pathological mechanisms of human pain. Karger, Base. *Pain and Headache*, vol 11, (Gildenberg, P. L., ed.), pp.
55. Blomqvist, A., Ma, W., and Berkley, K. J. (1989) Spinal input to the parabrachial nucleus in the cat. *Brain Res.* **480**, 29–36.

56. Cechetto, D. F., Standaert, D. G., and Saper, C. B. (1985) Spinal and trigeminal dorsal horn projections to the parabrachial nucleus in the rat. *J. Comp. Neurol.* **240,** 153–160.

57. McMahon, S. B. and Wall, P. D. (1985) Electrophysiological mapping of brainstem projections of spinal cord lamina I cells in the rat. *Brain Res.* **333,** 19–26.

58. Panneton, W. M. and Burton, H. (1985) Projections from the paratrigeminal nucleus and the medullary and spinal dorsal horn to the perabrachial area in the cat. *Neuroscience* **15,** 779–798.

59. Bernard, J. F., Huang, G. F., and Besson, J. M. (1994) The parabrachial area: electrophysiological evidence for an involvement in visceral nociceptive processes. *J. Neurophysiol.* **71,** 1646–1660.

60. Bester, H., Menendez, L., Besson, J. M., and Bernard, J. F. (1995) Spino (trigemino) parabrachiohypothalamic pathway: electrophysiological evidence for an involvement in pain processes. *J. Neurophysiol.* **73,** 568–585.

61. Foreman, R. D., Blair, R. W., and Weber, R. N. (1984) Viscerosomatic convergence onto T_2–T_4 spinoreticular, spinoreticular–spinothalamic, and spinothalamic tract neurons in the cat. *Exp. Neurol.* **85,** 597–619.

62. Yezerski, R. P. and Broton, J. C. (1991) Functional properties of spinomesencephalic tract (SMT) cells in the upper cervical spinal cord of the cat. *Pain* **45,** 187–196.

63. Yezierski, R. P. and Schwartz, R. H. (1986) Response and receptive-field properties of spinomesencephalic tract cells in the cat. *J. Neurophysiol.* **55,** 76–96.

64. Ménétrey, D. and Basbaum, A. I. (1987) Spinal and trigeminal projections to the nucleus of the solitary tract: a possible substrate for somatovisceral and viscerovisceral reflex activation. *J. Comp. Neurol.* **255,** 439–450.

65. Burstein, R. (1996) Somatosensory and visceral input to the hypothalamus and limbic system. *Prog. Brain Res.* **107,** 257–267.

66. Al-Chaer, E. D., Lawand, N. B., Westlund, K. N., and Willis, W. D. (1996) Pelvic visceral input into the nucleus gracilis is largely mediated by the postsynaptic dorsal column pathway. *J. Neurophysiol.* **76(4),** 2675–2690.

67. Al-Chaer, E. D., Lawand, N. B., Westlund, K. N., and Willis, W. D. (1996) Visceral nociceptive input into the ventral posterolateral nucleus of the thalamus: a new function for the dorsal column pathway. *J. Neurophysiol.* **76(4),** 2661–2674.

68. Al-Chaer, E. D., Westlund, K. N., and Willis, W. D. (1997) Sensitization of postsynaptic dorsals column neuronal responses by colon inflammation. *NeuroReport* **8(15),** 3267–3273.

69. Apkarian, A. V., Brüggemann, J. S. T., and Airapetian, L. R. (1995) A thalamic model for true and referred visceral pain, in *Visceral*

Note: M = male; F = female; CAD = coronary artery disease shown at angiography; RCA = right coronary artery; LAD = left anterior descending coronary artery; Cx = left circumflex coronary artery; diag = diagonal branch of LAD; 3V = three vessel coronary artery disease; new R occ = new occlusion of the right coronary artery; CABG = coronary artery bypass grafting; ETT = exercise treadmill test; + = ETT positive for ischemic changes; ECG = electrocardiogram; RBBB = right bundle branch block; old inf Qs = old inferior lead Q waves; dob = at peak effect of dobutamine infusion; √ST = ST segment depression; √T = T-wave inversion; inferolat = inferolateral; LBBB = left bundle branch block; HR = heart rate; SBP = systolic blood pressure; DBP = diastolic blood pressure; RPP = heart rate × systolic pressure product; Max dose dob = maximal dose of dobutamine; RWMA = echocardiographic regional wall motion abnormality; ant/lat = anterolateral; ant/ap = anteroapical; inf = inferior; inf/bas = inferobasal; lat = lateral; inf/lat = inferolateral; post/sep = posteroseptal.

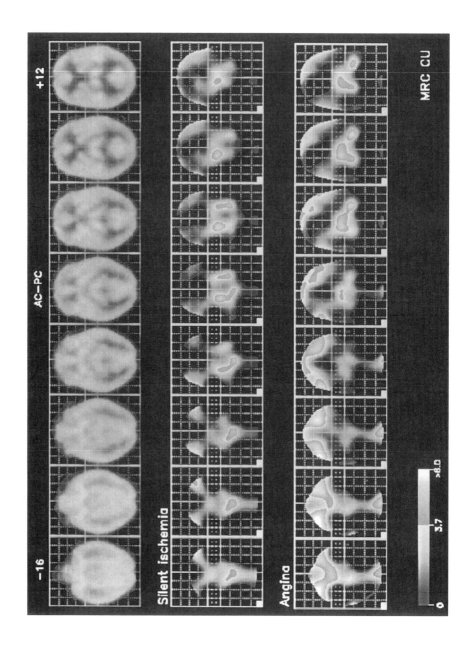

of painless events is estimated at ~30% *(32–36)*. Silent ischemia often coexists with painful ischemia in the same patient; this common observation precludes any simple explanation related to the particular characteristics of an individual patient.

Clinically, silent myocardial ischemia is important because of its association with a poor prognosis (e.g., after an episode of unstable angina *(33–37)* or myocardial infarction *(38,39)*. Most dramatically, silent ischemia has been assumed in patients in whom sudden cardiac death is the first presentation of coronary artery disease *(40)*. Silent ischemia has also been found during exercise in cardiac arrest survivors and in patients with life-threatening arrhythmias *(41)*.

The pathophysiological basis of silent ischemia has not been established. From the observation *(35)* that in stable angina, the number of painless episodes of ST segment depression can far exceed the number of painful ones, it was hypothesized that silent myocardial ischemia represented less severe ischemia *(33,35,36,42,43)*. A more recent study *(44)*, however, which assessed the significance of chest pain in coronary artery disease patients with a high *a priori* likelihood of inducible ischemia, found that the differences in objective measurements of ischemia (using ambulatory ECG monitoring and thallium-201 SPECT exercise testing) between patients with angina and silent ischemia patients were insignificant. The higher incidence in diabetics *(45)* implicated

---

Fig. 1. *(opposite page)* Cerebral areas activated during angina pectoris and silent ischemia. The top row shows averaged blood flow maps from all subjects and all conditions normalized into a standard stereotactic space. These pictures can be used for anatomical localization of the activation foci. The latter are displayed as statistical parametric maps in the same stereotactic anatomical space shown in the above averaged blood flow maps. Results for the silent ischemia patients are shown in the middle row and results for the angina pectoris patients are shown in the bottom row. The magnitude of the Z scores is displayed for both patients groups according to the same linear color scale (threshold for significance: 3.7). AC–PC indicates the intercommissural plane. Distances are expressed in millimeters from this reference (AC–PC) plane.

Table 2
Coordinates of Loci of Maximal Increases
in rCBF During Angina Pectoris

Brain region	Left				Right			
	x	y	z	Z score	x	y	z	Z score
Lateral basal frontal cortex	−32	26	−16	6.2	22	26	−8	5.7
Extrastriate cortex					2	−94	−4	5.3
Mesial orbitofrontal cortex	−8	56	0	4.6	8	54	−4	4.2
Ventral cingulate cortex	−14	8	−20	4.3	12	6	−16	4.4
Hippocampal gyrus	2	−6	8	4.7	28	−38	8	5.2
Thalamus	−10	−18	4	4.7	28	−38	8	5.2
Hypothalamus	−6	−2	−20	4.7				

Note: This table eports the coordinates in the x, y, and z axes of the significant rCBF increases with reference to the stereotactic space defined by the atlas of Talairach and Tournoux (26). Statistical magnitudes are expressed as Z scores. In addition to the loci presented, an additional brainstem locus, [−8 −36, −20; Z score 3.5] was found when the data were analyzed according to omnibus significance with 0.01 threshold. It was not included in the main table as it did not reach significance at the Bonferroni level.

peripheral neuropathy in the process; differences in autonomic nerve function have also been described in nondiabetic patients with silent myocardial ischemia (46). Conversely, silent ischemia can be shown in many nondiabetics with no evidence of neuropathy. With the discovery of the brain's endogenous opiate system (47), a higher pain threshold because of enhanced central opiate activity offered an explanation for the silence of silent myocardial ischemia. However, the opiate studies, often having been based on plasma β-endorphin measurements, have been equivocal (42,48–53). In addition, psychological and personality factors may play a role in the perception of angina (54).

With this background, we proceeded to study a series of patients with "pure" silent myocardial ischemia (i.e., no pain experienced despite reproducible ECG and echo signs of ischemia) according to the same study protocol as for our angina study *(see* Subheading 3.1.*).* A particular aspect of the angina study that encouraged us toward the study of patients with silent ischemia was the finding of persistence of thalamic activation after the cessation of the symptoms and signs of myocardial ischemia, inviting the hypothesis that editing [a phenomenon akin to gating *(55)*] of painful signals may occur at the thalamic level.

3.2.1. Study Population

Nine right-handed male patients (age 62 [7] yr) with significant CAD were studied. Five patients had three-vessel disease, two patients had two-vessel disease, and two patients had undergone previous coronary bypass grafting but had recently developed occlusion of important grafts. Eight of the patients were identified during the investigation of exertional breathlessness; in two of these cases, this symptom (breathlessness) was found in patients who had previously undergone coronary artery bypass surgery for breathlessness, mild angina, and reduced effort tolerance. One patient had previously sustained an inferior myocardial infarction. All exhibited painless myocardial ischemia demonstrable by the development of ischemic electrocardiographic changes and new regional wall motion abnormalities during dobutamine stress echocardiography in the complete absence of chest pain. As mentioned, none of the nine silent ischemia patients displayed a "mixed" clinical picture (i.e., of angina on some occasions and painless ischemia on others). Resting ventricular function was normal in all patients except the one who had sustained the infarct; in him, infero-lateral hypokinesia could be seen. No patient in either group was diabetic or had any systemic disease.

3.2.2. PET Scanning Protocol

The same protocol as that described earlier was employed to make the same six rCBF measurements. However, because of the absence of pain accompanying the ECG changes as an indication of myocardial ischemia, we were particular to include stress echocardiography during the scanning sequence as a means of demonstrating unequivocal ischemia in this patient group. An echocardiogram (using a Challenge 7000 echocardiograph, Esaote Biomedica, Florence, Italy) was recorded before the start of PET scanning and optimal echocardiographic views were chosen on the basis of the previous stress echocardiogram as those that best showed the development of a new wall motion abnormality. A brief echo was performed before each scan to allow for the effects of pressure of the transducer on the anterior chest wall. During the dobutamine infusion, ischemia was confirmed electrocardiographically and echocardiographically. In all silent ischemia patients, chest pain was obligatorily absent, however, awareness of an increase in heart rate and/or force of contraction was no obstacle to inclusion in the study.

3.2.3. Analysis of PET Images

This was performed as for the angina study presented earlier. The magnitude of rCBF changes induced by silent myocardial ischemia were compared to the mean of baselines 1 and 2. In addition, the rCBF changes induced by placebo and low-dose dobutamine were compared to baseline and, finally, rCBF in the postischemic phase (baseline 3) was compared to baselines 1 and 2 combined.

3.2.4. Results

3.2.4.1. CLINICAL OBSERVATIONS

No chest pain or other sensations of note were reported during the baseline scans, the placebo infusion, or the low-dose dobutamine infusion. During the high-dose dobutamine infusion, seven of the silent ischemia patients were aware of a rapid and more forceful heart beat, one patient experienced slight warmth of the chest wall, and one experienced no unusual sensations at all. All of the patients denied that any of the sensations they felt were in any way painful or uncomfortable. In all cases, the occurrence of silent myocardial ischemia was confirmed electrocardiographically and by the development of a new regional wall motion abnormality during real-time two-dimensional echocardiography. The final scan, baseline 3, was performed in all cases after the complete return of the echocardiogram and electrocardiogram to baseline.

3.2.4.2. Hemodynamic Effects
of the High-Dose Dobutamine Infusion

The silent ischemia patients received comparable doses of intravenous dobutamine for the induction of myocardial ischemia to those administered to the angina patients. There were significant increases in heart rate, systolic blood pressure, and product of heart rate and systolic blood pressure (rate–pressure product) in the silent ischemia patients, but the changes were comparable to those in the angina patients. The time to significant ischemic electrocardiographic changes and the extent of such changes were also comparable between the silent ischemia patients and the earlier group of patients with angina pectoris. The data are presented in detail in Table 1.

3.2.4.3. PET Findings

During myocardial ischemia, rCBF increased bilaterally in the brainstem, thalamus, hippocampal gyrus, and, to a lesser extent, the right and left dorsal and right lateral basal frontal cortical areas. (Fig. 1 and Table 3). The low-dose dobutamine infusion, although not producing echocardiographic or electrocardiographic changes of myocardial ischemia, was associated with a small increase in rCBF bilaterally in the thalami (Z scores, 4.7 [left] and 4.3 [right]) and in the left hippocampal and right anterior cingulate cortices (Z scores, 4.7 and 3.9, respectively). The placebo infusion produced a small activation in the right frontal cortex (Z score, 3.8). A comparison of the postischemic scan, baseline 3, to the previous baseline scans showed persistent increases in left thalamic and dorsal frontal cortical rCBF (Z scores, 3.8 and 3.9, respectively).

*3.2.5. A Comparison of Angina Pectoris
and Silent Ischemia*

After separate analysis of the PET data from the two patient groups, a direct comparison of the silent ischemia and

Table 3
Coordinates of Loci of Maximal Increases
in rCBF During Silent Myocardial Ischemia

Brain region	Left				Right			
	x	y	z	Z score	x	y	z	Z score
Lateral basal frontal cortex					36	24	−12	3.9
Hippocampal gyrus	−14	−40	0	4.1				
Dorsal frontal cortex	−2	−2	52	4.8				
Thalamus	−16	−20	4	4.9	22	−24	4	3.9
Cerebellum	0	−48	−16	4.0				

Note: This table reports the co-ordinates in the x, y, and z axes of the significant rCBF increases, with reference to the stereotactic space defined by the atlas of Talairach and Tournoux (26). Statistical magnitudes are expressed as Z scores.

angina pectoris data was performed. Differences between the two patient groups with respect to the areas of increased rCBF during myocardial ischemia were computed as interactions between the between-group factors (angina versus silent ischemia) and the within-group conditions (myocardial ischemia versus baselines 1 and 2). As the interaction effect could be predicted by the main effect (myocardial ischemia—baselines 1 and 2) in each group, a less harsh statistical threshold ($p < 0.01$, without Bonferroni correction) was used for the statistical maps.

An overall comparison of the results for myocardial ischemia/angina versus baseline in the two patient groups showed that angina was associated with greater rCBF increases bilaterally in the anterior and ventral cingulate cortex, mesial orbitofrontal, and basal frontal cortex and left temporal pole (Figs. 1 and 2 and Table 4).

3.2.6. Discussion: Angina Pectoris and Silent Ischemia

We believe that the areas identified in the angina study constitute the central components mediating perception of pain from the heart. An important finding was that thalamic

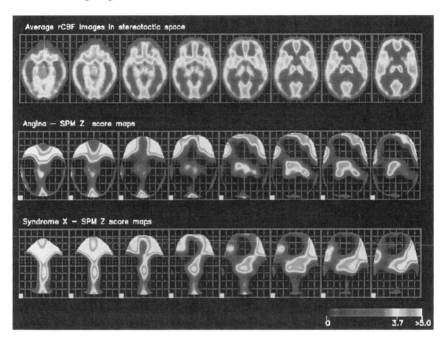

Fig. 2. Cerebral areas activated during chest pain in patients with syndrome X (bottom row) and angina pectoris resulting from coronary artery disease (middle row). The top row shows averaged blood flow maps from all subjects and all conditions normalized into a standard stereotactic space. These pictures can be used for anatomical localization of the activation foci. The latter are displayed as statistical parametric maps in the same stereotactic anatomical space shown in the above averaged blood flow maps. The magnitude of the Z scores is displayed for both patients groups according to the same linear color scale (threshold for significance: 3.7). AC–PC indicates the intercommissural plane. Distances are expressed in millimetres from this reference (AC–PC) plane.

but not frontal cortical activity persisted through the post angina scan, possibly indicating that the thalamus continues to receive inputs from the heart after angina ceases to be felt. However, although the thalamus is active, this less intense signal is not transmitted to the cerebral cortex and, consequently, conscious perception of angina does not occur. The silent ischemia study showed that during silent myocardial ischemia, significant rCBF increases are observed in subcorti-

Table 4

Coordinates of Loci of Significant Differences in Maximal
rCBF Increases During Myocardial Ischemia between Patients
with Angina Pectoris and Patients with Silent Myocardial Ischemia

Brain region	Left				Right			
	x	y	z	Z score	x	y	z	Z score
Mesial orbitofrontal cortex	−6	50	−4	3.2				
Basal frontal cortex	−4	18	−20	2.9				
Anterior cingulate cortex	−16	42	−4	2.8	6	42	−4	3.4
Ventral cingulate cortex	−12	22	−16	2.9	6	18	−16	2.7
Anterior temporal pole	−36	10	−20	3.4				

Note: This table reports the coordinates in the x, y, and z axes of the significant differences in rCBF increases between the patient groups. (Coordinates refer to the atlas of Talairach and Tournoux (26)]. Statistical magnitudes are expressed as Z scores. In this table, $Z > 2.3$ reflects $p < 0.01$. The table includes the temporal lobe locus, not included in Table 3 because although the omnibus significance of the result was $p < 0.001$, this did not withstand the more rigorous Bonferroni correction employed for all the other loci. It has been included in this table because of the adequate significance of its result according to the interaction test ([angina—baseline 2] – [placebo—baseline 1]).

cal structures, but that the degree and extent of cortical activation in silent ischemia is slight compared to overt cardiac pain. In the latter, a much more extensive pattern of activation was observed, especially at the cortical level in the ventral cingulate and basal frontal cortices. In the silent ischemia patients, as in those with angina pectoris, thalamic activity persisted through the postischemic scan.

These findings—that an equivalent stress on the hearts of silent ischemia patients produced the same degree of thalamic activation, but significantly less cortical activation, especially with respect to the anterior and ventral cingulate and basal frontal cortices—show that afferent stimuli from the heart *do* reach the central nervous system in patients with silent ischemia; that is, the absence of sensation of chest pain is unlikely to be the result of failure of transmission by the peripheral nerves. The results point to a difference in the central nervous handling of the afferent signals from the heart in the silent ischemia patients. One hypothesis to account for this would be editing or "gating" (55) of afferent stimuli at the thalamic level.

The differences between the silent ischemic and angina patients were, principally, the absence of activation of the basal frontal and anterior and ventral cingulate cortices and left temporal pole. Now, the two patient groups were closely matched with respect to resting ventricular function, dobutamine dose, hemodynamic changes as a result of dobutamine, and time to onset of, and extent of, ischemia. Therefore, it might be reasonable to suggest that as far as could be determined, the threshold for myocardial ischemia was similar in both groups.

The anterior cingulate has been associated with emotional responses to pain (56) and it has documented connections to the nucleus of the solitary tract (5–7,57), to the dorsal motor nucleus of the vagus, and to the sympathetic thoracic intermediolateral cell column (5–7,58). In addition, it is known from studies on the rhesus monkey that there are connections between the frontal cortex and the anterior cingulate (59,60). That perception of chest pain involves the cingulate cortex is, therefore, entirely consistent with current neuroanatomical data. A potential regulatory role for the frontal cortex (modifying the emotional response to angina in the light of previous subjective experience of it) is also possible.

Investigation of both patient groups indicated that the thalamus continues to receive inputs from the heart after the cessation of myocardial ischemia, consistent with the observation that metabolic disturbances continue in the heart hours after ischemia has apparently resolved (28). Presumably, the less intense signal is not transmitted further because it is below the necessary threshold (the Z scores for thalamic activation at this stage were substantially lower than during myocardial ischemia).

One hypothesis concerning silent ischemia referred to earlier (33,35,36,42,43) is that silent myocardial ischemia is merely milder than that which produces angina pectoris. This is not supported by our data, in which the silent ischemia patients had coronary artery disease of comparable if not greater severity (more vessels were diseased per patient) than the angina pectoris group. The maximal dobutamine dose and the increase in cardiac work produced by the latter were equivalent for the two patient groups. Finally, the fact that in the silent ischemia patients, even low-dose dobutamine infusion evoked a significant bilateral increase in thalamic rCBF, might suggest that there was a ready induction of myocardial ischemia in this patient group.

Our findings suggest that a stimulus of comparable intensity can induce myocardial ischemia, which, in certain circumstances (i.e., those that make the ischemia silent), may or may not be associated with a painful sensation. We are clearly far from being able to predict the code of afferent stimuli that represents an adequate algogenic signal. This absence of predictability might reflect a complex pattern of afferent impulses related to mechanical and/or chemical stimulation rather than the relatively simple involvement of a specific nociceptive pathway (61). It could still be claimed that the afferent signals that reach the thalamus during myocardial ischemia in silent ischemia patients (and which we assume to be gated from further transmission) are not painful signals but are proprioceptive inputs from mechanoceptors in the myocardium. In addition, as far as is known, there are no nerve endings in the myocardium whose specific function is the mediation of pain signals (61). If it were the case that proprioceptive inputs to the heart can be shown to be increased during silent myocardial ischemia, it would give further support to the argument that cardiac nociception depends on the intensity of general afferent signals from the heart rather than a specific pain pathway [the "intensity" rather than the 'specificity' theory of cardiac pain mediation (61)]. Our study does not address the precise mechanism of operation of the gating that we hypothesise to occur in the thalamus. Further research at the neurotransmitter level might elucidate this.

Table 5 *(continued)*

Syndrome X Patients' and Normal Controls' Characteristics, Hemodynamics, and Pain Responses

Patient	SBP (dob)	DBP (rest)	DBP (dob)	RPP (rest)	RPP (dob)	Max dose dob	Pain score	P; (L]
(a) Syndrome X								
1	130	80	60	10,150	18,200	30	6	
2	155	75	100	9800	18,600	25	9	
3	145	70	100	9100	17,400	30	9	
4	190	90	100	11,220	26,600	25	9	
5	153	60	95	7200	13,311	20	9	
6	120	65	95	8100	12,840	25	8	
7	197	70	113	11,200	26,792	25	8	
8	160	70	90	7800	16,640	45	3	
Mean (SD)	156 (27)	73 (9)	73 (13)	9321 (1531)	18,798 (5310)	28 (8)	7.6 (2.0)	1.6
(b) Normal controls								
1	116	77	75	9576	13,920	30	0	
2	138	63	94	7920	14,904	35	0	
3	117	67	59	10,120	15,912	30	0	
4	176	73	88	8946	21,120	30	1	
5	198	74	88	9222	22,272	25	1	
6	231	118	101	9672	18,480	25	0	
7	169	89	74	14,420	20,111	25	0	
8	173	65	70	8880	21,798	25	0	
Mean (SD)	165 (40)	78 (18)	81 (14)	9033 (1730)	17,060 (5394)	28 (4)	0.25 (0.46)	

Note: M = male; F = female; ECG = electrocardiogram; RBBB = right bundle branch block; old inf Qs = old inferior lead Q waves; d(peak effect of dobutamine infusion; √ST = ST segment depression; √T = T-wave inversion; Nonspec T = nonspecific ST-segment ch Nonsp ST/T inf = nonspecific ST- and T-wave changes in the inferior leads; HR = heart rate; SBP = systolic blood pressure; DBP = di blood pressure; RPP = heart rate × systolic pressure product; Max dose dob = maximal dose of dobutamine; LDD = low dose dobutal

The syndrome X patients all experienced severe chest pain in the high-dose dobutamine infusion scan. The pain was accompanied by rectilinear or down-sloping ST-segment depression ≥0.1 mV on the ECG. Three out of eight syndrome X patients experienced chest pain during the low-dose dobutamine infusion; one syndrome X patient felt chest pain during the placebo infusion.

3.3.4.3. PET FINDINGS

During the chest pain provoked by high-dose dobutamine, rCBF increased in the hypothalamus, cerebellum, thalamus (bilaterally), lateral orbitofrontal cortex bilaterally, right insula, and right premotor cortex (Table 6). Low-dose dobutamine produced an increase in rCBF in the right thalamus (18, –36, 4; Z=4.26) and right prefrontal cortex (46, 26, 8; Z=4.44). In baseline 3, the scan performed after the cessation of chest pain, rCBF was found to be still increased in the left thalamus (–20, –26, 8; Z=4.09). There were no differences in rCBF between the placebo infusion and the resting state.

3.3.4.4. SECONDARY COMPARISON OF SYNDROME X PET RESULTS WITH DATA FROM PATIENTS WITH ANGINA PECTORIS RESULTING FROM CORONARY ARTERY DISEASE

An overall comparison of the results for the dobutamine scans versus baseline in the syndrome X and CAD patient groups showed that during high-dose dobutamine, rCBF was significantly greater in the right insula in the syndrome X patients. To a lesser extent, the rCBF changes in the cerebellum, right thalamus, left orbitofrontal, right dorsal frontal, and bilateral prefrontal cortices were also significantly greater in the syndrome X patients (Fig. 2). During the low-dose dobutamine infusion, rCBF changes were significantly greater in the midbrain and right prefrontal and orbitofrontal cortices in the syndrome X patients (Table 7).

3.4. Normal Subjects

In addition to the above studies of patients, we have investigated a population of normal volunteers to estab-

Table 6

Coordinates of Loci of Maximal Increases in rCBF During Chest Pain
as a Result High-Dose Dobutamine in Syndrome X Patients

Brain region	Left				Right			
	x	*y*	*z*	Z score	*x*	*y*	*z*	Z score
Lateral orbitofrontal cortex	−28	26	−20	7.0	24	30	−20	7.24
Right insula					40	20	4	3.5
Premotor cortex	−56	6	20	4.6				
Thalamus	−22	−32	8	4.1				
Hypothalamus	−2	−6	−24	7.1				
Brainstem	−4	−96	−24	4.6				

Note: This table reports the coordinates in the *x*, *y*, and *z* axes of the significant rCBF increases, with reference to the stereotactic space defined by the atlas of Talairach and Tournoux (26). Statistical magnitudes are expressed as Z scores.

Table 7

Coordinates of Loci of Significant Differences
in Maximal rCBF Increases During Chest Pain Between Patients
with Syndrome X and Patients with Coronary Artery Disease

Brain region	Left				Right			
	x	*y*	*z*	Z score	*x*	*y*	*z*	Z score
Lateral orbitofrontal cortex	−28	18	−16	3.2	24	18	−20	2.9
Insula					34	2	12	4.8
Globus pallidus					24	−6	4	3.8
Thalamus					16	−6	0	3.6
Cerebellum					8	−54	−20	3.6

Note: This table reports the coordinates in the *x*, *y*, and *z* axes of the significant differences in rCBF increases between the patient groups. [Coordinates refer to the atlas of Talairach and Tournoux (26). Statistical magnitudes are expressed as Z scores. In this table, Z>2.3 reflects $p < 0.01$.

lish the central neural correlates of the dobutamine stress in health.

3.4.1. Study Population

Eight normal subjects were studied (five female, age 56 [11]; p = NS versus the syndrome X or the CAD patients). All these volunteers gave no history of cardiac or pulmonary disease, had no risk factors for coronary artery disease, and had normal resting and stress electrocardiograms and normal effort tolerance.

3.4.2. PET Scanning Protocol

The identical scanning protocol was followed for the normal controls, except that for this study we were able to use a Siemens 953B positron tomograph *(98)* (Erlangen, FRG) with intravenously infused $H_2{}^{15}O$ (infused at 10 mL/min and 55 MBq/mL activity over 2 min). For ethical reasons (the radiation exposure using the 953B scanner was approx 5.5 mSv compared to slightly more than 12 mSv for the same protocol performed on the 931-081/12 scanner), the studies of all the control subjects were performed on the 953B scanner. However, the method of analysis permitted a direct comparison of the various data sets. All subjects had the same series of measurements as the patient groups had undergone.

3.4.3. Analysis of PET Images

This process was essentially the same as the analyses described earlier.

3.4.4. Results

3.4.4.1. HEMODYNAMIC EFFECTS
OF THE HIGH-DOSE DOBUTAMINE INFUSION

The controls received comparable doses of intravenous dobutamine to those received by both the CAD and the syndrome X patients. There were significant increases in heart rate, systolic blood pressure, and RPP both at rest and during the peak dobutamine dose in both groups, but the changes were comparable to those of the patient groups. The data are presented in detail in Table 5.

3.4.4.2. SYMPTOMS EXPERIENCED

The controls described awareness of strong and fast heart beat (4/8) ± neck or throat tightness (2/8), shortness of breath (1/8), or no different sensation (2/8). Their ECGs remained

Table 8
Coordinates of Loci of Maximal Increases
in rCBF During High-Dose Dobutamine in Normal Controls

Brain region	Left				Right			
	x	y	z	Z score	x	y	z	Z score
Lateral orbitofrontal cortex	−24	40	0	3.9				
Anterior pole of temporal lobe	−38	20	−28	6.9	22	20	−28	7.3
Insula	−28	−6	20	5.9				
Dorsal cingulate cortex	−8	−30	36	5.2				
Thalamus	−22	−32	16	5.1	22	−38	8	3.9
Cerebellum	−40	−90	−30	4.7				

Note: This table reports the coordinates in the x, y, and z axes of the significant rCBF increases, with reference to the stereotactic space defined by the atlas of Talairach and Tournoux (26). Statistical magnitudes are expressed as Z scores.

normal. No controls experienced chest pain during the low-dose dobutamine infusion or during the placebo.

3.4.4.3. PET Findings

During high-dose dobutamine, the controls showed increases in rCBF in left cerebellum, bilaterally in the thalami, in the left dorsal cingulate and left insular cortices, and bilaterally in the anterior pole of the temporal lobes and in the orbitofrontal cortices (Table 8). Low-dose dobutamine produced an increase in rCBF in the right thalamus (14, −38, 12; Z=3.93), left orbitofrontal cortex (−38, 20, −28; Z=4.38), and right anterior temporal pole (28, 22, −24; Z=5.16). In baseline 3, rCBF was found still to be mildly increased in the left thalamus (18, −34, 8; Z=3.71).

3.4.4.4. Comparison of Areas of Activation Between Syndrome X Patients and Controls

The changes in rCBF evoked by high-dose dobutamine compared to baseline (the main effect studied) were noted and the findings for the syndrome X patients and the controls were contrasted. The areas in which comparable effects

Table 9
Coordinates of Loci of Maximal Increases
in rCBF During High-Dose Dobutamine Infusion, Common
to Both the Syndrome X Patients and to the Normal Control Subjects

Brain region	Left				Right			
	x	y	z	Z score	x	y	z	Z score
Lateral orbitofrontal cortex	−24	36	−16	6.70	24	34	−16	7.33
Anterior pole of temporal lobe	−34	20	−28	7.63	40	22	−20	7.27
Medial parietal cortex	−8	66	36	5.87				
Thalamus	−22	−30	8	5.62	18	−28	12	4.25
Hypothalamus	0	−6	−28	7.62				

Note: This table reports the coordinates in the x, y, and z axes of the significant rCBF increases with reference to the stereotactic space defined by the atlas of Talairach and Tournoux *(26)*. Statistical magnitudes are expressed as Z scores. Ant = anterior.

upon rCBF were found in both groups are listed in Table 9. However, the contrast showed significant differences for the right insular cortex (40, 20, 4; Z=4.7) and left orbitofrontal cortex (−28, 32, −16; Z=3.6), where rCBF changed during the main effect in patients but not in controls (Fig. 3) Conversely, significant differences were found for the anterior/mid cingulate cortex bilaterally ([−28, −6, 20; Z=4.7] and [18, 26, 16; Z=4.7]), in controls but not in patients.

3.4.5. Discussion

Considering the main effect investigated in the study of syndrome X patients and of controls, namely dobutamine stress compared to baseline, we have found comparable effects in both syndrome X patients and in normal controls for rCBF in the hypothalamus, thalami, right frontal cortex, and the anterior poles of the temporal poles. However, the contrast between the groups showed significant differences for the right insular cortex and left orbitofrontal cortex, where rCBF changed during the main effect in patients but not in controls. Conversely, significant differences were found for

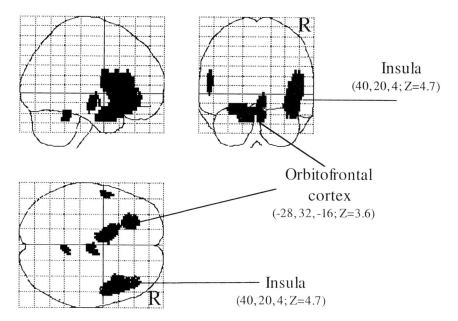

Fig. 3. Cerebral regions activated during high-dose dobutamine infusion in patients with syndrome X, but not activated in normal controls. The changes in rCBF evoked by high-dose dobutamine compared to baseline (the main effect studied) were noted and the findings for the patients and the controls were contrasted. This SPM{Z} map shows the areas (the right insular cortex [40, 20, 4; Z=4.7] and left orbitofrontal cortex [−28, 32, −16; Z=3.6]) where rCBF changed during the main effect in patients but not in controls. R = right; coordinates in the x, y, and z axes refer to the stereotactic space defined by the atlas of Talairach and Tournoux (26).

the anterior/mid cingulate cortex bilaterally in controls but not in patients. As noted in Subheading 3.3.4.4., a secondary comparison with our earlier published data from patients with angina as a result of CAD showed significant differences between the syndrome X patients and the CAD patients with respect to rCBF in the right insula and, to a lesser extent, the cerebellum, right thalamus, and bilaterally the prefrontal and orbitofrontal cortices.

3.4.5.1. Methodological Considerations:
The Effects of Dobutamine on the Study Groups

The dobutamine was administered in very similar doses to all groups and had comparable hemodynamic effects.

Symptomatically, each group behaved according to type: the normal subjects experienced a more powerful heart beat but were free of frank pain; the syndrome X patients, despite the absence of (echocardiographic) correlates of myocardial ischemia, all developed severe chest pain that persisted for many minutes after discontinuation of the dobutamine; and the symptomatic CAD patients developed quite severe chest pain, associated with regional wall motion abnormality on echo but that rapidly resolved on cessation of the dobutamine.

Associated with these clinical responses, the patterns of brain activation evoked show a commonality with respect to activation of the hypothalamus, the thalami, and parts of the prefrontal and frontal cortices. It, therefore, might be hypothesized that the cardiac afferent nerve → thalamus → prefrontal and frontal cortex pathway is common to all three groups. Alternatively, this pattern might be attributable to a common, nonspecific pharmacological effect of dobutamine upon these brain regions. However, it should be borne in mind that dobutamine (a β_1 agonist which acts by increasing cardiac work) does not cross the blood-brain barrier (24), precluding a direct pharmacological effect on central neurones. With regard to an indirect effect of dobutamine causing alteration of cerebral blood flow, this point might be refuted by our findings in the silent ischemia study. In the latter, comparable thalamic activation was demonstrated to that in the angina pectoris patients, but there was only trivial cerebral cortical activation in the silent ischemia patients; again, the dose of dobutamine administered to each group was equivalent.

A further feature of the use of dobutamine stress was the opportunity it afforded to assess the effects on regional myocardial function, a sensitive index of ischemia. In all the syndrome X patients, left ventricular function was normal at rest and unchanged, or even enhanced during dobutamine stress. In contrast, patients with CAD showed the development of regional wall motion abnormalities in the territories subtended by stenosed coronary arteries.

3.4.5.2. IMPLICATIONS OF THE PRESENT STUDY FOR THE ETIOLOGY OF CHEST PAIN IN SYNDROME X

As indicated earlier and reviewed extensively elsewhere *(99)*, the case for myocardial ischemia being the cause of chest pain in syndrome X has become severely undermined. In contrast, a number studies have shown many syndrome X patients to have an abnormal sensitivity to stimuli from the heart *(88–90)*, whether in response to mechanical stimulation (inflation of a balloon in the right atrium or injection of the coronary arteries with contrast medium), electrical stimulation (pacing of the right atrium), or pharmacological challenge (intravenous or intracoronary adenosine) *(77,93)*. In view of these demonstrable abnormalities of visceral pain perception, we sought to employ a direct approach to investigate the neurophysiology of chest pain in syndrome X; the study outlined above was the outcome.

There is clearly an extensive commonality between the syndrome X patients and the normal controls with respect to rCBF changes in several cerebral regions (Table 9) including some which have important connections to the limbic system. This is consistent with both study groups sharing the experience of a rapid or powerful heart beat in response to inotropic stimulation by the dobutamine. The distinguishing feature for the syndrome X patients was the perception of severe central chest pain. When the findings for the syndrome X patients were compared to those of our earlier CAD study population (Table 7), left frontal and right insular activation was noticeably greater in the syndrome X patients, despite the absence of any sign of myocardial pathology in the latter group. Thus, the unpleasant sensation of pain in syndrome X is associated with right insula activation beyond that in angina because of CAD and yet it occurs in the absence of any signs of cardiac dysfunction.

The significance of the insular and prefrontal activation during chest pain in syndrome X invites further consideration. Thirty years ago, Luria and Simernitskaya *(100)* proposed a relatively more important role for the right hemisphere in the perception of visceral changes and suggested that feedback loop activity involving this region may be critical for emotional experience. Subsequent physiological and anatomic data have also pointed to the insula being involved in monitoring common visceral sensations and in modifying and integrating autonomic responses (5–7). Animal studies have also demonstrated projections from the insula to the orbitofrontal cortex and to the primary somatosensory cortex. In addition, the former regions have connections to nuclei involved in efferent autonomic activity.

This may account for a number of the findings reported of abnormal autonomic neural activity in patients with syndrome X. Such abnormal autonomic neural regulation in syndrome X would include (1) a blunting of the day–night difference in and (2) an absence of effect of orthostasis on the low frequency (LF) spectral component of heart rate variability, a quantity which reflects sympathetic nervous activity (85). In addition, the discovery of abnormal activation of the right insula and prefrontal cortex may also offer an explanation for the prolongation of maximal corrected QT interval that has been described in syndrome X (101). Oppenheimer et al. have mapped out primary chronotropic areas in both the rat (102) and human (103) insula bilaterally. Stimulation of the right anterior insula was shown to have the greatest effect in producing changes consistent with sympathetic activation. Strokes involving this region have been associated with QT prolongation and an associated excess of life-threatening arrhythmias in patients with such a cerebral lesion (104,105).

Finally, this neurophysiological view of the etiology of chest pain in syndrome X might also account for one outstanding puzzling clinical feature in syndrome, namely the electrocardiographic ST depression during exercise stress. Thus, besides the more obvious common causes of a false-positive exercise ECG (106) [e.g., overactivity of the sympathetic nervous system (80,84–86), abnormal transmembrane potassium flux (107), and hyperventilation (108)], an efferent neural action upon the ECG during chest pain in syndrome X patients might also be hypothesised to contribute to the ECG's "ischemic-like" appearance.

4. Hypothesis

An overall view of the interpretation of signals from the heart might therefore be as follows. Normally, at rest or during physiological exertion, although a continuous stream of afferent stimuli from the heart reach the brain, these do not reach consciousness (i.e., there is no percept). With myocardial dysfunction (e.g., during ischemia in CAD), there is a greater intensity of afferent signaling from the heart and a correspondingly greater extent of cortical activation, such that the chest pain percept is generated. In syndrome X, one might also have expected that the percept of chest pain would be accompanied by extensive cerebral cortical activation and the present study shows this to be so. In fact, the percept of pain in syndrome X is accompanied by greater and more extensive cortical activation than in angina resulting from CAD, despite there being no discernible myocardial pathology. Syndrome X might therefore be thought of as a "top-down" process, a cortical pain syndrome, in contrast with the "bottom-up" generation of a pain percept resulting from myocardial ischemia in CAD.

5. Conclusion

We conclude from these studies that in the patients with coronary artery disease, the central structures activated in angina pectoris but not in silent ischemia constitute the pathways involved in the perception of anginal pain. It is also hypothesised that the thalamus may have a key role in the perception of pain from the heart, acting as a gate to afferent pain signals, with cortical activation being necessary for the sensation of pain. From the silent ischemia study, it might be concluded that altered central nervous handling of afferent signals from the heart (an "overactive gate") contributes to the lack of perception of chest pain in this group of patients. In syndrome X, the right insula activation that exceeds that in angina because of CAD, might point to syndrome X being a "visceral cortical pain syndrome." The application of functional neuroimaging has therefore produced a number of new insights into the etiology of cardiological symptoms and offers the prospect of more to come.

References

1. Opie, L. H. (1991) *The Heart. Physiology and Metabolism.* Raven, New York, pp. 52–66.
2. Hoffman, J. I. E. (1987) Transmural myocardial perfusion. *Prog. Cardiovasc. Dis.* **29,** 429–464.
3. Uren, N. G., Melin, J. A., De Bruyne, B., Wijns, W., Baudhuin, T., and Camici, P. G. (1994) Relation between myocardial blood flow and the severity of coronary artery stenosis. *N. Engl. J. Med.* **330,** 1782–1788.
4. Malliani, A. (1995) The conceptualisation of cardiac pain as a non-specific and unreliable alarm system, in *Visceral Pain,* Progress in Pain Research and Management, vol. 5 (Gebhart, G. F., ed.), IASP, Seattle, WA, pp. 63–74.
5. Spyer, K. M. (1992) Central nervous control of the cardiovascular system, in *Autonomic Failure. A Textbook of Clinical Disorders of the Autonomic Nervous System.* (Bannister, R. and Mathias, C. J., eds.), Oxford University Press, Oxford, pp. 54–77.
6. Cechetto, D. F. (1995) Supraspinal mechanisms of visceral representation, in *Visceral Pain, Progress in Pain Research and Management,* vol. 5 (Gebhart, G. F., ed.), IASP, Seattle, WA, pp. 261–290.
7. Meller, S. T. and Gebhart, G. F. (1992) Visceral pain: a review of experimental studies. *Neuroscience* **48,** 501–524.
8. Mancia, G. and Mark, A. L. (1983) Arterial baroreflex in humans, in *Handbook of Physiology. The Cardiovascular System III* (Shepherd, J. T., Abboud, F. M., and Geiger, S. R., eds.), American Physiological Society, Bethesda, MD, pp. 755–793.
9. Pagani, M., Somers, V., Furlan, R., Dell'Orto, S., Conway, J., Baselli, G., et al. (1988) Changes in autonomic regulation induced by physical training in mild hypertension. *Hypertension* **12,** 600–612.
10. Dampney, R. A. L. (1994) Functional organization of central pathways regulating the cardiovascular system. *Physiol. Rev.* **74,** 323–364.
11. White, J. C. (1957) Cardiac pain. Anatomic pathways and physiologic mechanisms. *Circulation* **16,** 644–655.
12. François-Franck, C. A. (1899) Signification physiologique de la résection du sympathetique dans la maladie de Basedow, l'épilepsie, l'idiotie et le glaucome. *Bull. Acad. Med. Paris* **41,** 565–574.
13. Mannheimer, C., Augustinsson, L. E., Carlsson, C. A., Manhem, K., and Wilhelmsson, C. (1988) Epidural spinal electrical stimulation in severe angina pectoris. *Br. Heart J.* **59,** 56–61.
14. Hill, J. A. and Pepine, C. J. (1986) Myocardial ischaemia and chest pain: a misunderstood and oversimplified relationship? *Cardiol. Clin.* **4,** 621–625.

15. Rosen, S. D., Paulesu, E., Frith, C. D., Jones, T., Davies, G. J., Frackowiak, R. S. J., et al. (1994) Central neural correlates of angina pectoris as a model of visceral pain. *Lancet* **344,** 147–150.

16. Rosen, S. D., Paulesu, E., Nihoyannopoulos, P., Tousoulis, D., Frackowiak, R. S. J., Frith, C. D., et al. (1996) Silent ischaemia as a central problem: regional brain activation compared in silent and painful myocardial ischaemia. *Ann. Intern. Med.* **124,** 939–949.

17. Fox, P. T., Raichle, M. E., Mintun, M. A., and Dence, C. (1988) Nonoxidative glucose consumption during focal physiologic neural activity. *Science* **241,** 462–464.

18. Raichle, M. (1987) Circulatory and metabolic correlates of brain function in normal humans, in *Handbook of Physiology. Section 1: The Nervous System. Vol. V. Higher Functions of the Brain Part 2* (Mountcastle, V. B., Plum, F., and Geiger, S. R., eds.), American Physiological Society, Bethesda, MD, pp. 643–674.

19. Mata, M., Fink, D. G., Ganier, H., Smith, C. B., Davidsen, L., Sawaki, H., et al. (1980) Activity-dependent energy metabolism in rat posterior pituitary primarily reflects sodium pump activity. *J. Neurochem.* **34,** 213–215.

20. Friston, K. J. and Frackowiak, R. S. J. (1991) Imaging functional anatomy, in *Brain Work and Mental Activity, Alfred Benzon Symposium* Vol. 31 (Lassen, N. A. Ingvar, D. H., Raichle, M. E., and Friberg, L., eds.), Munksgaard, Copenhagen, pp. 267–279.

21. Friston, K. J., Frith, C. D., Liddle, P. F., Lammertsma, A. A., Dolan, R. D., and Frackowiak, R. S. J. (1990) The relationship between local and global changes in PET scans. *J. Cereb. Blood Flow Metab.* **10,** 458–466.

22. Friston, K. J., Frith, C. D., Liddle, P. F., and Frackowiak, R. S. J. (1991) Comparing functional (PET) images: assessment of significant change. *J. Cereb. Blood Flow Metab.* **11,** 690–699.

23. Spinks, T. J., Jones, T., Bailey, D. L., et al. (1992) Physical performance of a positron tomograph for brain imaging with retractable septa. *Phys. Med. Biol.* **37,** 1637–1655.

24. Takao, Y., Kamisaki, Y., and Itoh, T. (1992) Beta adrenergic regulation of amine precursor amino-acid transport across the blood-brain barrier. *Eur. J. Pharmacol.* **215,** 245–251.

25. Opie, L. H. (1991) *Drugs and the Heart.* W. B. Saunders, Philadelphia, p. 143.

26. Talairach, J. and Tournoux, P. (1988) *A Co-planar Stereotactic Atlas of the Human Brain.* Thieme, Stuttgart.

27. Friston, K. J., Passingham, R. E., Nutt, J. G., Heather, J. D., Sawle, G. V., and Frackowiak, R. S. J. (1989) Localisation in PET images: direct fitting of the intercommissural (AC–PC) line. *J. Cereb. Blood Flow Metab.* **9,** 690–695.

28. Camici, P. G., Araujo, L. I., Spinks, T., Lammertsma, A. A., Kaski, J. C., Shea, M. J., et al. (1986) Increased uptake of 18F-fluorodeoxyglucose

in postischemic myocardium of patients with exercise-induced angina. *Circulation* **74**, 81–88.

29. Heberden, W. (1772) Some account of a disorder of the breast. *Med. Trans. Roy. Coll. Phys. London* **2**, 59–67.

30. Warren, J. (1812) Remarks on angina pectoris. *N. Engl. J. Med. Surg.* **1**, 1–11.

31. Babey, A. M. (1939) Painless acute infarction of the heart. *N. Engl. J. Med.* **220**, 410–412.

32. Kannel, W. B. and Abbott, R. D. (1984) Incidence and prognosis of unrecognised myocardial infarction. An update on the Framingham study. *N. Engl. J. Med.* **311**, 1144–1147.

33. Epstein, S. E., Quyyumi, A. A., and Bonow, R. O. (1988) Current concepts, myocardial ischemia: silent or symptomatic. *N. Engl. J. Med.* **318**, 1038–1043.

34. Schang, S. J. and Pepine, C. J. (1977) Transient asymptomatic ST segment depression during daily activity. *Am. J. Cardiol.* **39**, 396–402.

35. Deanfield, J. E., Maseri, A., Selwyn, A. P., Ribeiro, P., Chierchia, S., Krikler, S., et al. (1983) Myocardial ischaemia during daily life in patients with stable angina: its relation to symptoms and heart rate changes. *Lancet* **2**, 753–758.

36. Quyyumi, A. A., Mockus, L., Wright, C., and Fox, K. M. (1985) Morphology of ambulatory ST segment changes in patients with varying severity of coronary artery disease: investigation of the frequency of nocturnal ischaemia and coronary artery spasm. *Br. Heart J.* **53**, 186–193.

37. Gottlieb, S. O., Weisfeldt, M. L., Ouyang, P., Mellits, E. D., and Gerstenblith, G. (1986) Silent ischemia as a marker for early unfavorable outcome in patients with unstable angina. *N. Engl. J. Med.* **314**, 1214–1219.

38. Tzivoni, D., Gavish, A., Zin, D., Gottlieb, S., Moriel, M., Keren, A., et al. (1988) Prognostic significance of ischemic episodes in patients with previous myocardial infarction. *Am. J. Cardiol.* **62**, 661–664.

39. Gottlieb, S. O., Gottlieb, S. H., Achuff, S. C., Baumgardner, R., Mellits, E. D., Weisfeldt, M. L., et al. (1988) Silent ischemia on Holter monitoring predicts mortality in high risk post infarction patients. *J. Am. Med. Assoc.* **259**, 1030–1035.

40. Warnes, C. A. and Roberts, W. C. (1984) Sudden coronary death: relation of amount and distribution of coronary narrowing at necropsy to previous symptoms of myocardial ischemia, left ventricular scarring and heart weight. *Am. J. Cardiol.* **54**, 65–73.

41. Hong, R. A., Bhandari, A. K., McKay, C. R., Au, P. K., and Rahimtoola, S. H. (1987) Life threatening ventricular tachycardia and fibrillation induced by painless myocardial ischemia during exercise testing. *J. Am. Med. Assoc.* **257**, 1937–1940.

42. Glazier, J. J., Chierchia, S., Brown, M. J., and Maseri, A. (1986) Importance of generalized defective perception of painful stimuli

as a cause of silent myocardial ischemia in chronic stable angina pectoris. *Am. J. Cardiol.* **58,** 667–672.

43. Chierchia, S., Lazzari, M., Freedman, S. B., Bencivelli, W., and Maseri, A. (1983) Impairment of myocardial perfusion and function during painless myocardial ischemia. *J. Am. Coll. Cardiol.* **1,** 924–930.

44. Klein, J., Chao, S. Y., Berman, D. S., and Rozanski, A. (1994) Is 'silent' myocardial ischemia really as severe as symptomatic ischemia? The analytical effect of patient selection biases. *Circulation* **89,** 1958–1966.

45. Langer, A., Freeman, M., Josse, R., Steiner, G., and Armstrong, P. (1991) Detection of silent myocardial ischemia in diabetes mellitus. *Am. J. Cardiol.* **67,** 1073–1078.

46. Shakespeare, C. F., Katritsis, D., Crowther, A., Cooper, I. C., Coltart, J. C., and Webb-Peploe, M. M. (1994) Differences in autonomic function in patients with silent and symptomatic myocardial ischaemia. *Br. Heart J.* **71,** 22–29.

47. Woolf, C. J. and Wall, P. D. (1983) Endogenous opioid peptides and pain mechanisms: a complex relationship. *Nature* **306,** 739–740.

48. Sheps, D. S., Maixner, W., and Hinderliter, A. L. (1989) Mechanisms of pain perception in patients with silent myocardial ischemia. *Am. Heart J.* **119,** 983–987.

49. Droste, C. and Roskamm, H. (1990) Pain perception and endogenous pain modulation in angina pectoris, in *Silent Myocardial Ischemia: A Critical Appraisal* (Kellerman, J. J. and Braunwald, E., eds.), Advances in Cardiology Vol. 37, Karger, Basel, pp. 142–164.

50. Van Rijn, T. and Rabkin, S. W. (1986) Effect of naloxone on exercise-induced angina pectoris: a randomized, double blind crossover trial. *Life Sci.* **38,** 609–615.

51. Ellestad, M. H. and Kuan, P. (1984) Naloxone and asymptomatic ischemia: failure to induce angina during exercise testing. *Am. J. Cardiol.* **54,** 982–984.

52. Heller, G. V., Garber, C. E., Connolly, M. J., Allen-Rowlands, C. F., Siconolfi, S. F., Gann, D. S., et al. (1987) Plasma β-endorphin levels in silent myocardial ischemia induced by exercise. *Am. J. Cardiol.* **59,** 735–739.

53. Falcone, C., Specchia, G., Rondanelli, R., Guasti, L., Corsico, G., Codega, S., et al. (1988) Correlation between beta-endorphin plasma levels and anginal symptoms in patients with coronary artery disease. *J. Am. Coll. Cardiol.* **11,** 719–723.

54. Barsky, A. J., Hochstrasser, B., Coles, A., Zisfein, J., O'Donnell, C., and Eagle, K. A. (1990) Silent myocardial ischemia: Is the person or the event silent? *J. Am. Med. Assoc.* **264,** 1132–1135.

55. Wall, P. D. (1978) The gate control theory of pain mechanisms. A re-examination and a restatement. *Brain* **101,** 1–18.

56. Neafsey, E. J., Terreberry, R. R., Hurley, K. M., Ruit, K. G., and Frysztak, R. J. (1993) Anterior cingulate cortex in rodents: connec-

tions, visceral control functions and implications for emotion, in *Neurobiology of Cingulate Cortex and Limbic Thalamus: A Comprehensive Handbook* (Vogt, B. A. and Gabriel, M., eds.), Birkhäuser, Boston, pp. 206–223.

57. Terreberry, R. R. and Neafsey, E. J. (1983) Rat medial frontal cortex: a visceral motor region with a direct projection to the solitary nucleus. *Brain Res.* **278,** 245–249.

58. Hurley, K. M., Herbert, H., Moga, M. M., and Saper, C. B. (1991) Efferent projections of the inferolimbic cortex of the rat. *J. Comp. Neurol.* **308,** 249–276.

59. Vogt, B. A. and Pandya, D. N. (1987) Cingulate cortex of the rhesus monkey: II. cortical afferents. *J. Comp. Neurol.* **262,** 271–289.

60. Van Hoesen, G. W., Morecraft, R. J., and Vogt, B. A. (1993) Connections of the monkey cingulate cortex, in *Neurobiology of Cingulate Cortex and Limbic Thalamus: A Comprehensive Handbook* (Vogt, B. A. and Gabriel, M., eds.), Birkhäuser, Boston, pp. 249–284.

61. Malliani, A. (1987) Pathophysiology of ischemic cardiac pain, in *Silent Ischemia* (von Arnim, T. and Maseri, A., eds.), Steinkopff, Darmstadt, pp. 19–24.

62. Jones, A. K. P., Brown, W. D., Friston, K. J., Qi, L. Y., and Frackowiak, R. S. J. (1991) Cortical and subcortical localization of response to pain in man using positron emission tomography. *Proc. Roy. Soc. Lond. B* **244,** 39–44.

63. Talbot, J. D., Marrett, S., Evans, A. C., Meyer, E., Bushnell, M. C., and Duncan, G. H. (1991) Multiple representations of pain in human cerebral cortex. *Science* **251,** 1355–1358.

64. Morecraft, R. J., Geula, C., and Mesulam, M. M. (1992) Cytoarchitecture and neural afferents of orbitofrontal cortex in the brain of the monkey. *J. Comp. Neurol.* **323,** 341–358.

65. Gabriel, M., Kubota, Y., Sparenborg, S., Straube, K., and Vogt, B. A. (1991) Effects of cingulate cortical lesions on avoidance learning and training-induced activity in rabbits. *Exp. Brain Res.* **86,** 585–600.

66. Keefer, C. S. and Resnik, W. H. (1928) Angina pectoris: a syndrome caused by anoxemia of the myocardium. *Arch. Intern. Med.* **41,** 769–807.

67. Cannon, R. O., Camici, P. G., and Epstein, S. E. (1992) Pathophysiological dilemma of syndrome X. *Circulation* **85,** 883–892.

68. Rosen, S. D. and Camici, P. G. (1994) Syndrome X: background clinical aspects, pathophysiology and treatment. *G. Ital. Cardiol.* **24,** 779–790.

69. Epstein, S. E. and Cannon, R. O. (1986) Site of increased resistance to coronary flow in patients with angina pectoris and normal epicardial coronary arteries. *J. Am. Coll. Cardiol.* **8,** 459–461.

70. Cannon, R. O., Schenke, W. H., Leon, M. B., Rosing, D. R., Urqhart, J., and Epstein, S. E. (1987) Limited coronary flow reserve after dipyridamole in patients with ergonovine-induced coronary vasoconstriction. *Circulation* **75,** 163–174.

71. Green, L. H., Cohn, P. F., Holman, B. L., Adams, D. F., and Markis, J. E. (1978) Regional myocardial blood flow in patients with chest pain syndromes and normal coronary arteriograms. *Br. Heart J.* **40**, 242–249.
72. Opherk, D., Zebe, H., Weihe, E., Mall, G., Dürr, C., Gravert, B., et al. (1981) Reduced coronary dilatory capacity and ultrastructural changes in the myocardium in patients with angina pectoris but normal coronary arteriograms. *Circulation* **63**, 817–825.
73. Chauhan, A., Mullins, P. A., Taylor, G., Petch, M. C., and Schofield, P. M. (1993) Effect of hyperventilation and mental stress on coronary blood flow in syndrome X. *Br. Heart J.* **69**, 516–524.
74. Holdright, D. R., Lindsay, D. C., Clarke, D., Fox, K., Poole-Wilson, P. A., and Collins, P. (1993) Coronary flow reserve in patients with chest pain and normal coronary arteries. *Br. Heart J.* **70**, 513–519.
75. Geltman, E. M., Henes, C. G., Sennef, M. J., Sobel, B. E., and Bergman, S. R. (1990) Increased myocardial perfusion at rest and diminished perfusion reserve in patients with angina and angiographically normal coronary arteries. *J. Am. Coll. Cardiol.* **16**, 586–595.
76. Camici, P. G., Gistri, R., Lorenzoni, R., Sorace, O., Michelassi, C., Bongiorni, M. G., et al. (1992) Coronary reserve and exercise ECG in patients with chest pain and normal coronary angiograms. *Circulation* **86**, 179–186.
77. Rosen, S. D., Uren, N. G., Kaski, J.-C., Tousoulis, D., Davies, G. J., and Camici, P. G. (1994) Coronary vasodilator reserve, pain perception and gender in patients with syndrome X. *Circulation* **90**, 50–60.
78. Nihoyannopoulos, P., Kaski, J.-C., Crake, T., and Maseri, A. (1991) Absence of myocardial dysfunction during pacing stress in patients with syndrome X. *J. Am. Coll. Cardiol.* **18**, 1463–1470.
79. Panza, J. A., Laurienzo, J. M., Curiel, R. V., Unger, E. F., Quyyumi, A. A., Dilsizian, V., et al. (1997) Investigation of the mechanism of chest pain in patients with angiographically normal coronary arteries using transesophageal dobutamine stress echocardiography. *J. Am. Coll. Cardiol.* **29**, 293–301.
80. Camici, P. G., Marraccini, P., Lorenzoni, R., Buzzigoli, G., Pecori, N., Perissinotto, A., et al. (1991) Coronary hemodynamics and myocardial metabolism in patients with syndrome X: response to pacing stress. *J. Am. Coll. Cardiol.* **17**, 1461–1470.
81. Rosano, G. M., Kaski, J. C., Arie, S., Pereira, W. I., Horta, P., Collins, P., et al. (1996) Failure to demonstrate myocardial ischaemia in patients with angina and normal coronary arteries. Evaluation by continuous coronary sinus pH monitoring and lactate metabolism. *Eur. Heart J.* **17**, 1175–1180.
82. Tousoulis, D., Crake, T., Lefroy, D., Galassi, A. R., and Maseri, A. (1993) Left ventricular hypercontractility and ST segment depression in patients with syndrome X. *J. Am. Coll. Cardiol.* **22**, 1607–1613.

83. Spinelli, L., Ferro, G., Genovese, A., Cinquegrana, G., Spadafora, M., and Condorelli, M. (1990) Exercise-induced impairment of diastolic time in patients with X syndrome. *Am. Heart J.* **119,** 829–833.

84. Rosano, G. M., Ponikowski, P., Adamopoulos, S., Collins, P., Poole-Wilson, P. A., Coates, A. J. S., et al. (1994) Abnormal autonomic control of the cardiovascular system in syndrome X. *Am. J. Cardiol.* **73,** 1174–1179.

85. Rosen, S. D., Guzzetti, S., Cogliati, C., Lombardi, F., Camici, P. G., and Malliani, A. (1996) Autonomic dysregulation in syndrome X: power spectral analysis of the ambulatory ECG. *J. Amb. Monit.* **9,** 119–131.

86. Rosen, S. D., Boyd, H., Rhodes, C. G., Kaski, J.-C., and Camici, P. G. (1996) Myocardial β-adrenoceptor density and plasma catecholamines in patients with Syndrome X. *Am. J. Cardiol.* **78,** 37–42.

87. Meeder, J. G., Blanksma, P. K., van der Wall, E. E., Willemsen, A. T. M., Pruim, J., Anthonio, R. L., et al. (1997) Coronary vasomotion in patients with syndrome X: evaluation with positron emission tomography and parametric myocardial perfusion imaging. *Eur. J. Nucl. Med.* **24,** 530–537.

88. Shapiro, L. M., Crake, T., and Poole-Wilson, P. (1988) A. Is altered cardiac sensation responsible for chest pain in patients with normal coronary arteries? Clinical observation during cardiac catheterisation. *Br. Med. J.* **296,** 170–171.

89. Cannon, R. O., Quyyumi, A. A., Schenke, W. H., Fananapazir, L., Tucker, E. E., Gaughan, A. M., et al. (1990) Abnormal cardiac sensitivity in patients with chest pain and normal coronary arteries. *J. Am. Coll. Cardiol.* **16,** 1359–1366.

90. Chauhan, A., Mullins, P. A., Thuraisingham, S. I., Taylor, G., Petch, M. C., and Schofield, P. M. (1994) Abnormal cardiac pain perception in syndrome X. *J. Am. Coll. Cardiol.* **24,** 329–335.

91. Lagerqvist, B., Sylvén, C., Beerman, B., Helmius, G., and Waldenstrom, A. (1990) Intracoronary adenosine causes angina pectoris like pain—an inquiry into the nature of visceral pain. *Cardiovasc. Res.* **24,** 609–613.

92. Eriksson, B., Svedenhag, J., Martinsson, A., and Sylvén, C. (1995) Effect of epinephrine infusion on chest pain in syndrome X in the absence of signs of myocardial ischemia. *Am. J. Cardiol.* **75,** 241–245.

93. Lagerqvist, B., Sylvén, C., and Waldenstrom, A. (1992) Lower threshold for adenosine-induced chest pain in patients with angina and normal coronary angiograms. *Br. Heart J.* **68,** 282–285.

94. Picano, E., Lattanzi, F., Masini, M., Distante, A., and L'Abbate, A. (1987) Usefulness of a high dose dipyridamole echocardiography test for diagnosis of syndrome X. *Am. J. Cardiol.* **60,** 508–512.

95. Lucarini, A., Picano, E., Marini, C., Favilla, S., Salvetti, A., and Distante, A. (1992) Activation of sympathetic tone during dipyridamole test. *Chest* **102,** 444–447.

1.2. Local Tissue Renin–Angiotensin Systems

In addition to the synthesis of Ang II as a circulating hormone, Ang II is also synthesized in numerous peripheral tissues (6,7). Moreover, all components of the RAS have been localized in the CNS, including renin, angiotensinogen, ACE and Ang II (6–8), although these components do not always illustrate an overlapping distribution. Immunoreactive renin has been localized to the magnocellular neurons of the paraventricular hypothalamic nucleus (PVN) and the supraoptic nucleus (SON), the median eminence, as well as the posterior pituitary (9). Dzau and colleagues have detected the expression of renin mRNA in the brain (10), further supporting the concept of an independent renin–angiotensin system in the brain. Angiotensinogen expression was localized to the mediobasal hypothalamus by use of antisera directed against rat plasma angiotensinogen, but it was not associated with the PVN or the SON (9). Hybridization histochemistry for angiotensinogen mRNA revealed a more ubiquitous distribution, including the inferior olive, the reticular formation, the nucleus tractus solitarius (NTS), reuniens nucleus, and the superior colliculus, among others (11). Interestingly, the mRNA for angiotensinogen has been found to be associated only with astrocytes, not with neurons. In the brain, ACE activity has been reported to be higher than in plasma and has been localized to the periventricular organs, subfornical organ (SFO) and the area postrema (AP), among others (12). The definitive demonstration for the synthesis of Ang II in the brain was provided by Ganten and colleagues (13). Later studies established that the concentration of Ang II in the brain ranges from femtomoles to picomoles per gram of brain tissue. However, local concentrations of Ang II in some neuronal populations may exceed this amount (12).

1.3. Physiology of the RAS: Peripheral Actions

The actions of Ang II in the periphery and the brain are distinct, yet serve a collective purpose, namely body fluid and cardiovascular homeostasis. In the periphery, Ang II produces a potent constrictor effect on smooth muscle (14), thereby increasing blood pressure. Ang II increases the synthesis and secretion of aldosterone from the adrenal cortex (15). Aldosterone acts upon the renal distal tubule of the kidney to promote sodium reabsorption, which indirectly enhances Ang II-mediated homeostatic processes. At the kidney, Ang II produces vasoconstriction of renal efferent arterioles leading to an increase in filtration fraction, creating an environment that promotes ion and water reabsorption from the tubular lumen into the blood (16,17). Ang II has also been shown to promote sodium and water reabsorption from the small intestine (18,19). Ang II stimulates the release of catecholamines from the adrenal medulla by depolarizing adrenal chromaffin cells (1,20). Moreover, Ang II potentiates the release of norepinephrine from sympathetic nerve terminals (21) and has been reported to increase the synthesis of norepinephrine (1).

1.4. Physiology of the RAS: Ingestive Behaviors

All of the actions of Ang II in the periphery appear to augment the reabsorption of sodium and water, which is essential under physiological or pathophysiological conditions of extracellular volume depletion, such as hemorrhage, dehydration, or sodium depletion. However, in addition to the conservation of body fluids, the central actions of Ang II serve to restore fluid volume by evoking two ingestive behaviors, namely thirst and sodium appetite. The original proposal for a central mechanism in Ang II-induced drinking behavior was provided by Epstein and colleagues, in which they demonstrated that intracerebroventricular (icv) administration of Ang II elicits drinking behavior (22). However, increased circulating levels of hormone may also contribute to Ang II-induced thirst by activating Ang II receptors localized to those neuronal regions lacking a blood-brain barrier (BBB), namely the circumventricular organs (CVOs). The SFO appears to be a major integration center for coordinating Ang II actions in the periphery and the CNS. In this regard, Simpson and colleagues demonstrated that microinjection of Ang II into the SFO elicits drinking *(23,24)*. Furthermore, SFO lesions inhibited drinking responses to peripheral Ang II *(25)*, as did knife cuts of SFO efferents *(26)*. However, icv administration of Ang II produced drinking even in the presence of SFO lesions *(27)*. Jensen et al. have demonstrated that microinjection of Ang II into the PVN produced a drinking response *(28)*. One of the two major SFO efferent pathways projects to the PVN *(29)*. Therefore, increased circulating levels of hormone may activate Ang II receptors expressed in the SFO, which project their signal to the hypothalamus to mediate drinking behavior.

The initial description of sodium appetite induced by Ang II was provided by Fisher and Buggy *(30)*. Epstein and colleagues confirmed and extended these results by demonstrating that continuous central infusions of Ang II stimulates rats to ingest 3% NaCl solutions, as would peripheral administration of renin *(31)*. Fluharty and Epstein later proposed that central Ang II and peripheral mineralocorticoids act in a synergistic fashion in the mediation of sodium appetite *(32)*. Sakai et al. *(33)* reported that central blockade of mineralocorticoid receptors combined with ACE inhibition completely suppressed sodium appetite in sodium-depleted rats. Taken together, these results illustrated that central Ang II and mineralocorticoids are necessary for the arousal of sodium appetite. (*See* Fig. 1.)

2. Characterization of Angiotensin Receptor Subtypes

2.1. Pharmacology of Angiotensin Receptor Subtypes

The multiplicity of responses mediated by Ang II led to the proposal of multiple Ang II receptor subtypes, a hypothesis strengthened by pharmacological data from numerous investigators *(34–37)*. The unequivocal demonstration for the existence of Ang II receptor subtypes came with the development of subtype selective antagonists *(38)*. The nonpeptide antagonist DuP 753, now known as losartan, exhibits high affinity for a population of Ang II binding sites that are now

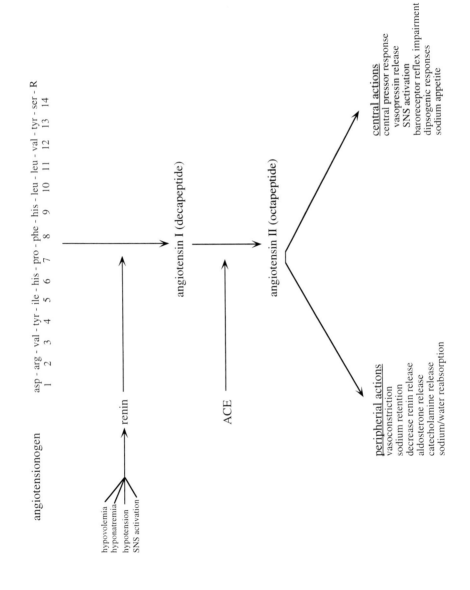

angiotensionogen   asp - arg - val - tyr - ile - his - pro - phe - his - leu - leu - val - tyr - ser - R

1   2   3   4   5   6   7   8   9   10   11   12   13   14

hypovolemia
hyponatremia
hypotension
SNS activation

renin

angiotensin I (decapeptide)

ACE

angiotensin II (octapeptide)

peripherial actions
vasoconstriction
sodium retention
decrease renin release
aldosterone release
catecholamine release
sodium/water reabsorption

central actions
central pressor response
vasopressin release
SNS activation
baroreceptor reflex impairment
dipsogenic responses
sodium appetite

referred to as angiotensin Type 1 or AT_1 receptors. Angiotensin Type 2 (AT_2) receptors have low affinity for losartan but exhibit high affinity for the nonpeptide compound PD 123319 and the peptide compound CGP 42112A. The development of subtype selective antagonists has facilitated the analysis of the cellular and pharmacologic properties of Ang II receptor subtypes, including the localization of AT_1 and AT_2 receptors in the periphery and the CNS.

2.2. Angiotensin Receptor Subtypes and Ingestive Behaviors

Many of the physiological actions of Ang II have been shown to be mediated through the AT_1 receptor subtype, in that these responses are blocked by the AT_1 receptor antagonist losartan. In the CNS, AT_1 receptors expressed in the CVOs respond to circulating Ang II to elicit ingestive behaviors. In this regard, intravenous or subcutaneous administration of losartan has been shown to inhibit Ang II-induced increases in water consumption (39). The Ang II receptor subtypes that contribute to homeostatic mechanisms in the brain beyond the BBB remains much more equivocal. Johnson and colleagues have demonstrated that losartan inhibited the pressor and drinking response induced by icv administration of Ang II, indicating that these responses were mediated through the AT_1 subtype (40). These results were confirmed by Fregly and Rowland, in that losartan blocked Ang II-mediated drinking (41). However, these same investigators later

---

Fig. 1. *(opposite page)* The renin–angiotensin System: synthesis and physiology. Several physiological stimuli lead to the release of renin from the kidney. Upon release into circulation, renin will cleave the prohormone angiotensinogen to the biologically inactive decapeptide, Ang I. The biologically active octapeptide is formed by the actions of angiotensin-converting enzyme (ACE). Once formed, Ang II mediates the physiological effects of the RAS by activating membrane-associated receptors in both the periphery and the CNS. In addition to blood-borne hormone, local renin–angiotensin systems have also been identified in the periphery and the brain. (Adapted from ref. 220.)

reported that the AT_2 receptor antagonist PD 123319 also inhibited Ang II-induced drinking, albeit at higher doses (42). Phillips and colleagues reported that the AT_1 receptor blockade abolished dipsogenic responses, whereas PD 123317 merely attenuated drinking (43). Utilization of antisense oligonucleotides has further examined the role of the AT_1 receptor subtype in Ang II-induced drinking behavior. Sakai et al. demonstrated that antisense oligonucleotides attenuated drinking behavior elicited by administration of central Ang II (44). Gyurko and co-workers (45) confirmed and extended these results by demonstrating that AT_1 antisense oligonucleotides inhibited Ang II drinking responses and significantly reduced blood pressure in hypertensive rats (see Subheading 4.2.).

The role of the Type 2 receptors in the elicitation of thirst has also been examined. For example, Rowland and Fregly have reported that icv injection of PD 123319 attenuated drinking induced by several experimental paradigms, such as hypertonic NaCl, hypovolemia, and water deprivation. These investigators proposed a model of drinking behavior in which AT_1 receptors are responsible for the Ang II-induced drinking pathway, whereas AT_2 receptors serve as the integrator in a final common pathway for both Ang and non-Ang drinking pathways (46). The development of AT_2 receptor knockout mice has provided some provocative data on the role of the Type 2 receptor in dipsogenic responses. For example, AT_2 knockout mice exhibited impaired dipsogenic responses following 40-h water deprivation compared to wild-type mice (47). Such results strongly suggested that Type 2 receptors are an essential component of dipsogenic responses induced by hypovolemia.

Several studies have investigated the role of Ang II receptor subtypes in sodium appetite, again with paradoxical results. For example, Thunhorst and Johnson (48) demonstrated that sodium appetite elicited by combined treatment of the diuretic furosemide and the ACE inhibitor captopril is mediated through the AT_1 receptor subtype. Conversely, Rowland et al. examined the role of Ang II receptor subtypes on salt appetite in several experimental paradigms *(42)*. These studies revealed that icv administration of losartan inhibited sodium ingestion in all of these paradigms, whereas PD 123319 and CGP 42112A only partially inhibited sodium appetite in some experimental conditions. Therefore, unlike Ang II dipsogenic responses, the elicitation of sodium appetite by the central RAS appears to be mediated solely through the AT_1 receptor subtype. Collectively, these results illustrate that the AT_1 receptor subtype plays an important role in the elicitation of ingestive behaviors. These studies have also provided provocative evidence for participation of Type 2 receptors in dipsogenic responses, although the exact role of AT_2 receptors in thirst and sodium appetite remains to be identified.

2.3. Distribution of Angiotensin Receptor Subtypes in the Brain

2.3.1. Quantitative Autoradiographic Studies

The development of subtype specific antagonists has facilitated the localization of Ang II receptor subtypes by quantitative autoradiographic techniques in the brain. The collective results from these studies have been largely consistent, but in some instances, they have revealed different patterns of receptor expression in the CNS. A complete overview of Ang II receptor expression in the brain as described by quantitative autoradiography is beyond the scope of this chapter (*see* ref. *49*). Nevertheless, it is important to note that AT_1 receptor expression in the brain is associated with regions known to mediate many of the central actions of Ang II. For example, the CVOs express a high density of AT_1 receptors *(50–53)*. In addition, AT_1 receptors are expressed in brainstem structures such as the AP, the dorsal motor nucleus of the vagus (dmnX), and the NTS. Hypothalamic structures, such as the SON and the PVN, have also been shown to express AT_1 receptors. The expression of AT_2 receptors in these hypothalamic structures remains controversial, however, in that some investigators have predicted a low to moderate expression of AT_2 receptors *(54)*; other studies have revealed the exclusive expression of the AT_1 subtype *(50–52)*. Quantitative autoradiographic techniques have been consistent in the demonstration of AT_2 receptor expression in somatic sensory-motor areas such as the locus coeruleus (LC), lateral septal nucleus, inferior olive, the medial geniculate nucleus, the superior colliculus, and the cerebellum *(50–53,55)*.

2.3.2. Immunohistochemical Localization of Angiotensin Receptor Subtypes

Although it is generally true that the development of selective antagonists has facilitated the localization of Ang II receptor subtypes in the CNS, autoradiographic studies may not possess the anatomical resolution necessary to identify or differentiate among all populations of Ang II receptor subtypes. The development of subtype selective antisera for Ang II receptors has overcome some of the limitations of autoradiography, thus allowing for a more precise localization of Ang II receptor subtypes in the brain. In this regard, immunohistochemical localization of the AT_1 receptor subtype in rat brain was largely consistent with previous autoradiographic studies *(56)*. AT_1 receptor immunoreactivity was detected in the CVOs, such as the SFO and organum vasculosum lamina terminalis (OVLT), as well as in brainstem structures such as the NTS and the nucleus ambiguous. In the hypothalamus, AT_1 receptor immunoreactivity in the PVN and the SON appeared to be associated with oxytocin- and vasopressin-containing lateral magnocellular neurons. AT_1 immunoreactivity was not detected in the suprachiasmatic nucleus, as predicted by autoradiographic analysis, indicating potential heterogeneity within the AT_1 receptor subtype. AT_1 receptor heterogeneity has been confirmed by the cloning of two distinct genes for the AT_1 subtype, referred to as AT_{1A} and AT_{1B} receptors *(57,58)*.

Immunohistochemical localization of the AT_2 receptor subtype has also been performed *(59)*. As was observed with the AT_1 receptor subtype, AT_2 immunoreactivity was largely consistent with previous autoradiographic analyses. In particular, AT_2 receptor immunoreactivity was observed in the

LC, cerebellum, and the central amygdaloid nucleus. AT_2 receptor immunoreactivity was also detected in the lateral magnocellular neurons of the PVN and SON. Interestingly, AT_2 receptor immunoreactivity was not detected in the inferior olive, a region previously shown to express AT_2 receptors. These results supported the hypothesis of AT_2 receptor heterogeneity, as suggested by earlier reports *(60)*. Indeed, ensuing functional, biochemical, pharmacological, immunological, and molecular studies have strengthened the hypothesis of AT_2 receptor heterogeneity *(61–67)*.

3. Centrally Mediated Cardiovascular Actions of the RAS

3.1. Angiotensin II Pressor Responses

In their seminal publication, Bickerton and Buckley provided evidence for a central mechanism in Ang II-induced increases in blood pressure in dogs *(20)*. Moreover, these investigators proposed that increases in blood pressure mediated by the central RAS involved activation of the sympathetic nervous system (SNS). Indeed, subsequent investigations confirmed the role of the SNS in blood pressure increases induced by Ang II *(68–70)*; they also identified vasopressin release as an equal and independent contributor in cardiovascular responses of the central RAS *(69,71)* (*see* Subheading 3.2.). Following these initial reports, the sites of Ang II cardiovascular pressor responses in the brain have been identified. In this regard, pressor and dipsogenic responses produced by injection of Ang II into the cerebral ventricles identified the anterior third ventricle, in particular the OVLT, as an angiotensin responsive site *(72)*. Microinjection of Ang II into the PVN elicited increases in blood pressure and drinking, an effect blocked by nonselective receptor antagonists *(28)*. The medulla has also been identified as a brain region that actively participates in the cardiovascular actions of Ang II, such as increased blood pressure and heart rate *(73,74)*. These studies also proposed the AP as a potential site for mediating the central actions of

Ang II, a hypothesis later confirmed by / subsequent investigations *(75)*. The SFO has also been identified as a site of action for the pressor responses of the central RAS *(24)*.

As described earlier, the early studies examining blood pressure and heart rate responses suggested that the central RAS elevates these cardiovascular indices. However, later studies have indicated that Ang II produces biphasic effects dependent on the dose of agonist used, as well as the population of brain Ang II receptors activated. For example, Diz and co-workers reported that microinjection of low doses of Ang II into the dmnX produced bradycardia and decreased blood pressure *(76)*. Conversely, higher doses of Ang II elevated blood pressure without producing any changes in heart rate when microinjected into the dmnX or the NTS *(76)*. Casto and Phillips reported that microinjection of Ang II into the NTS and the AP produced dose-dependent increases in blood pressure that were accompanied by small decreases in heart rate *(77)*. In agreement with this observation, Rettig et al. described that similar concentrations of Ang II microinjected into the NTS increased blood pressure without affecting heart rate *(78)*. However, these same investigators observed that low doses of Ang II reduced blood pressure and heart rate. The disparity between the results may be related to the doses of Ang II administered, because low-dose Ang II evoked depressor responses, whereas higher doses of Ang II increased blood pressure. Nonetheless, the results from these studies, along with others *(79,80)*, identified the medulla in general, and the AP, NTS, and the dmnX in particular, as brain regions intimately involved in central Ang II cardiovascular responses.

More recent studies have determined that the biphasic nature of Ang II cardiovascular responses in the medulla results from activation of Ang II receptor populations, that are anatomically and functionally distinct. For example, Sasaki and Dampney demonstrated that activation of Ang II receptors in the caudal ventrolateral medulla (CVLM) produced dose-dependent decreases in blood pressure and heart rate *(81)*. Conversely, Ang II microinjected into the rostral

Studies by Allen and co-workers identified other brain regions essential for the Ang II-mediated release of AVP *(111)*. In particular, microinjection of Ang II into the caudal ventrolateral medulla (CVLM) increased plasma AVP levels in a dose-dependent fashion, an effect blocked by prior administration of the nonselective receptor antagonist [Sar^1–Thr^8]-angiotensin II (sarthran). Interestingly, these studies also revealed that microinjection of Ang II into the CVLM generated depressor responses and bradycardia, in agreement with earlier reports *(81)*. These results identified the CVLM as a brain region important for the completion of central Ang II cardiovascular actions, in general, and the Ang II stimulated release of AVP, in particular.

Collectively, these results demonstrated that central Ang II mediates the release of vasopressin from the magnocellular neurons of the hypothalamus. Stimulation of Ang II receptors in the CVOs, which respond to circulating Ang II, as well as Ang II receptor fields beyond the BBB, is necessary for the release of AVP. However, functional studies were not able to establish the relative contributions of angiotensin receptor subtypes in this central action of the RAS. More recent studies have attempted to identify the Ang II receptor subtypes involved in the release of vasopressin from the magnocellular neurons of the hypothalamus. In this regard, Hogarty et al. reported that lateral ventricle injections of Ang II increased MAP and increased plasma levels of AVP *(43)*. Subtype selective antagonists determined that both AT$_1$ and AT$_2$ receptors are involved in the Ang II-mediated release of AVP. In particular, PD 123177 was as effective as losartan in attenuating the Ang II-induced release of vasopressin from the hypophysis. In agreement with this study, Veltmar et al. reported that losartan attenuated but did not eliminate Ang II-induced release of vasopressin from the PVN *(112)*. Conversely, Qadri and co-workers reported that exclusive blockade of AT$_1$ receptors abolishes vasopressin release in response to microinjection of Ang II into the SON *(113)*. Subsequent studies confirmed and extended these earlier observations in that losartan inhibited Ang II-induced AVP release in a dose-dependent fashion *(114)*. Interestingly, AT_2 receptor antagonism with PD 123177 actually potentiated Ang II-mediated increases in plasma AVP concentrations, suggesting that AT_2 receptors tonically inhibit the release of vasopressin.

Similarly, localization studies have been unable to accurately define the role of AT_1 and AT_2 receptors in the release of AVP. As described, the majority of receptor autoradiographic studies predicted the exclusive expression of the AT_1 receptor subtype in the PVN and the SON. Immunohistochemical analysis has also revealed that AT_1 receptor immunoreactivity is associated with magnocellular neurons of the PVN and SON *(56)*. More recently, *in situ* hybridization histochemistry has detected AT_1 receptor mRNA in the SON and PVN *(66,115)*. Taken together, these results predict that AT_1 receptors mediate the release of vasopressin, because AT_1 receptor binding, immunoreactivity, and mRNA are expressed in hypothalamic magnocellular neurons. However, colocalization studies have demonstrated that AT_{1A} and AT_{1B} receptor mRNAs are not expressed in AVP positive neurons in the hypothalamus *(116)*. The localization of AT_2 receptors in the hypothalamus has been more controversial. As described earlier, although the majority of quantitative autoradiographic studies have predicted the exclusive expression of AT_1 receptors in the hypothalamus, some investigators demonstrated AT_2 receptor binding activity in the PVN and the SON *(54)*. Moreover, immunohistochemical analysis has revealed the expression of AT_2 receptors in the magnocellular neurons of the PVN and SON *(59)*. Most recently, AT_2 receptor immunoreactivity has been colocalized with AVP immunopositive magnocellular neurons of the PVN and SON *(117)*. Nonetheless, in this same study, AT_2 receptor binding activity was not detected in the hypothalamus.

In summary, functional studies have illustrated that subtype selective antagonists attenuate but do not eliminate Ang II-induced release of vasopressin. This suggests that multiple Ang II receptor subtypes may be involved in mediating the release of AVP from the hypothalamus. Receptor autoradiography, immunohistochemistry, and *in situ* hybridization histochemistry analyses have also failed to reach a consensus regarding the localization of Ang II receptor subtypes in vasopressinergic neurons of the hypothalamus. Future investigations will be required to more accurately define the nature of the functional interactions between AT_1 and AT_2 receptors that leads to the release of AVP.

3.3. Baroreceptor Reflex Function

In order to compensate for transient increases in blood pressure and cardiac output, baroreceptors located in the carotid sinus and the aortic arch are activated to initiate decreases in total peripheral resistance and bradycardia. The baroreceptor reflex is produced by modulation of the autonomic nervous system via sympathoinhibition and stimulation of the parasympathetic outflow. Pressor responses mediated by the RAS are unique, however, in that increases in total peripheral resistance are not accompanied by reflex bradycardia, suggesting that Ang II opposes baroreceptor activity. Inhibition of the baroreceptor reflex by the central RAS was first proposed by Sweet and Brody *(118)*. These investigators also postulated that the failure of baroreceptor compensatory mechanisms may contribute to the pathogenesis of hypertension. Subsequent studies have illustrated that the inhibition of baroreceptor reflexes can be mediated by Ang II of peripheral origin, but it requires the participation of central mechanisms *(119–125)*. Stein and co-workers confirmed and extended earlier observations by providing the first direct evidence for a central mechanism in the attenuation of reflex bradycardia *(126)*. In particular, Ang II was shown to oppose baroreceptor reflex by increasing sympathetic outflow. More recently, inhibition of central RAS activity by ACE inhibitors and by nonselective receptor antagonists has been shown to potentiate phenylephrine-induced bradycardia in both normotensive and hypertensive rats, suggesting that Ang II exerts tonic inhibitory control over baroreceptor reflex activity *(127)*. However, baroreceptor reflex activity also suppresses the cardiovascular responses of the RAS *(128)*. Specifically, elimination of baroreceptor activity by sinoaortic baroreceptor denervation dramatically potentiates the pressor responses of peripheral and central Ang II, an observation confirmed by other investigators *(81,129–131)*. Therefore, these results suggest that the baroreceptor reflex arc may act to suppress Ang II pressor responses at the same time that Ang II opposes baroreceptor reflex-induced bradycardia.

Following the demonstration that the central RAS actively participates in the inhibition of baroreceptor reflex activity, subsequent studies have attempted to identify the brain regions involved in this response. The existing literature offered the cardiovascular centers of the brainstem as the sites where the central RAS acts to attenuate baroreflex activity. To begin, noradrenergic neurons in the brainstem, which represent an important component in the pressor response of the central RAS, are also involved in autonomic cardiovascular responses *(132–134)*. In addition, studies have previously identified the NTS as the first synapse of the baroreceptor reflex arc *(135,136)*. Indeed, tracing studies have identified the projections from the NTS, that subserve baroreceptor reflexes *(137)*. Collectively, these observations identified the NTS as a region intimately involved in the Ang II inhibition of baroreceptor reflex function. This hypothesis was confirmed by investigations in which subpressor doses of Ang II microinjected into the NTS inhibited phenylephrine-induced bradycardia *(138)*. Interestingly, the hypertensive rat exhibited attenuated baroreceptor sensitivity when compared to normotensive rats, supporting the hypothesis that baroreceptor activity is impaired in the hypertensive state *(see* Section 4b). The nonselective receptor antagonist sarthran was shown to inhibit endogenous Ang II opposition of baroreceptor activity by potentiating phenylephrine-induced bradycardia *(139,140)*. Microinjection of the nonselective receptor antagonist [Sar^1–Ala^8]-angiotensin II (saralasin) into the NTS has produced similar effects on baroreceptor reflex activity in conscious, freely moving rats *(141)*. The area postrema has also been identified as a brain region that participates in Ang II attenuation of baroreceptor reflexes.

Peripheral administration of Ang II elevated baroreceptor pressure levels without altering baroreceptor sensitivity, an effect that was eliminated in animals with AP lesions *(142)*. This study predicted that resetting of baroreflex activity in the AP may represent a mechanism through which central Ang II inhibits baroreceptor function. Collectively, these results identified the NTS and the AP as brain regions where central Ang II exerts tonic inhibitory control over baroreceptor activity.

Most recently, the neuropharmacology of Ang II suppression of baroreceptor activity has been examined. For example, Wong et al. demonstrated that losartan reversed Ang II-induced impairment of baroreceptor reflex activity and also inhibited the activity of endogenous Ang II *(143)*. The authors concluded that AT_1 receptors exert tonic control over baroreceptor function by resetting the baroreceptor setpoint. Bendle and co-workers reported that fourth ventricle administration of losartan reversed endogenous Ang II opposition to renal sympathetic baroreceptor functions by modulating sympathoinhibitory and sympathoexcitatory activities. The AT_2 receptor blocker PD 123319 had no effect on baroreceptor function, suggesting that AT_1 receptors are exclusively responsible for inhibition of baroreceptor reflexes *(144)*. Conversely, Lin et al. observed that both AT_1 and AT_2 receptors are involved in the Ang II attenuation of baroreceptor activity *(145)*. In particular, the nonselective antagonist [Sar^1–Ile^8]-angiotensin II (sarile) as well as the selective antagonists losartan and PD 123319 were equally effective at restoring baroreceptor reflexes induced by subpressor doses of Ang II. However, microinjection of PD 123319 was able to potentiate phenylephrine-induced increases in baroreceptor activity, whereas losartan had no effect.

In summary, Ang II opposes baroreceptor reflex bradycardia, producing in little or no change in heart rate resulting from the pressor actions of the RAS. As has been established for the central pressor response, the NTS and the AP are critically involved in the Ang II impairment of baroreceptor activity. Pharmacological analysis has revealed that Ang II exerts tonic inhibitory control over baroreflex function and has suggested that both AT_1 and AT_2 receptors are involved in the Ang II opposition to baroreceptor reflex activity. Nonetheless, future investigations will be required to more accurately define the pharmacology and physiology of Ang II receptor subtypes that oppose baroreceptor reflex activity. (*See* Fig. 2.)

4. The Spontaneously Hypertensive Rat and the RAS

4.1. Cardiovascular Studies

Neurohormonal systems, including the RAS, are believed to contribute to the pathogenesis of essential hypertension in humans (*See* Section 5). The spontaneously hypertensive rat (SHR) was developed as an experimental system to examine the etiology of hypertension *(146)*, but it has also been recognized as an excellent model system to provide correlative information in the pathophysiology of essential hypertension in man *(147)*. This section summarizes our current understanding of the critical role of the RAS in the development and maintenance of hypertension in the SHR. The characterization of the neuropharmacology of the central RAS in the hypertensive rat has provided insights into the etiology and treatment of essential hypertension in man, which will be described in ensuing sections.

Analysis of the development and maintenance of elevated blood pressure in the SHR has confirmed the hypothesis that hyperactivity of the RAS is an essential component in this experimental model of hypertension. Hoffman et al. examined the cardiovascular responses mediated by the central RAS in the hypertensive rat *(148)*. In particular, icv injections of Ang II produced greater increases in blood pressure in SHRs when compared to normotensive Wistar Kyoto (WKY) rats, whereas other cardiovascular indices, such as bradycardia, AVP release, as well as the elicitation of dipsogenic responses were similar in the SHR and the WKY rat. In subsequent investigations, microinjection of Ang II into the NTS of the hypertensive rat was shown to yield angiotensin II (octapeptide)

central actions	central localization	subtype(s)
central pressor response	CVOs/brainstem/hypothalamus	AT_1/AT_2
AVP release	CVOs/hypothalamus	AT_1/AT_2
SNS component	CVOs/brainstem	AT_1
baroreceptor reflex impairment	CVOs/NTS/AP	$AT_1/AT_2(?)$
dipsogenic responses	CVOs/hypothalamus	$AT_1/AT_2(?)$
sodium appetite	CVOs/hypothalamus	AT_1

Fig. 2. Summary of the cardiovascular and body fluid homeostatic mechanisms of the central RAS including the brain regions involved in the cardiovascular actions of the RAS, as well as the pharmacology of central Ang II responses. See text for details. CVOs = Circumventricular organs; NTS = nucleus tractus solitarius; AP = area postrema.

potentiated pressor responses and increases in heart rates compared to normotensive WKY rats or Sprague–Dawley (SD) rats. Moreover, microinjection of vasopressin into the NTS produced similar results *(149)*. Collectively, this study predicted that hyperactivity of these peptidergic systems was present in the SHR and also identified the NTS as a region where the increased sensitivity of the central RAS may reside. Subsequent studies by Ferrario and colleagues identified the ventrolateral medulla (VLM) as another site of Ang II pressor actions in the SHR *(150)*. Interestingly, this study revealed that the VLM produced biphasic changes in blood pressure. In particular, Ang II microinjected into the rostral ventrolateral medulla (RVLM) produced the expected dose-dependent increases in MAP, an effect that was abolished by ganglionic blockade. However, in the caudal ventrolateral medulla (CVLM), Ang II significantly decreased blood pressure and heart rate in the SHR, in agreement with previous observations in normotensive rats *(76,81)*. Collectively, these reports identified central sites in the medulla that mediate Ang II pressor responses in the SHR.

Pharmacologic manipulation of the central RAS strengthened the hypothesis that Ang II contributes to the maintenance of increased blood pressure in the SHR. For instance, Phillips and colleagues *(151)* demonstrated that peripheral and central administration of the nonselective receptor antagonist saralasin reduced blood pressure in the SH-stroke prone (SH-SP) rat. In addition, elimination of the peripheral component of the RAS by nephrectomy had no effect on central saralasin reductions in blood pressure in the SH-SP rat, suggesting that increased activity of the central RAS plays an important role in the maintenance of the hypertensive state. Similar findings were reported by McDonald et al. using the nonselective antagonist sarile *(152)*. The nonselective antagonist saralasin was also shown to reduce MAP in several different models of experimental hypertension *(153)*. The results from these early studies suggested that hyperactivity of the central RAS plays a role in the development and maintenance of hypertension. More recently, Jensen et al. demon-

strated that icv injection of the nonselective receptor antagonist sarthran significantly decreased MAP in hypertensive
rats, an effect also observed in normotensive WKY rats and
SD rats *(154)*. Microinjection of the Ang II receptor antagonist sarile into the RVLM has also been shown to produce
dose-dependent decreases in blood pressure in both SHRs
and WKY rats *(155)*. Reductions in arterial blood pressure
elicited by sarile microinjection were greater in the SHR compared to normotensive controls. In addition, sarile was more
efficacious in reducing the firing rate of RVLM cardiovascular neurons in the SHR, suggesting that these neurons are
more sensitive in the hypertensive state. Collectively, these
results indicated that central Ang II contributes to tonic regulation of blood pressure and strengthened the hypothesis of
increased activity of the RAS in the SHR. In support of this
hypothesis, microinjection of sarthran has been shown to
eliminate the tonic activity of CVLM neurons and RVLM
neurons in the SHR *(156)*. Conversely, some researchers have
reported that blockade of central angiotensin receptors does
not lower mean arterial pressure in the SHR *(131,157)*. Nonetheless, while the discrepancies between these observations
remain to be clarified, the large majority of studies provided
further evidence for increased activity of the central RAS,
such as increased Ang II receptor sensitivity, in the hypertensive state.

More recent investigations examined the contributions
of AT_1 and AT_2 receptors in the development and maintenance of hypertension in the SHR. In this regard, DePasqulae
and co-workers reported that icv administration of losartan
eliminated blood pressure increases elicited by central Ang
II in the SHR *(85)*. However, central losartan administration
alone did not reduce blood pressure in the SHR. In agreement with this report, Bunting and Widdop reported that
acute icv injection of the AT_1 receptor antagonists losartan
or CV-11974 eliminated increases in MAP and HR produced
by central administration of Ang II, but were ineffective at
reducing cardiovascular parameters when administered
alone *(66)*. Similarly, chronic CV-11974 administration had

no effect on resting levels, but did inhibit Ang II-induced increases in MAP and HR in the SHR. Therefore, unlike nonselective Ang II receptor antagonists such as sarile and sarthran, AT_1 receptor antagonists were incapable of reducing blood pressure in the SHR in these studies.

The expression of AT_2 receptors are developmentally regulated in that Type 2 receptor expression is high in the neonate but steadily declines to adult levels during maturation *(52,158)*. Accordingly, Toney and Porter investigated the pressor responses mediated by AT_1 and AT_2 receptors in both young and adult SHRs *(159)*. These investigators reported that icv administration of losartan but not PD 123319 inhibited Ang II mediated increases in MAP in young SHRs, indicating that this cardiovascular response was a result of AT_1 receptor activation *(159)*. However, losartan was more efficacious at each dose tested when combined with PD 123319. In addition, when the SNS component and the AVP component of central RAS cardiovascular responses were examined individually, blockade of both AT_1 and AT_2 receptors was required for elimination of the vasopressin-mediated pressor responses. These results intimate that unlike the AT_1-mediated SNS component, the vasopressin component of the Ang II central pressor response requires the activation of both AT_1 and AT_2 receptors in the young SHR. Conversely, when similar studies were performed in adult SHRs, AT_2 receptor blockade had no effect on either component of the central pressor responses *(160)*. In view of the developmental profile of AT_2 receptors, these results indicate that both AT_1 and AT_2 receptors may be involved in the development of increased blood pressure, whereas hypertension is maintained in the adult SHR exclusively by AT_1 receptors.

4.2. Neurochemistry and Neuropharmacology of the Spontaneously Hypertensive Rat

The results of studies examining the cardiovascular responses in the SHR predicted that increased activity of the central angiotensin system contributes to the etiology of the hypertensive state. However, the neuropharmacological and neurochemical changes in the RAS associated with hypertension still needed to be identified. A pharmacological change in SHRs that could contribute to the development and maintenance of hypertension is an increase in Ang II receptor expression. The first study to examine receptor binding activity in the SHR predicted that Ang II receptor density and affinity were unchanged in the SHR when compared to normotensive WKY rats *(161)*. However, subsequent studies began to identify regions where Ang II binding activity was increased in the spontaneously hypertensive rat. For example, Stamler et al. reported that Ang II receptor binding activity in the organum vasculosum of the lamina teminalis (OVLT) was increased in SHRs compared to WKY rats *(162)*. This increase in Ang II receptor binding in the OVLT was not associated with changes in receptor affinity. Similar increases in Ang II receptor densities in the absence of changes in receptor affinity were described by Sumners and colleagues in neuronal cultures prepared from neonatal SHRs *(163)*. Angiotensin receptor binding has also been shown to be increased in the SFO of the hypertensive rat compared to aged-matched WKY rats *(164,165)*. However, unlike the previous studies, the increase in Ang II binding activity was associated with increases in receptor affinity in the SHR. A more comprehensive study by Gehlert and co-workers confirmed and extended earlier reports *(166)*. Ang II receptor binding in the SHR was increased in the OVLT and the SFO, as described previously. In addition, this study identified other regions that exhibited increased Ang II receptor densities in the SHR, including the NTS, the dmnX, the LC, and the SON. Moreover, increases in receptor density in the SFO and the SON were accompanied by increases in receptor affinity in the SHR. Conversely, Healy and Zhang reported that Ang II receptor affinity was decreased in the solitary-vagal area (SVA) of the hypertensive rat *(167)*. Ang II binding activity was increased in the SHR compared to WKY rats in the SVA, which includes the NTS and the dmnX. However, more discrete examination of the NTS has predicted that Ang II binding capacity in the NTS is unchanged in the SHR, whereas Ang II binding activity was increased in the AP in the hypertensive rat compared to normotensive controls (168).

Angiotensin II receptor subtype binding activity and mRNA expression have also been analyzed in the hypertensive rat. For instance, the preoptic area (POA) has been shown to exhibit changes in AT_1 receptor message levels in the SHR. This increase was selective for AT_{1A} receptor mRNA in that AT_{1B} mRNA was unchanged in the POA in the hypertensive compared to normotensive controls (169). Northern blot analysis has illustrated that AT_1 receptor mRNA expression is increased in the hypothalamus and brainstem of SHRs, a change resulting from elevated expression of both AT_{1A} and AT_{1B} receptor mRNAs (170).

These same investigators described similar results in primary neuronal cultures prepared from hypothalamus and brainstem (171). In addition, primary neuronal cultures from the SHR expressed higher densities of AT_1 receptor binding activity, increases that were not accompanied by changes in receptor affinity. In a related study, AT_2 receptor binding activity was not increased in primary neuronal cultures prepared from SHRs compared to cultures from WKY rats (172). Succeeding reports have also illustrated elevated AT_1 receptor expression in the SHR. For example, quantitative autoradiographic analysis has revealed increased AT_1 receptor expression in the NTS, the dmnX, the AP, and the spinal trigeminal nucleus in the SHR (173). Collectively, these results suggest that elevated Ang II receptor densities, as well as alterations in receptor affinity, are important factors in the development and maintenance of hypertension. Indeed, increased sensitivity of septal neurons to Ang II in SHRs may result from these pharmacological changes (174).

Evidence to support the hypothesis of increased Ang II receptor sensitivity in the hypertensive state has been provided through the use of antisense oligonucleotides (AS-ODNs). For example, central administration of AS-ODNs designed against the AT_1 receptor or angiotensinogen significantly reduce MAP in hypertensive rats (45). The antihypertensive activity of the AS-ODNs resulted from decreases in AT_1 receptor binding activity and Ang II concentrations. Subsequent studies provided similar results and also demonstrated that AS-ODNs against the AT_1 receptor reduced blood pressure in the SHR for up to 7 d following a single central administration (175). Most recently, these same investigators reported that prolonged reductions in blood pressure were achieved in the SHR by administering AS-ODNs in a vector delivery system. In particular, adeno-associated viral vectors packaged with AT_1 receptor antisense significantly reduced blood pressure in the SHR up to 9 wk following a single central administration (176). Therefore, these results illustrate that antisense technology may eventually provide a novel therapeutic approach in the treatment of hypertension.

In addition to changes in Ang II receptor binding characteristics, increased activity of other members of the central RAS have been identified in the hypertensive rat. For instance, increases in renin activity have been reported in several brain regions, including the NTS, the A5 area, and the neurohypophysis in young SHRs compared to aged-matched WKY rats (177). Furthermore, this study indicated that angiotensinase activity was decreased in the SON, the pineal gland, and the neurohypophysis of young SHRs. These observations indicated that increased Ang II peptide levels may also contribute to hypertension in the SHR. In support of this hypothesis, Ang II levels were found to be higher in selected brain nuclei of SHRs (178). A subsequent study by Ganten and colleagues, which was the first to provide unequivocal evidence for the synthesis of Ang II in the brain, also demonstrated increased turnover of Ang II in the brain of SHRs (13). The use of ACE inhibitors such as captopril has provided further evidence to support the theory of increased activity of the central RAS in the hypertensive rat (179–182). Taken together, these results demonstrate that Ang II receptor binding, receptor affinity, and receptor sensitivity, as well as renin activity and Ang II synthesis are increased in the SHR and support the hypothesis that increased activity of the central RAS is a contributing factor in the development and maintenance of hypertension.

As described previously, numerous studies have predicted that baroreceptor reflex activity is impaired in hypertension *(118,148,183,184)*. In addition to enhanced activity of the central RAS in the hypertensive rat, Ang II opposition to baroreceptor reflex activity may also contribute to the development and maintenance of the hypertensive state. Indeed, impaired baroreceptor activity can be restored via pharmacological interruption of endogenous central Ang II activity. For example, angiotensin-converting-enzyme inhibitors *(127,182,185,186)* as well as angiotensin receptor antagonists *(127,187)* have been shown to restore baroreceptor function in the SHR. Collectively, these results provide evidence that baroreceptor reflex activity is impaired in the SHR, an effect reversed by pharmacological interruption of the central RAS.

In summary, the spontaneously hypertensive rat has been extensively studied in order to achieve a greater understanding of the pathophysiological changes that occur in hypertension. The above-described studies illustrate that the central renin–angiotensin system contributes to the development and maintenance of the hypertensive state. Indeed, pharmacologic intervention of the RAS with ACE inhibitors and Ang II receptor antagonists produce positive hemodynamic effects in the SHR. The results from experimental studies have fostered the development of pharmacological strategies in the treatment of hypertension and congestive heart failure in man, as will be described in the following section.

5. Clinical Considerations for the RAS

As described in Section 1.3, Ang II induces the constriction of vascular smooth muscle, producing a subsequent rise in systemic blood pressure. Therefore, blockade or inhibition of the renin–angiotensin system may have therapeutic benefits in the treatment of heart failure and hypertension. Indeed, increased activity of the renin–angiotensin system has been shown to participate in the etiology of these pathophysiological conditions. Initial clinical investigations focused on Ang II receptor blockade utilizing the peptide antagonist saralasin, which was able to reduce pressor responses to Ang II *(188)*. However, as a peptide, this compound had limited oral bioavailability. In addition, saralasin and other Ang II peptide antagonists exhibited partial agonist activity. Nonetheless, although saralasin had limited efficacy, it did illustrate that modulation of the renin–angiotensin system could have clinical applications in the treatment of CHF and hypertensin.

An alternative approach in the modulation of the renin–angiotensin system would be to decrease circulating levels of Ang II by inhibiting the activity of ACE. Earlier studies demonstrated that the venoms of pit vipers of the species *Bothrops jararaca* were shown to contain a substance that inhibited degradation of bradykinin *(189)* and were referred to as bradykinin potentiating factors (BPFs). It was later demonstrated that BPFs also blocked ACE activity, thus facilitating the development of converting enzyme inhibitors. In the clinical setting, ACE inhibitors such as captopril have been shown to serve as balanced vasodilators having effects on both arteries and veins *(190)*. Decreases in blood pressure and total peripheral resistance were not accompanied by increases in heart rate or cardiac output in hypertensive patients. However, ACE inhibition is associated with increases in cardiac output in patients with CHF *(190–192)*. These patients also experienced decreases in MAP and systemic vascular resistance, as well as reduced afterload and decreased heart rate. As has been shown with hypertensive patients, the positive hemodynamic effects of ACE inhibitors in the treatment of CHF are largely the result of the balanced vasodilation of both arterial and venous beds *(190)*. ACE inhibition has also been shown to improve cardiac function and hemodynamics following myocardial infarction *(190)*. ACE inhibitors are well tolerated in most patients, but they are associated with a cough reflex with a clinical incidence ranging from 1% to 33%, most often occurring in older patients *(193,194)*. Consequently, ACE inhibitors have become one of the most often prescribed agents in the treatment of CHF and hypertension.

One of the major concerns prior to and during the treatment of hypertension and CHF is blood flow distribution. Cardiac output and organ blood flow may not be substantially effected in mild forms of these diseases, but in more severe forms of hypertension and heart failure, cardiac output is reduced. Blood flow distribution is also effected, but with the exception of the most severe cases of heart failure and hypertension, the brain and heart still receive normal blood flow, often to the detriment of other organs *(195)*. Coronary flow reserve, also referred to as coronary vascular capacity, is known to be impaired in hypertension. Antihypertensive therapy, including the use of ACE inhibitors, has been shown to restore coronary reserve *(196)*. For example, in patients with mild hypertension without ventricular hypertrophy, captopril restores hemodynamic parameters and coronary flow reserve reduced by diuretic treatment *(197)*. Acute ACE inhibition with cilazapril has also been shown to produce sustained increases in coronary hemodynamics, such as coronary blood flow, in hypertensive patients *(198)*. More recently, long-term therapy of hypertensive patients with the ACE inhibitor enalapril has been shown to lower systolic and diastolic pressures, as well as improve coronary reserve *(199)*. The RAS is also believed to contribute to ventricular hypertrophy associated with heart failure and hypertension *(200)*. In this regard, long-term therapy with ACE inhibitors reversed left ventricular hypertrophy in hypertensive patients *(201,202)*. Moreover, long-term treatment with enalapril not only improved cardiac hemodynamics but also reduced left ventricular mass *(199)*. Therefore, the hemodynamic benefits of ACE inhibitors may also include the ability of these antihypertensive agents to decrease arterial stiffness, thereby increasing arterial dilation *(203)*.

Clinical studies have indicated that neuroendocrine activation, including increased activity of the RAS, is also involved in the pathogenesis of heart failure *(204–206)*. The RAS is proposed to contribute to the development of reduced cardiovascular parameters in CHF, such as reduced coronary blood flow and reserve, ventricular hypertrophy, and increased myocardial oxygen demand. Appropriately, the clinical use of ACE inhibitors has been shown to provide beneficial effects on cardiac hemodynamics in heart failure patients *(206,207)*. For example, as described for hypertensive patients, heart failure patients receiving ACE-inhibitor therapy experienced improvement of cardiac hemodynamics, including redistribution of regional blood flow *(208)*. Moreover, intracoronary administration of enalaprilat to specifically target the cardiac RAS produces cardiac vasodilation and also elicited negative inotropic effects in heart failure patients *(209)*. More recent clinical findings suggest that in addition to improving cardiovascular indices, a 6-mo treatment with cilazapril also reduces left ventricular mass, supporting evidence that the RAS participates in the development of ventricular hypertrophy in CHF *(210)*. Experimental studies have also examined the role of the RAS in heart failure. In particular, central blockade of AT_1 receptors produced significant improvement in hemodynamic parameters in experimentally induced heart failure *(211)*. Therefore, in addition to the well-defined role of the peripheral RAS, these results suggest that the central RAS may also contribute to the pathogenesis of congestive heart failure.

In addition to improving cardiac hemodynamics, ACE inhibitors have also been shown to increase cerebral blood flow in heart failure *(212)*. For example, decreases in blood pressure produced by captopril in CHF patients were not accompanied by decreases in cerebral blood flow *(213)*. Indeed, reductions in cerebral blood flow observed in the most severe cases of heart failure are restored by captopril treatment *(214)*. More recent clinical trials have shown that enalapril increases cerebral blood flow in patients with heart failure *(215)*, as well as in patients with chronic cerebral infarction *(216)*. Collectively, these clinical studies demonstrate that the RAS plays an important role in cerebral blood flow regulation, an effect that in experimental studies has been shown to be mediated through the AT_2 receptor subtype *(217)*.

More recently, attention has been focused on the development of nonpeptide angiotensin receptor antagonists

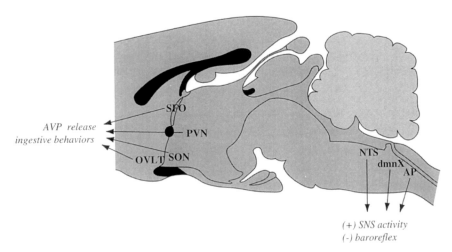

Fig. 3. Sagittal rat brain section highlighting Ang II receptor populations involved in the cardiovascular and body fluid homeostatic mechanisms of the central RAS. See text and Fig. 2 for details. SFO = Subfornical
organ; OVLT = organum vasculosum lateral teminalis; SON = supraoptic nucleus; PVN = paraventricular nucleus; AP = area postrema; NTS =
nucleus tractus solitarius; dmnX = dorsal motor nucleus of the vagus.

(190,193,218), as well as the development of renin inhibitors
(190,193,218). These compounds represent the next generation
of pharmaceuticals used in the treatment of CHF and hypertension. However, angiotensin receptor blockade is associated with both an increase in circulating levels of Ang II and
plasma renin activity *(219)*, which may potentially produce
deleterious physiological side effects and therefore make
these compounds less desirable than the well-tolerated ACE
inhibitors. Accordingly, long-term clinical studies will be necessary to evaluate the efficacy of angiotensin receptor antagonists,
such as losartan, compared to ACE inhibitors in the treatment
of hypertension and congestive heart failure. (*See* Fig. 3.)

6. Conclusions and Future Perspectives

The combined actions of the peripheral and central
renin–angiotensin systems results in the regulation of body
fluid and cardiovascular homeostasis. In the periphery, Ang

II evokes pressor responses and promotes sodium and fluid retention. The discovery of a central RAS has resulted in a greater understanding of the physiological as well as the pathophysiological activities of Ang II. The central RAS mediates a pressor response that is produced by the equal and independent contributions of the SNS and vasopressin. In addition, the central RAS contributes to the restoration of body fluids during pathophysiological events such as hemorrhage or dehydration by eliciting ingestive behaviors. The development of subtype selective antagonists facilitated investigations into the cardiovascular responses mediated by the central RAS and has allowed for the localization of Ang II receptor subtypes in the brain. The use of powerful molecular tools, such as the development of receptor knockout mice and the use of antisense technology, provides new avenues of research to investigate the actions of Ang II. Elevated activity of the RAS is now accepted to contribute to the development and maintenance of hypertension in animals and in man. Accordingly, angiotensin-converting enzyme inhibitors and angiotensin Type 1 receptor antagonists are currently being employed in the clinical setting in the treatment of hypertension and heart failure. The exciting challenge now facing investigators is to achieve an even greater understanding of the actions of the central and peripheral renin–angiotensin systems in both the physiological and pathophysiological settings. Such investigations would hopefully produce novel therapeutic approaches to combat hypertension and congestive heart failure in man.

Acknowledgments

The author would like to thank Dr. Steven Fluharty for helpful comments and suggestions, Dr. Louis Lucas for assistance in the preparation of figures, and Jocelyn Gnirrep for assistance in the final preparation of this chapter.

References

1. Peach, M. J. (1977) Renin-angiotensin system: biochemistry and mechanism of action. *Physiol. Rev.* **57,** 313–370.

2. Catanzaro, D. F., Mullins, J. J., and Morris, B. J. (1983) The biosynthetic pathway of renin in mouse submandibular gland. *J. Biol. Chem.* **258,** 7364–7368.

3. Taugner, R., Buhrle, C. P., Nobling, R., and Kirschke, H. (1985) Coexistence of renin and cathepsin in epithelial cell secretory granules. *Histochemistry* **83,** 103–108.

4. Matsuba, H., Watanabe, T., Watanabe, M., Ishii, Y., Waguri, S., Kominami, E., et al. (1989) Immunohistochemical localization of prorenin, renin and cathepsins B, H, and L in juxtaglomerular cells of the rat kidney. *J. Histochem. Cytochem.* **37,** 1689–1697.

5. Zehr, J. E., Kurz, K. D., Seymour, A. A., and Schultz, H. D. (1980) Mechanisms controlling renin release. *Adv. Exp. Med. Biol.* **130,** 135–170.

6. Ganong, W. F. (1994) Origin of the angiotensin II secreted by cells. *Proc. Soc. Exp. Biol. Med.* **205,** 213–219.

7. Phillips, M. I., Speakman, E. A., and Kimura, B. (1993) Levels of angiotensin and molecular biology of the tissue renin angiotensin systems. *Regul. Pept.* **43,** 1–20.

8. Phillips, M. I., Weyhenmeyer, D., and Ganten, D. (1979) Evidence for an endogenous brain renin angiotensin system. *Fed. Proc.* **38,** 2260–2266.

9. Healy, D. P. and Printz, M. P. (1984) Distribution of immunoreactive angiotensin II, angiotensin I, angiotensinogen, and renin in the central nervous system of intact and nephrectomized rats. *Hypertension* **6(Suppl. I),** I-130–I-136.

10. Dzau, V. J., Ingelfinger, J., Pratt, R. E., and Ellison, K. E. (1986) Identification of renin and angiotensinogen messenger RNA sequences in mouse and rat brains. *Hypertension* **8,** 544–548.

11. Lynch, K. R., Hawelu-Johnson, C. L., and Guyenet, P. G. (1987) Localization of brain angiotensinogen mRNA by hybridization histochemistry. *Mol. Brain Res.* **2,** 149–158.

12. Ganten, D. and Speck, G. (1978) The brain renin-angiotensin system: a model for the synthesis of peptides in the brain. *Biochem. Pharmacol.* **27,** 2379–2389.

13. Ganten, D., Hermann, K., Bayer, C., Unger, T., and Lang, R. E. (1983) Angiotensin synthesis in the brain and increased turnover in hypertensive rats. *Science* **221,** 869–871.

14. Morgan, K. G. (1987) Calcium and smooth muscle tone. *Am. J. Med.* **82(Suppl. 3B),** 9–15.

15. Aguilera, G. and Marusic, E. T. (1971) Role of the renin–angiotensin system in the biosynthesis of aldosterone. *Endocrinology* **89,** 1524–1529.

16. Loudon, M., Bing, R. F., Thurston, H., and Swales, J. D. (1983) Arterial wall uptake of renal renin and blood pressure control. *Hypertension* **5,** 629–634.

17. Navar, L. G. and Rosivall, L. (1984) Contribution of the renin-angiotensin system to the control of intrarenal hemodynamics. *Kidney Int.* **25,** 857–868.

18. Levens, N. R., Peach, M. J., and Carey, R. M. (1981) Interactions between angiotensin peptides and the sympathetic nervous system mediating intestinal sodium and water absorption in the rat. *J. Clin. Invest.* **67,** 1197–1207.
19. Levens, N. R., Peach, M. J., Carey, R. M., Poat, J. A., and Munday, K. A. (1981) Response of the rat jejunum to angiotensin II: role of norepinephrine and prostaglandins. *Am. J. Physiol.* **240,** G17–G24.
20. Bickerton, R. K. and Buckley, J. P. (1961) Evidence for a central mechanism in angiotensin induced hypertension. *Proc. Soc. Exp. Biol. Med.* **106,** 834–836.
21. Malik, K. U. and Nasjletti, A. (1976) Facilitation of adrenergic transmission by locally generated angiotensin II in rat mesenteric arteries. *Circ. Res.* **38,** 26–30.
22. Epstein, A. N., Fitzsimons, J. T., and Rolls, B. J. (1970) Drinking induced by injection of angiotensin into the brain of the rat. *J. Physiol. (Lond.)* **210,** 457–474.
23. Simpson, J. B. and Routtenberg, A. (1973) Subfornical organ: site of drinking elicitation by angiotensin II. *Science* **181,** 1172–1175.
24. Mangiapane, M. L. and Simpson, J. B. (1980) Subfornical organ: forebrain site of pressor and dipsogenic action of angiotensin II. *Am. J. Physiol.* **239,** R382–R389.
25. Simpson, J. B. and Routtenberg, A. (1975) Subfornical lesions reduce intravenous angiotensin-induced drinking. *Brain Res.* **88,** 154–161.
26. Lind, R. W. and Johnson, A. K. (1882) On the separation of functions mediated by the AV3V region. *Peptides* **3,** 495–499.
27. Lind, R. W., Thunhorst, R. L., and Johnson, A. K. (1984) The subfornical organ and the integration of multiple factors in thirst. *Physiol. Behav.* **32,** 69–74.
28. Jensen, L. L., Harding, J. W., and Wright, J. W. (1992) Role of paraventricular nucleus in control of blood pressure and drinking in rats. *Am. J. Physiol.* **262,** F1068–F1075.
29. Miselis, R. R., Shapiro, R. E., and Hand, P. J. (1979) Subfornical organ efferents to neural systems for control of body water. *Science* **205,** 1022–1025.
30. Buggy, J. and Fisher, A. E. (1974) Dual role for angiotensin in thirst and salt appetite. *Nature* **250,** 735–737.
31. Bryant, R. W., Epstein, A. N., Fitzsimons, J. T., and Fluharty, S. J. (1980) Arousal of a specific and persistent sodium appetite in rat with continuous intracerebroventricular infusion of angiotensin II. *J. Physiol. (Lond.)* **301,** 365–382.
32. Fluharty, S. J. and Epstein, A. N. (1983) Sodium appetite elicited by intracerebroventricular infusion of angiotensin II in the rat: II Synergistic interaction with systemic mineralcorticoids. *Behav. Neurosci.* **97,** 746–758.
33. Sakai, R. R., Nicolaidis, S., and Epstein, A. N. (1986) Salt appetite is suppressed by interference with angiotensin II and aldosterone. *Am. J. Physiol.* **251,** R762–R768.

34. Peach, M. J. and Levens, N. R. (1980) Molecular approaches to the study of angiotensin receptors. *Adv. Exp. Med. Biol.* **130,** 171–194.
35. Trachte, G. J. and Peach, M. J. (1983) A potent noncompetitive angiotensin II antagonist induces only competitive inhibition of angiotensin III responses. *J. Cardiovasc. Pharmacol.* **5,** 1025–1033.
36. Douglas, J. G. (1987) Angiotensin receptor subtypes of the kidney cortex. *Am. J. Physiol.* **253,** F1–F7.
37. Reagan, L. P., Ye, X. H., Mir, R., DePalo, L. R., and Fluharty, S. J. (1990) Up-regulation of angiotensin II receptors by *in vitro* differentiation of murine N1E-115 neuroblastoma cells. *Mol Pharmacol.* **38,** 878–886.
38. Bumpus, F. M., Catt, K. J., Chiu, A. T., DeGasparo, M., Goodfriend, T., Husain, A., et al. (1991) Nomenclature for angiotensin receptors. A report of the Nomenclature Committee of the-Council for High Blood Pressure Research. *Hypertension.* **17,** 720–721.
39. Wong, P. C., Price, W. A., Chiu, A. T., Duncia, J. V., Carini, D. J., Wexler, R. R., et al. (1991) *In vivo* pharmacology of DuP 753. *Am. J. Hypertens.* **4,** 288S–298S.
40. Kirby, R. F., Thunhorst, R. L., and Johnson, A. K. (1992) Effects of a non-peptide angiotensin receptor antagonist on drinking and blood pressure responses to centrally administered angiotensins in the rat. *Brain Res.* **576,** 348–350.
41. Fregly, M. J. and Rowland, N. E. (1991) Effect of nonpeptide angiotensin II receptor antagonist, DuP 753, on angiotensin-related water intake in rats. *Brain Res. Bull.* **27,** 97–100.
42. Rowland, N. E., Rozelle, A., Riley, P. J., and Fregly, M. J. (1992) Effect of nonpeptide angiotensin receptor antagonists on water intake and salt appetite in rats. *Brain Res. Bull.* **29,** 389–393.
43. Hogarty, D. C., Speakman, E. A., Puig, V., and Phillips, M. I. (1992) The role of angiotensin, AT_1 and AT_2 receptors in the pressor, drinking and vasopressin responses to central angiotensin. *Brain Res.* **586,** 289–294.
44. Sakai, R. R., He, P. F., Yang, X. D., Ma, L. Y., Guo, Y. F., Reilly, J. J., et al. (1994) Intracerebroventricular administration of AT_1 receptor antisense oligonucleotides inhibits the behavioral actions of angiotensin-II. *J. Neurochem.* **62,** 2053–2056.
45. Gyurko, R., Wielbo, D., and Phillips, M. I. (1993) Antisense inhibition of AT_1 receptor mRNA and angiotensinogen mRNA in the brain of spontaneously hypertensive rats reduces hypertension of neurogenic origin. *Regul. Pept.* **49,** 167–174.
46. Rowland, N. E. and Fregly, M. J. (1993) Brain angiotensin AT-2 receptor antagonism and water intake. *Brain Res. Bull.* **32,** 391–394.
47. Hein, L., Barsh, G. S., Pratt, R. E., Dzau, V. J., and Kobilka, B. K. (1995) Behavioural and cardiovascular effects of disrupting the angiotensin II type-2 receptor gene in mice. *Nature* **377,** 744–747.

48. Thunhorst, R. L. and Johnson, A. K. (1994) Renin–angiotensin, arterial blood pressure and salt appetite in rats. *Am. J. Physiol.* **266,** R458–R465.
49. Steckelings, U. M., Bottari, S. P., and Unger, T. (1992) Angiotensin receptor subtypes in the brain. *Trends Pharmacol. Sci.* **13,** 365–368.
50. Song, K., Allen, A. M., Paxinos, G., and Mendelsohn, F. A. O. (1992) Mapping of angiotensin II receptor subtype heterogeneity in rat brain. *J. Comp. Neurol.* **316,** 467–484.
51. Aldred, G. P., Chai, S. Y., Song, K., Zhuo, J., MacGregor, D. P., and Mendelsohn, F. A. O. (1993) Distribution of angiotensin II receptor subtypes in the rabbit brain. *Regul. Pept.* **44,** 119–130.
52. Tsutsumi, K. and Saavedra, J. M. (1991) Characterization and development of angiotensin II receptor subtypes (AT_1 and AT_2) in rat brain. *Am. J. Physiol.* **261,** R209–R216.
53. Gehlert, D. R., Gackenheimer, S. L., and Schober, D. A. (1991) Autoradiographic localization of subtypes of angiotensin II antagonist binding in the rat brain. *Neuroscience* **44,** 501–514.
54. Obermuller, N., Unger, T., Gohlke, P., de Gasparo, M., and Bottari, S. P. (1991) Distribution of angiotensin II receptor subtypes in rat brain nuclei. *Neurosci. Lett.* **132,** 11–15.
55. Allen, A. M., Paxinos, G., McKinley, M. J., Chai, S. Y., and Mendelsohn, F. A. O. (1991) Localization and characterization of angiotensin II receptor binding sites in the human basal ganglia, thalamus, midbrain pons, and cerebellum. *J. Comp. Neurol.* **312,** 291–298.
56. Phillips, M. I., Shen, L., Richards, E. M., and Raizada, M. K. (1993) Immunohistochemical mapping of angiotensin AT_1 receptors in the brain. *Regul. Pept.* **44,** 95–107.
57. Griendling, K. K., Murphy, T. J., and Alexander, R. W. (1993) Molecular biology of the renin-angiotensin system. *Circulation* **87,** 1816–1828.
58. Iwai, N. and Inagami, T. (1992) Identification of two subtypes in the rat type I angiotensin II receptor. *FEBS Lett.* **298,** 257–260.
59. Reagan, L. P., Flanagan-Cato, L. M., Yee, D. K., Ma, L.-Y., Sakai, R. R., and Fluharty, S. J. (1994) Immunohistochemical mapping of angiotensin type 2 (AT_2) receptors in rat brain. *Brain. Res.* **662,** 45–59.
60. Tsutsumi, K. and Saavedra, J. M. (1992) Heterogeneity of angiotensin II AT_2 receptors in the rat brain. *Mol. Pharmacol.* **41,** 290–297.
61. Xiong, H. and Marshall, K. C. (1994) Angiotensin II depresses glutamate depolarizations and excitatory postsynaptic potentials in the locus coeruleus through angiotensin II subtype 2 receptors. *Neuroscience* **62,** 163–175.
62. Ambuhl, P., Felix, D., Imboden, H., Khosla, M. C., and Ferrario, C. M. (1992) Effects of angiotensin II and its selective antagonists on inferior olivary neurones. *Regul. Pept.* **41,** 19–26.
63. Siemens, I. R., Reagan, L. P., Yee, D. K., and Fluharty, S. J. (1994) Biochemical characterization of two distinct angiotensin AT_2

receptor populations in murine neuroblastoma N1E-115 cells. *J. Neurochem.* **62,** 2106–2115.

64. Reagan, L. P., Sakai, R. R., and Fluharty, S. J. (1996) Immunological analysis of Angiotensin AT_2 receptors in peripheral tissues of developing and adult rats. *Regul. Pept.* **65,** 159–164.

65. Yee, D. K., He, P.,, Yang, X.-D., Reagan, L. P., Hines, J., Siemens, I. R., et al. (1997) Cloning and expression of angiotensin II Type 1 and Type 2 receptors from murine neuroblastoma N1E-115 cells. *Mol. Brain Res.* **45,** 108–116.

66. Johren, O., Inagami, T., and Saavedra, J. M. (1995) AT_{1A}, AT_{1B}, and AT_2 angiotensin II receptor subtype gene expression in rat brain. *NeuroReport* **6,** 2549–2552.

67. Johren, O., Inagami, T., and Saavedra, J. M. (1996) Localization of AT_2 angiotensin II receptor gene expression in rat brain by *in situ* hybridization histochemistry. *Mol. Brain Res.* **37,** 192–200.

68. Smookler, H. H., Severs, W. B., Kinnard, W. J., and Buckley, J. P. (1966) Centrally mediated cardiovascular effects of angiotensin II. *J. Pharmacol. Exp. Ther.* **153,** 485–494.

69. Falcon, J. C., II, Phillips, M. I., Hoffman, W. E., and Brody, M. J. (1978) Effects of intraventricular angiotensin II mediated by the sympathetic nervous system. *Am. J. Physiol.* **235,** H392–H399.

70. Scholkens, B. A., Jung, W., Rascher, W., Dietz, R., and Ganten, D. (1982) Intracerebroventricular angiotensin II increases arterial blood pressure in rhesus monkeys by stimulation of pituitary hormones and the sympathetic nervous system. *Experientia* **38,** 469–470.

71. Unger, T., Rascher, W., Schuster, C., Pavlovitch, R., Schomig, A., Dietz, R., et al. (1981) Central blood pressure effects of substance P and angiotensin II: role of the sympathetic nervous system and vasopressin. *Eur. J. Pharmacol.* **71,** 33–42.

72. Hoffman, W. E. and Phillips, M. I. (1976) Regional study of cerebral ventricle sensitive sites to angiotensin II. *Brain Res.* **110,** 313–330.

73. Joy, M. D. and Lowe, R. D. (1970) Evidence for a medullary site of action in the cardiovascular response to angiotensin II. *J. Physiol. (Lond.)* **206,** 41P–42P.

74. Joy, M. D. and Lowe, R. D. (1970) The site of cardiovascular action of angiotensin II in the brain. *Clin. Sci.* **39,** 327–336.

75. Joy, M. D. (1971) The intramedullary connections of the area postrema involved in the central cardiovascular response to angiotensin II. *Clin. Sci.* **41,** 89–100.

76. Diz, D. I., Barnes, K. L., and Ferrario, C. M. (1984) Hypotensive actions of microinjections of angiotensin II into the dorsal motor nucleus of the vagus. *J. Hypertens.* **2(Suppl. 3),** 53–56.

77. Casto, R. and Phillips, M. I. (1984) Cardiovascular actions of microinjections of angiotensin II in the brain stem of rats. *Am. J. Physiol.* **246,** R811–R816.

78. Rettig, R., Healy, D. P., and Printz, M. P. (1986) Cardiovascular effects of microinjections of angiotensin II into the nucleus tractus solitarii. *Brain Res.* **364,** 233–240.

79. Allen, A. M., Dampney, R. A., and Mendelsohn, F. A. (1988) Angiotensin receptor binding and pressor effects in cat subretrofacial nucleus. *Am. J. Physiol.* **255,** H1011–H1017.

80. Andreatta, S. H., Averill, D. B., Santos, R. A. S., and Ferrario, C. M. (1988) The ventrolateral medulla: a new site of action of the renin-angiotensin system. *Hypertension* **11(Suppl. I),** I-163–I-166.

81. Sasaki, S. and Dampney, R. A. L. (1990) Tonic cardiovascular effects of angiotensin II in the ventrolateral medulla. *Hypertension* **15,** 274–283.

82. Agarwal, S. K., Gelsema, A. J., and Calaresu, F. R. (1989) Neurons in rostral VLM are inhibited by chemical stimulation of caudal VLM in rats. *Am. J. Physiol.* **257,** R265–R270.

83. Ito, S. and Sved, A. F. (1996) Blockade of angiotensin receptors in rat rostral ventrolateral medulla removes excitatory vasomotor tone. *Am. J. Physiol.* **270,** R1317–R1323.

84. Wong, P. C., Price, W. A., Chiu, A. T., Duncia, J. V., Carini, D. J., Wexler, R. R., et al. (1990) Nonpeptide angiotensin II receptor antagonists. VIII. Characterization of functional antagonism displayed by DuP 753, an orally active antihypertensive agent. *J. Pharmacol. Exp. Ther.* **252,** 719–725.

85. DePasquale, M. J., Fossa, A. A., Holt, W. F., and Mangiapane, M. L. (1992) Central DuP 753 does not lower blood pressure in spontaneously hypertensive rats. *Hypertension* **19,** 668–671.

86. Fow, J. E., Averill, D. B., and Barnes, K. L. (1994) Mechanisms of angiotensin-induced hypotensin and bradycardia in the medial solitary tract nucleus. *Am. J. Physiol.* **276,** H259–H266.

87. Collister, J. P., Hornfeldt, B. J., and Osborn, J. W. (1996) Hypotensive response to losartan in normal rats. Role of ang II and the area postrema. *Hypertension* **27,** 598–606.

88. Collister, J. P. and Osborn, J. W. (1998) Area postrema lesion attenuates the long-term hypotensive effects of losartan in salt-replete rats. *Am. J. Physiol.* **274,** R357–R366.

89. Bui, J. D., Kimura, B., and Phillips, M. I. (1992) Losartan potassium, a nonpeptide antagonist of angiotensin II, chronically administered p.o. does not readily cross the blood-brain barrier. *Eur. J. Pharmacol.* **219,** 147–151.

90. Li, Z., Bains, J. S., and Ferguson, A. V. (1993) Functional evidence that the angiotensin antagonist losartan crosses the blood-brain barrier in the rat. *Brain Res. Bull.* **30,** 33–39.

91. Gorbea-Opplinger, V. J., and Fink, G. D. (1995) Cerebroventricular injections of angiotensin II antagonist: Effects on blood pressure responses to central and systemic angiotensin II. *J. Pharmacol. Exp. Ther.* **273,** 611–616.

92. Lowes, V. L., McLean, L. E., Kasting, N. W., and Ferguson, A. V. (1993) Cardiovascular consequences of microinjection of vasopressin and angiotensin II in the area postrema. *Am. J. Physiol.* **265,** R625–R631.

93. Song, K., Zhou, J., and Mendelsohn, F. A. O. (1991) Access of peripherally administered DuP 753 to rat brain angiotensin II receptors. *Br. J. Pharmacol.* **104,** 771–772.

94. Zhuo, J., Song, K., Abelrahman, A., and Mendelsohn, F. A. O. (1994) Blockade by intravenous losartan of AT_1 angiotensin II receptors in rat brain, kidney and adrenals demonstrated by *in vitro* autoradiography. *Clin. Exp. Pharmacol. Physiol.* **21,** 557–567.

95. Toney, G. M. and Porter, J. P. (1993) Functional role of brain AT_1 and AT_2 receptors in the central angiotensin II pressor response. *Brain Res.* **603,** 57–63.

96. Widdop, R. E., Gardiner, S. M., Kemp, P. A., and Bennett, T. (1993) Central administration of PD 123319 or EXP-3174 inhibits effects of angiotensin II. *Am. J. Physiol.* **264,** H117–H125.

97. Widdop, R. E., Gardiner, S. M., Kemp, P. A., and Bennett, T. (1993) Differential blockade of central effects of angiotensin II by AT_2-receptor antagonists. *Am. J. Physiol.* **265,** H226–H231.

98. Ichiki, T., Labosky, P. A., Shiota, C., Okuyama, S., Imagawa, Y., Fogo, A., et al. (1995) Effects on blood pressure and exploratory behavior of mice lacking angiotensin II type-2 receptor. *Nature* **377,** 748–750.

99. Szczepanska-Sadowska, E. (1996) Interaction of vasopression and angiotensin in the central control of blood pressure and thirst. *Regul. Pept.* **66,** 65–71.

100. Liard, J. F. (1984) Vasopressin in cardiovascular control: role of circulating vasopressin. *Clin. Sci.* **67,** 473–481.

101. Severs, W. B. and Daniels-Severs, A. E. (1973) Effects of angiotensin on the central nervous system. *Pharmacol. Rev.* **25,** 415–449.

102. Keil, L. C., Summy Long, J., and Severs, W. B. (1975) Release of vasopressin by angiotensin II. *Endocrinology.* **96,** 1063–1065.

103. Sterling, G. H., Chee, O., Riggs, R. V., and Keil, L. C. (1980) Effect of chronic intracerebroventricular angiotensin II infusion on vasopressin release in rats. *Neuroendocrinology* **31,** 182–188.

104. Bealer, S. L., Phillips, M. I., Johnson, A. K., and Schmid, P. G. (1979) Anteroventral third ventricle lesions reduce antidiuretic responses to angiotensin II. *Am. J. Physiol.* **236,** E610–E615.

105. Mangiapane, M. L., Thrasher, T. N., Keil, L. C., Simpson, J. B., and Ganong, W. F. (1983) Deficits in drinking and vasopressin secretion after lesions of the nucleus medianus. *Neuroendocrinology* **37,** 73–77.

106. Lind, R. W., Swanson, L. W., and Ganten, D. (1984) Angiotensin II immunoreactivity in the neural afferents and efferents of the subfornical organ of the rat. *Brain Res.* **321,** 209–215.

107. Lind, R. W., Swanson, L. W., and Ganten, D. (1985) Organization of angiotensin II immunoreactive cells and fibers in the rat central nervous system. *Neuroendocrinology* **40,** 2–24.
108. Jhamandas, J. H., Lind, R. W., and Renaud, L. P. (1989) Angiotensin II may mediate excitatory neurotransmission from the subfornical organ to the hypothalamic supraoptic nucleus: an anatomical and electrophysiological study in the rat. *Brain Res.* **487,** 52–61.
109. Ferguson, A. V. and Kasting, N. W. (1986) Electrical stimulation of the subfornical organ increases plasma vasopressin concentrations in the conscious rat. *Am. J. Physiol.* **251,** R425–R428.
110. Shoji, M., Share, L., and Crofton, J. T. (1989) Effect on vasopressin release of microinjection of angiotensin II into the paraventricular nucleus of conscious rats. *Neuroendocrinology* **50,** 327–333.
111. Allen, A. M., Mendelsohn, F. A. O., Gieroba, Z. J., and Blessing, W. W. (1990) Vasopressin release following microinjection of angiotensin II into the caudal ventrolateral medulla oblongata in the anesthetized rabbit. *J. Neuroendocrinol.* **2,** 867–873.
112. Veltmar, A., Culman, J., Qadri, F., Rascher, W., and Unger, T. (1992) Involvement of adrenergic and angiotensinergic receptors in the paraventricular nucleus in the angiotensin II-induced vasopressin release. *J. Pharmacol. Exp. Ther.* **263,** 1253–1260.
113. Qadri, F., Culman, J., Veltmar, A., Maas, K., Rascher, W., and Unger, T. (1993) Angiotensin II-induced vasopressin release is mediated through alpha-1 adrenoceptors and angiotensin II AT_1 receptors in the supraoptic nucleus. *J. Pharmacol. Exp. Ther.* **267,** 567–574.
114. Holhe, S., Spitznagel, H., Rascher, W., Culman, J., and Unger, T. (1995) Angiotensin AT_1 receptor-mediated vasopressin release and drinking are potentiated by an AT_2 receptor antagonist. *Eur. J. Pharmacol.* **275,** 277–282.
115. Bunnemann, B., Iwai, N., Metzger, R., Fuxe, K., Inagami, T., and Ganten, D. (1992) The distribution of angiotensin II AT_1 receptor subtype mRNA in the rat brain. *Neurosci. Lett.* **142,** 155–158.
116. Lenkei, Z., Corvol, P., and Llorens-Cortes, C. (1995) Comparative expression of vasopressin and angiotensin type-1 receptor mRNA in rat hypothalamic nuclei: a double *in situ* hybridization study. *Mol. Brain Res.* **34,** 135–142.
117. Shelat, S. G., Reagan, L. P., King, J. L., Fluharty, S. J., and Flanagan-Cato, L. M. (1998) Analysis of angiotensin type 2 receptors in vasopressinergic neurons and pituitary in the rat. *Regul. Pept.* **73,** 103–112.
118. Sweet, C. S. and Brody, M. J. (1970) Central inhibition of reflex vasodilation by angiotensin and reduced renal pressure. *Am. J. Physiol.* **219,** 1751–1758.
119. Scroop, G. C. and Lowe, R. D. (1968) Central pressor effect of angiotensin mediated by the parasympathetic nervous system. *Nature* **220,** 1331–1332.

120. Barrett, J. P., Ingenito, A. J., and Procita, L. (1971) Influence of the carotid sinus on centrally mediated peripheral cardiovascular effects of angiotensin II. *J. Pharmacol. Exp. Ther.* **176,** 692–700.
121. Lumbers, E. R., McCloskey, D. I., and Potter, E. K. (1979) Inhibition by angiotensin II of baroreceptor-evoked activity in cardiac vagal efferent nerves in the dog. *J. Physiol. (Lond.)* **294,** 69–80.
122. Lee, W. B., Ismay, M. J., and Lumbers, E. R. (1980) Mechanisms by which angiotensin II affects the heart rate of the conscious sheep. *Circ. Res.* **47,** 286–292.
123. Matsuo, H., Ichikawa, S., Sakamaki, T., Tajima, Y., Kogure, M., and Murata, K. (1981) The effect of central iso-renin angiotensin system on pressor responsiveness to angiotensin II. *Life Sci.* **28,** 2329–2336.
124. Matsumura, Y., Hasser, E. M., and Bishop, V. S. (1989) Central effect of angiotensin II on baroreflex regulation in conscious rabbits. *Am. J. Physiol.* **256,** R694–R700.
125. Reid, I. A. and Chou, L. (1990) Analysis of the action of angiotensin II on the baroreflex control of heart rate in conscious rabbits. *Endocrinology* **126,** 2749–2756.
126. Stein, R. D., Stephenson, R. B., and Weaver, L. C. (1984) Central actions of angiotensin II oppose baroreceptor-induced sympatho-inhibition. *Am. J. Physiol.* **246,** R13–R19.
127. Berecek, K. H., Robertson, J. D., and Thorstad, M. H. (1991) Central administration of a specific angiotensin II receptor antagonist on baroreflex function in spontaneously hypertensive rats. *J. Hypertens.* **9,** 365–371.
128. Barron, K. W., Trapani, A. J., Gordon, F. J., and Brody, M. J. (1989) Baroreceptor denervation profoundly enhances cardiovascular responses to central angiotensin II. *Am. J. Physiol.* **257,** H314–H323.
129. Head, G. A., Elghozi, J.-L., and Korner, P. I. (1988) Baroreflex modulation of central angiotensin II pressor responses in conscious rabbits. *J. Hypertens.* **6(Suppl. 4),** S505–S507.
130. Elghozi, J.-L. and Head, G. A. (1990) Spinal noradrenergic pathways and pressor responses to central angiotensin II. *Am. J. Physiol.* **258,** H240–H246.
131. Paull, J. R. A., Bunting, M. W., and Widdop, R. E. (1997) Role of the brain renin–angiotensin system in the maintenance of blood pressure in conscious spontaneously hypertensive and sinoaortic baroreceptor-denervated rats. *Clin. Exp. Pharmacol. Physiol.* **24,** 667–672.
132. Blessing, W. W. and Reis, D. J. (1982) Inhibitory cardiovascular function of neurons in the caudal ventrolateral medulla of the rabbit: relationship to the area containing A1 noradrenergic cells. *Brain Res.* **253,** 161–171.
133. West, M. J., Blessing, W. W., and Chalmers, J. (1981) Arterial baroreceptor reflex function in the conscious rabbit after brainstem lesions coinciding with the A1 group of catecholamine neurons. *Circ. Res.* **49,** 959–970.

134. Blessing, W. W., West, M. J., and Chalmers, J. (1981) Hypertension, bradycardia, and pulmonary edema in the conscious rabbit after brainstem lesions coinciding with the A1 group of catecholamine neurons. *Circ. Res.* **49,** 949–958.

135. Seller, H. and Illert, M. (1969) The localization of the first synapse in the carotid sinus baroreceptor reflex pathway and its alteration of the afferent input. *Pflugers Arch.* **306,** 1–19.

136. Reis, D. J. and Cuenod, M. (1965) Central neural regulation of carotid baroreceptor reflexes in the cat. *Am. J. Physiol.* **209,** 1267–1279.

137. Ross, C. A., Ruggiero, D. A., and Reis, D. J. (1985) Projections from the nucleus tractus solitarii to the rostral ventrolateral medulla. *J. Comp. Neurol.* **242,** 511–534.

138. Casto, R. and Phillips, M. I. (1986) Angiotensin II attenuates baroreflexes at the nucleus tractus solitarius of rats. *Am. J. Physiol.* **250,** R193–R198.

139. Campagnole-Santos, M. J., Diz, D. I., and Ferrario, C. M. (1988) Baroreceptor reflex modulation by angiotensin II at the nucleus tractus solitarii. *Hypertension* **11(Suppl. I),** I-167–I-171.

140. Guo, G. B. and Abboud, F. M. (1984) Angiotensin II attenuates baroreflex control of heart rate and sympathetic activity. *Am. J. Physiol.* **246,** H80–H89.

141. Michelini, L. C. and Bonagamba, L. G. H. (1990) Angiotensin II as a modulator of baroreceptor reflexes in the brainstem of conscious rats. *Hypertension* **15(Suppl. I),** I-45–I-50.

142. Matsukawa, S. and Reid, I. A. (1990) Role of the area postrema in the modulation of the baroreflex control of heart rate by angiotensin II. *Circ. Res.* **67,** 1462–1473.

143. Wong, J., Chou, L. and Reid, I. A. (1993) Role of AT_1 receptors in the resetting of the baroreflex control of heart rate by angiotensin II in the rabbit. *J. Clin. Invest.* **91,** 1516–1520.

144. Bendle, R. D., Malpas, S. C., and Head, G. A. (1997) Role of endogenous angiotensin II on sympathetic reflexes in conscious rabbits. *Am. J. Physiol.* **272,** R1816–R1825.

145. Lin, K. S., Chan, J. Y. H., and Chan, S. H. H. (1997) Involvement of AT_2 receptors at NRVL in tonic baroreflex suppression by endogenous angiotensins. *Am. J. Physiol.* **272,** H2204–H2210.

146. Okamoto, K. and Aori, K. (1963) Development of a strain of spontaneously hypertensive rats *Jpn. Circ. J.,* **27,** 282–293.

147. Trippodo, N. C. and Frohlich, E. D. (1981) Similarities of genetic (spontaneous) hypertension man and rat. *Circ. Res.* **48,** 309–319.

148. Hoffman, W. E., Phillips, M. I., and Schmid, P. G. (1977) Central angiotensin II-induced responses in spontaneously hypertensive rats. *Am. J. Physiol.* **232(4),** H426–H433.

149. Casto, R. and Phillips, M. I. (1985) Neuropeptide action in the nucleus tractus solitarius: angiotensin specificity and hypertensive rats. *Am. J. Physiol.* **249,** R341–R347.

150. Muratani, H., Averill, D. B., and Ferrario, C. M. (1991) Effect of angiotensin II in the ventrolateral medulla of spontaneously hypertensive rats. *Am. J. Physiol.* **260,** R977–R984.
151. Phillips, M. I., Mann, J. F. E., Haebara, H., Hoffman, W. E., Schelling, P., and Ganten, D. (1977) Lowering of hypertensin by central saralasin in the absence of plasma renin. *Nature* **270,** 445–447.
152. McDonald, W., Wickre, C., Aumann, S., Ban, D., and Moffitt, B. (1980) The sustained antihypertensive effect of chronic cerebro-ventricular infusion of angiotensin antagonist in spontaneously hypertensive rats. *Endocrinology* **107,** 1305–1308.
153. Mann, J. F. E., Phillips, M. I., Dietz, R., Haebara, H., and Ganten, D. (1978) Effects of central and peripheral angiotensin blockade in hypertensive rats. *Am. J. Physiol.* **234,** H629–H637.
154. Jensen, L. L., Harding, J. W., and Wright, J. W. (1988) Central effects of a specific angiotensin receptor antagonist, sarthran (Sar^1, Thr^{8}AII) in normotensive and spontaneously hypertensive rat strains. *Brain. Res.* **448,** 359–363.
155. Chan, R. K. W., Chan, Y. S., and Wong, T. M. (1994) Effects of [Sar^1, Ile^8]-angiotensin II on rostral ventrolateral medulla neurons and blood pressure in spontaneously hypertensive rats. *Neuroscience* **63,** 267–277.
156. Muratani, H., Ferrario, C. M., and Averill, D. B. (1993) Ventrolateral medulla in spontaneously hypertensive rats: role of angiotensin II. *Am. J. Physiol.* **264,** R388–R395.
157. Elghozi, J.-L., Altman, J., Devynck, M. A., Liard, J. F., Grunfeld, J. P., and Meyer, P. (1976) Lack of hypotensive effect on central injection of angiotensin inhibitors in spontaneously hypertensive (SH) and normotensive rats. *Clin. Sci. Mol. Med.* **51,** 385s–389s.
158. Tsutsumi, K. and Saavedra, J. M. (1991) Differential development of angiotensin II receptor subtypes in the rat brain. *Endocrinology* **128,** 630–632.
159. Toney, G. M. and Porter, J. P. (1993) Functional roles of brain AT$_1$ and AT$_2$ receptors in the central angiotensin II pressor response in conscious young spontaneously hypertensive rats. *Dev. Brain Res.* **71,** 193–199.
160. Toney, G. M. and Porter, J. P. (1993) Effects of blockade of AT$_1$ and AT$_2$ receptors in brain on the central angiotensin II pressor response in conscious spontaneously hypertensive rats. *Neuropharmacology* **32,** 581–589.
161. Cole, F. E., Frohlich, E. D., and Macphee, A. A. (1978) Angiotensin binding affinity and capacity in the midbrain area of spontaneously hypertensive rats. *Brain Res.* **154,** 178–181.
162. Stamler, J. F., Raizada, M. K., Fellows, R. E., and Phillips, M. I. (1980) Increased specific binding of angiotensin II in the organum vasculosum of the laminae terminalis area of the spontaneously hypertensive rat brain. *Neurosci. Lett.* **17,** 173–177.

163. Raizada, M. K., Muther, T. F., and Sumners, C. (1984) Increased angiotensin II receptors in neuronal cultures from hypertensive rat brain. *Am. J. Physiol.* **247,** C364–C372.

164. Saavedra, J. M., Correa, F. M., Plunkett, L. M., Israel, A., Kurihara, M., and Shigematsu, K. (1986) Binding of angiotensin and atrial natriuretic peptide in brain of hypertensive rats. *Nature* **320,** 758–760.

165. Saavedra, J. M., Correa, F. M. A., Kuriha, M., and Shigematsu, K. (1986) Increased number of angiotensin II receptors in the subfornical organ of spontaneously hypertensive rats. *J. Hypertens.* **4(Suppl. 5),** S27–S30.

166. Gehlert, D. R., Speth, R. C., and Wamsley, J. K. (1986) Quantitative autoradiography of angiotensin II receptors in the SHR brain. *Peptides* **7,** 1021–1027.

167. Healy, D. P. and Zhang, N. (1992) Angiotensin II receptors in the solitary-vagal area of hypertensive rats. *Hypertension* **19,** 355–361.

168. Andrews, C. O., Crim, J. W., and Hartle, D. K. (1993) Angiotensin II binding in area postrema and nucleus tractus solitarius of SHR and WKY rats. *Brain Res. Bull.* **32,** 419–424.

169. Komatus, C., Shibata, K., and Furukawa, T. (1996) The developmental increase of the AT_{1A}, but not the AT_{1B}, receptor mRNA level at the preoptic are in spontaneously hypertensive rats. *Life Sci.* **58,** 1109–1121.

170. Raizada, M. K., Sumners, C., and Lu, D. (1993) Angiotensin II type 1 receptor mRNA levels in the brains of normotensive and spontaneously hypertensive rats. *J. Neurochem.* **60,** 1949–1952.

171. Raizada, M. K., Lu, D., Tang, W., Kurian, P., and Sumners, C. (1993) Increased angiotensin II type 1 receptor gene expression in neuronal cultures from spontaneously hypertensive rats. *Endocrinology* **132,** 1715–1722.

172. Sumners, C., Richards, E. M., Tang, W., and Raizada, M. K. (1993) Angiotensin type 2 receptor expression in neuronal cultures from spontaneously hypertensive rat brain. *Regul. Pept.* **44,** 181–188.

173. Song, K., Kurobe, Y., Kanehara, H., Okunishi, H., Wada, T., Inada, Y., et al. (1994) Quantitative localization of angiotensin receptor subtypes in spontaneously hypertensive rats. *Blood Press.* **5(Suppl.),** 21–26.

174. Felix, D. and Schelling, P. (1982) Increased sensitivity of neurons to angiotensin II in SHR as compared to WKY rats. *Brain Res.* **252,** 63–69.

175. Gyurko, R., Tran, D., and Phillips, M. I. (1997) Time course of inhibition of hypertension by antisense oligonucleotides targeted to AT_1 angiotensin receptor mRNA in spontaneously hypertensive rats. *Am. J. Hypertens.* **10,** 56S–62S.

176. Phillips, M. I., Mohuczy-Dominiak, D., Coffey, M., Galli, S. M., Kimura, B., Wu, P., et al. (1997) Prolonged reduction of high blood pressure with an *in vivo*, nonpathogenic, adeno-associated viral vector delivery of AT_1-R mRNA antisense. *Hypertension* **29(Pt. 2),** 374–380.

177. Schelling, P., Meyer, D., Loos, H. E., Speck, G., Phillips, M. I., Johnson, A. K., et al. (1982) A micromethod for the measurement of renin in brain nuclei: its application in spontaneously hypertensive rats. *Neuropharmacology* **21**, 455–463.
178. Phillips, M. I. and Kimura, B. (1986) Converting enzyme inhibitors and brain angiotensin. *J. Cardiovasc. Pharmacol.* **8(Suppl. 10)**, S82–S90.
179. Mann, J. F., Rascher, W., Dietz, R., Schomig, A., and Ganten, D. (1979) Effects of an orally active converting-enzyme inhibitor, SQ 14225, on pressor responses to angiotensin administered into the brain of spontaneously hypertensive rats. *Clin. Sci.* **56**, 585–589.
180. Ferrario, C. M., Gildenberg, P. L., and McCubbin, J. W. (1972) Cardiovascular effects of angiotensin mediated by the central nervous system. *Circ. Res.* **30**, 257–262.
181. Okuno, T., Nagahama, S., Lindheimer, M. D., and Oparil, S. (1983) Attenuation of the development of spontaneous hypertension in rats by chronic central administration of captopril. *Hypertension* **5**, 653–662.
182. Berecek, K. H., Okuno, T., and Oparil, S. (1983) Altered vascular reactivity and baroreflex sensitivity induced by chronic central administration of captopril in the spontaneously hypertensive rat. *Hypertension* **5**, 698–700.
183. Gonzalez, E. R., Krieger, A. J., and Sapru, H. N. (1983) Central resetting of baroreflex in the spontaneously hypertensive rat. *Hypertension* **5**, 346–352.
184. Widdop, R. E., Verberne, J. M., Jarrot, B., and Louis, W. J. (1990) Impaired arterial baroreceptor reflex and cardiopulmonary vagal reflex in conscious spontaneously hypertensive rats. *J. Hypertens.* **8**, 269–275.
185. Cheng, S. W. T., Kirk, K. A., Robertson, J. D., and Berecek, K. H. (1989) Brain angiotensin II and baroreceptor reflex function in spontaneously hypertensive rats. *Hypertension* **14**, 274–281.
186. Head, G. A. and Adams, M. A. (1992) Characterization of the baroreceptor heart rate reflex during development in spontaneously hypertensive rats. *Clin. Exp. Pharmacol. Physiol.* **19**, 587–597.
187. Bartholomeusz, B. and Widdop, R. E. (1995) Effect of acute and chronic treatment with the angiotensin II subtype 1 receptor antagonist EXP 3174 on baroreflex function in conscious spontaneously hypertensive rats. *J. Hypertens.* **13**, 219–225.
188. Brunner, H. R., Gavras, H., Laragh, J. H., and Keenan, R. (1973) Angiotensin II blockade in man by Sar[1]-ala[8]-angiotensin II for understanding and treatment of high blood pressure. *Lancet* **ii**, 1045–1048.
189. Ferreira, S. H. (1965) A bradykinin-potentiating factor (BPF) present in the venom of *Bothrops jararaca*. *Br. J. Pharmacol.* **24**, 163–169.
190. Fouad-Tarazi, F. M. (1994) Hemodynamic effects of inhibitors of the renin-angiotensin system. *J. Hypertens.* **12(Suppl. 2)**, S25–S29.

191. LeJemtel, T. H., Keung, E., Frishman, W. H., Ribner, H. S., and Sonnenblick, E. H. (1982) Hemodynamic effects of captopril in patients with severe chronic heart failure. *Am. J. Cardiol.* **49,** 1484–1488.

192. Curtiss, C., Cohn, J. N., Vrobel, T., and Franciosa, J. A. (1978) Role of the renin–angiotensin system in the systemic vasoconstriction of chronic congestive heart failure. *Circulation* **58,** 763–770.

193. Brunner, H. R., Nussberger, J., and Waeber, B. (1993) Angiotensin II blockade compared with other pharmacological methods of inhibiting the renin-angiotensin system. *J. Hypertens.* **11(Suppl. 3),** S53–S58.

194. Morice, A. H., Brown, M. J., Lowry, R., and Higenbottam, T. (1987) Angiotensin-converting enzyme and the cough reflex. *Lancet* **2(8568),** 1116–1118.

195. Saxena, P. R. and Schoemaker, R. G. (1993) Organ blood flow protection in hypertension and congestive heart failure. *Am. J. Med.* **94(Suppl. 4A),** 4A-4S–4A-12S.

196. Motz, W. and Strauer, B. E. (1994) Organ protection: benefit from antihypertensive treatment? *J. Cardiovasc. Pharmacol.* **24(Suppl. 2),** S50–S54.

197. Magrini, F., Reggiani, P., Roberts, N., Meazza, R., Ciulla, M., and Zanchetti, A. (1988) Effects of angiotensin and angiotensin blockade on coronary circulation and coronary reserve. *Am. J. Med.* **84(Suppl. 3A),** 55–60.

198. Magrini, F., Reggiani, P., Fratianni, G., Morganti, A., and Zanchetti, A. (1993) Coronary blood flow in renovascular hypertension. *Am. J. Med.* **94(Suppl. 4A),** 4A-45S–4A-48S.

199. Motz, W. and Strauer, B. E. (1996) Improvement of coronary flow reserve after long-term therapy with enalapril. *Hypertension* **27,** 1031–1038.

200. Falkenhahn, M., Gohlke, P., Paul, M., Stoll, M., and Unger, T. (1994) The renin–angiotensin system in the heart and vascular wall: new therapeutic aspects. *J. Cardiovasc. Pharmacol.* **24(Suppl. 2),** S6–S13.

201. Nakashima, Y., Fouad, F. M., and Tarazi, R. C. (1984) Regression of left ventricular hypertrophy from systemic hypertension by enalapril. *Am. J. Cardiol.* **53,** 1044–1049.

202. Cruickshank, J. M., Lewis, J., Moore, V., and Dodd, C. (1992) Reversibility of left ventricular hypertrophy by differing types of hypertensive therapy. *J. Hum. Hypertens.* **6,** 85–90.

203. London, G. M. (1995) Large artery function and alterations in hypertension. *J. Hypertens.* **13(Suppl. 2),** S35–S38.

204. Zelis, R., Sinoway, L. I., Musch, T. I., Davis, D., and Just, H. (1988) Regional blood flow in congestive heart failure: concept of compensatory mechanisms with short and long term constants. *Am. J. Cardiol.* **62,** 2E–8E.

205. Francis, G. S., Benedict, C., Johnstone, D. E., Kirlin, P. C., Nicklas, J., Liang, C.-S., et al. (1990) Comparison of neuroendocrine activa-

tion in patients with left ventricular dysfunction with and without congestive heart failure. *Circulation* **82**, 1724–1729.

206. Kubo, S. H. (1990) Neurohormonal activation and the response to converting enzyme inhibitors in congestive heart failure. *Circulation* **81(Suppl. III)**, III-107–III-114.

207. Chatterjee, K. (1996) Inhibitors of the renin–angiotensin system in established cardiac failure. *Heart* **76(Suppl. 3)**, 83–91.

208. Levine, T. B., Olivari, M. T., Garberg, V., Sharkey, S. W., and Cohn, J. N. (1984) Hemodynamic and clinical response to enalapril, a long acting converting enzyme inhibitor, in patients with congestive heart failure. *Circulation* **3**, 548–553.

209. Foult, J.-M., Tavolaro, O., Antony, I., and Nitenberg, A. (1988) Direct myocardial and coronary effects of enalaprilat in patients with dilated cardiomyopathy: assessment by a bilateral intracoronary infusion technique. *Circulation* **77**, 337–344.

210. Dietz, R., Waas, W., Susselbeck, T., Willenbrock, R., and Osterziel, K. J. (1993) Improvement of cardiac function by angiotensin converting enzyme inhibition. Sites of action. *Circulation* **87(Suppl. IV)**, IV-108–IV-116.

211. Rademaker, M. T., Fitzpatrick, M. A., Charles, C. J., Frampton, C. M., Richards, A. M., Nichols, M. G., et al. (1995) Central angiotensin II AT_1-receptor antagonism in normal and heart-failed sheep. *Am. J. Physiol.* **269**, H425–H432.

212. Squire, I. B. (1994) Actions of angiotensin on cerebral blood flow autoregulation in health and disease. *J. Hypertens.* **12**, 1203–1208.

213. Paulson, O. B., Jarden, J. O., Godtfredsen, J., and Vorstrup, S. (1984) Cerebral blood flow in patients with congestive heart failure treated with captopril. *Am. J. Med.* **76(5B)**, 91–95.

214. Rajagopalan, B., Raine, A. E. G., Cooper, R., and Ledingham, J. G. G. (1984) Changes in cerebral blood flow in patients with severe congestive cardiac failure before and after captopril treatment. *Am. J. Med.* **76(5B)**, 86–90.

215. Kamishirado, H., Inoue, T., Fujito, T., Kase, M., Shimizu, M., Sakai, Y., et al. (1997) Effect of enalapril maleate on cerebral blood flow in patients with chronic heart failure. *Angiology* **48**, 707–713.

216. Kobayashi, S., Yamaguchi, S., Okada, K., Suyama, N., Bokura, K., and Murao, M. (1992) The effect of enalapril maleate on cerebral blood flow in chronic cerebral infarction. *Angiology* **43**, 378–388.

217. Naveri, L., Stromberg, C., and Saavedra, J. M. (1994) Angiotensin II AT_2 receptor stimulation extends the upper limit of cerebral blood flow autoregulation: agonist effects of CGP 42112 and PD 123319. *J. Cereb. Blood Flow Metab.* **14**, 38–44.

218. Foote, E. F. and Halstenson, C. E. (1993) New therapeutic agents in the management of hypertensin: angiotensin II-receptor antagonists and renin inhibitors *Ann. Pharmacother.* **27**, 1495–1503.

219. Christen, Y., Waeber, B., Nussberger, J., Lee, R. J., Timmermans, P. B. M. W. M., and Brunner, H. R. (1991) Dose-response relations following oral administration of DuP 753 to normal humans. *Am. J. Hypertens.* **4,** 350S–353S.

220. Fluharty, S. J., and Sakai, R. R. (1995) Behavioral and cellular analysis of adrenal steroid and angiotensin interactions mediating salt appetite, in *Progress in Psychobiology and Physiological Psychology* (Fluharty, S. J., Morrison, A. R., Sprague, J. M., and Stellar, E., eds.), Academic, New York, pp. 177–212.

CHAPTER 12

Mediators of Inflammation in Patients with Coronary Artery Disease

Mike J. L. DeJongste and Gert J. Ter Horst

1. Rationale

During the last century, in spite of the tremendous increase in theoretical knowledge and practical opportunities in medical science, the rate and number of diseases have not been decreased. This unexpected effect is related to the creation of new conditions for illness, which often results from changes in the environment. So, on the one hand, environmental modifications have increased life expectancy through expansion of and improvement in both hygienic and medical strategies. On the other hand, culture influences have yield to unhealthy habits like sedentary lifestyles, "fast food" meals, stressful jobs, and so forth. Subsequently, the illness pattern of the Western population changed from infectious diseases to more "culture" diseases, such as gastric ulcers and coronary artery disease (CAD). Ischemic coronary artery disease usually results from plaque formation in the coronary arteries. To date, in spite of thorough investigations, no evidence is available that "cultural" influences, such as smoking and unhealthy food (high energetic, fatty and salty meals) habits, are the sole initiators in the process of atherosclerotic

From: *The Nervous System and the Heart*
Ed: G. J. Ter Horst © Humana Press Inc.

plaque formation. Albeit that atherosclerotic plaque formation is likely to be multifactorial, the search for the initial trigger is ongoing. Such a trigger might very well be a chronic inflammatory state or an occasionally exaggerated inflammatory response. During the last years, more and more evidence is becoming available that in CAD an inflammatory response, whether or not related to an infectious trigger, plays a key role in the progression of the atherosclerotic plaque formation.

It is the purpose of this chapter to discuss newer insights in the pathophysiology of angina resulting from ischemic coronary artery disease and to suggest some potential ensuing therapies. Finally, in this chapter, we will discuss a putative, novel, humoral route of communication between the heart and the brain. This system, involving mediators of inflammation, may interact with signal transduction in the limbic forebrain (Chapter 2) by inducing a selective endothelial leakage at sites participating in the perception of anginal pain and initiation of the behavioral and cardiovascular responses. Potentially, this humoral mechanism could offer an explanation for the increased risk of cardiovascular events in patients suffering of a postmyocardial depression (Chapter 13).

2. Angina Pectoris and Myocardial Ischemia

Angina pectoris can be defined as the result of a disease of the coronary arteries causing momentary pain in the chest, sometimes spreading to arm(s), throat, and neck. Heberden first recognized angina pectoris as a clinical identity. In his classic article, he defined the strangling sensation with a feeling of anxiety, provoked through exercise and vanishing during rest, as "angor" onto the chest or "pectoris" (1). Angina pectoris may presents itself in a variety of forms of different duration and various initiating, aggravating, and relieving factors. To date, angina pectoris is usually characterized by a discomfort in the chest or associated adjacent areas of the body that is accompanied with myocardial ischemia (2). When myocardial cell damage (necrosis) is involved, the angina is termed "infarction pain."

Angina is a sensitive parameter for myocardial ischemia. On the other hand, angina is not a landmark of an occlusive coronary disease *(3)*. The specificity of angina for CAD is low, because the myocardial ischemic threshold is determined at a minimum of 60% reduction of the diameter of a coronary artery *(4)*, whereas the narrowing may be as large as 75% before either anginal complaints or symptoms of ischemia occur *(5)*. Regional or global myocardial ischemia occurs when the oxygen and nutrients supply from the coronary arteries does not meet the myocardial metabolic demand. Because a deficient nutrient supply is a more or less unknown element, it is used to define myocardial ischemia in terms of an oxygen deficit.

3. Tools for the Assessment of Angina Pectoris Resulting from Myocardial Ischemia

In addition to the relatively sensitive anamnesis, with an unfortunately low specificity, several tools for the investigation of myocardial ischemia are available. Because a normal electrocardiogram (ECG) does not exclude coronary artery disease, the standard 12-lead resting ECG is of little value for detection of stable angina resulting from occlusive coronary artery disease. Only abnormal ST segments or signs of an old myocardial infarction are valuable indicators for the detection of myocardial ischemia. Depending on the initial conditions, various influences can induce ECG changes (Fig. 1). Angina pectoris, the main clinical symptom accompanying ischemic heart diseases, is associated with an impaired residual coronary flow reserve *(6)*. When a patient with an ischemic heart disease experiences effort angina, the product of heart rate and systolic blood pressure increases and the coronary flow reserve no longer match the myocardial oxygen consumption. Stable angina pectoris is considered a symptomatic expression of a discrepancy between a reduced myocardial oxygen supply, usually the result of the formation of an atherosclerotic plaque and the myocardial oxygen consumption. Parameters determining the oxygen

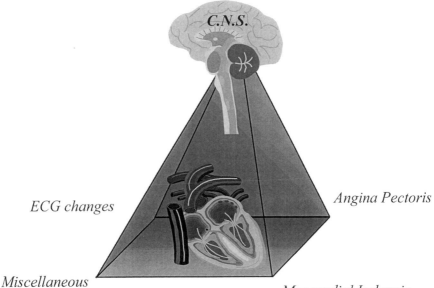

ECG changes   *Angina Pectoris*

Miscellaneous
influences (K, drugs etc)   *Myocardial Ischemia*

Fig. 1. Schematic relationship among the ST–T segment on the ECG, the occurrence of angina pectoris, and myocardial ischemia. Patients may experience anginal complaints without myocardial ischemia during esophagus spasm or with myocardial ischemia as a symptom of coronary artery disease. Myocardial ischemia and ST–T segment changes are not directly associated. There may be myocardial ischemia without ECG changes during conduction disturbances or cancellation. On the other hand, ST–T segment changes are not always delineating myocardial ischemia, as is the case in syndrome X (normal coronary arteries with typical angina and ST–T segment depression during exercise). All types of influences can affect the relationship among others, potassium, medication, and so on.

supply are the mean arterial blood pressure, the oxygen saturation of the blood, and the coronary vascular resistance (tonus of the coronary arteries, vasodilatation capacity). The myocardial oxygen demand is determined, among others, by heart rate, wall stress, and contractility force (afterload).

However, tachycardias "provoke myocardial ischemia more easily than increases in blood pressure" (7). Therefore, tests that combine both determinants of myocardial oxygen requirements usually are more reliable indicators for ischemia. In the sequence of events following changes in coronary blood flow, both anginal pain and ST-segment changes in the ECG are relatively late, inconsistent, and nonspecific phenomena of myocardial ischemia *(8)*. To illustrate the latter, the ECG does not necessarily show ST-segment changes in patients with a severe coronary artery disease during painful ischemic episodes. In contrast, the ST-segment changes may occur without concomitant angina pectoris ("silent ischemia") as has often been demonstrated during 48-h ambulatory ECG recordings. Moreover, patients with apparently unaffected coronary arteries may experience chest pain, with concomitant ST-segment changes on exercise ECG. This type of angina has been described as "syndrome X" *(9)* and may be a consequence of noncardiac diseases *(10)*. The above-mentioned discordance between angina and ST-segment changes may find its origin in the central nervous system (CNS) and, in particular, in circuitry for the regulation of myocardial blood flow.

Laboratory investigations (hypercholesterolemia) and chest X-rays (cardiomegaly) may give some indirect information on the existence of coronary heart disease. The exercise ECG is as a provocation test, a sensitive and relatively specific method for detection of ischemia. Forty-eight-hour ECG (Holter) recordings, on the other hand, supply information about among others occurrence of myocardial ischemia in daily life. Coronary and cine angiography are very useful methods for mapping the anatomy of the coronary arteries and the wall motions of the left ventricle, respectively. However, functional morphological aspects, important for treatment of CAD patients, are not covered by cine angiography. This may lead to interpretation problems with the cineangiogram, either in the case of longstanding reduced coronary flow resulting in "hibernation" *(11)* of the myocardium or move after short-term intermittent coronary artery occlusions "stunning" *(12)*. Both of these forms of ischemia are reversible. Especially in these stunned and hibernating conditions, radionuclides such as thallium-201 and technetium Sesta-MIBI scintigraphy, stress echocardiography and positron emission tomography (PET) have proven to be useful tools in the detection of viable myocardial tissue *(13)*. To date in clinical practice, the viability of the myocardium has become a major determinant in considering a patient for a revascularization procedure. Preconditioning is the term reserved for the protective effect (during a couple of hours) of brief periods (2–10 min) of myocardial ischemia on subsequent ischemic events *(14)*. Repetitive transient myocardial ischemic events improve cardiac function, when compared to the functioning of the heart in unconditioned controls *(15)*. This preconditioning effect may involve different chemical and physical factors that are associated with myocardial ischemia and fulfills a role in myocardial protection against environmental stress. The A1-adenosine receptors have been reported to attribute importantly to the induction of cardiac preconditioning, although the underlying mechanisms await further basic investigation *(16)*.

To date, the sequence of events during myocardial ischemia that triggers stimulation of both cardiac chemical and mechanical receptors has not yet been unraveled. However, it has been proposed and demonstrated clinically that adenosine plays a key role in cardiac nociceptor activation during ischemia (Chapter 7). Myocardial ischemia is associated with a release of various compounds from the myocardium into the circulation, which all potentially induce or modulate cardiac nociceptor activation. The soup of compounds initiating an inflammatory response may be comprised of adenosine, bradykinin, endothelin, histamine, 5-hydroxytryptine (serotonin), neurpeptide Y, and prostaglandins *(17)*. In a study performed to evaluate the relationship between cardiac receptor expression and anginal pain intensity, the level of cardiac bradykinin receptor density, and not the adenosine receptor expression, was found to correlate with the characteristics of anginal pain perception *(18)*.

4. The Inflammatory Response in Atherosclerosis

During the last decade, gradual awareness has been created in the literature for the concept that the process of atherogenesis is reflecting the general pathology of a chronic inflammatory tissue response against injury *(19)*. However, debate is ongoing about whether or not the inflammatory response is induced by a chronic external stimulus (for instance, by an infection) or results from an altered internal stimulus, such as mechanical stress-induced collagen production to maintain cell integrity *(20)*.

Evidence that a chronic inflammation promotes coronary atherosclerotic disease is provided by, among others, the increased release of free radicals during angina. The absence of plasma troponin-T, excluding myocardial cell necrosis as a course of the inflammatory response, and the activation of systemic markers of inflammation (neutrophils, lymphocytes, C-reactive protein, acute-phase proteins, interleukin-1 and -6, and tumor necrosis factor-alpha) are indicative of coronary endothelial inflammatory reactions in patients with unstable angina *(21)*. Finally, myocardial infarction is also associated with an inflammatory response that encompasses increased activity of leukocytes and immune activation.

The integrity of the endothelial cell layer and optimal endothelial cell function are critical factors for the protection of the vessel from thrombosis; it prevents adhesion of blood cells, inhibits smooth-muscle proliferation, and sustains vasodilatation. Different noxious stimuli can either activate or damage the coronary endothelium, such as mechanical (shear stress), chemical (oxidized low-density lipoproteins), immunological (sensitized lymphocytes), infectious (*Chlamydia pneumoniae*, Cytomegalovirus, herpes virus), and anoxic (ischemic) *(22)* stimuli. Myocardial hypoxia leads to endothelial damage, whether or not in conjunction with smooth-muscle cell impairment. The injury will alter the antiadhesive function of endothelial cells by triggering the expression of selective cellular adhesion molecules (CAMs) on the cell membrane *(23)*. These CAMs play a key role in the cardiovascular pathology of both cell–cell and cell–extracellular matrix interactions. Several CAMs have been identified, such as selectins, integrins, and immunoglobulins. The latter molecules, involved in the adhesion of leukocytes, consist of intracellular adhesion molecules (ICAM), vascular cell adhesion molecules (VCAM), and platelet-endothelial cell adhesion molecules (PECAM). Ligands expressed at the cell membrane of immune activated blood cells will recognize these CAMs and enable the docking of these cells to the affected endothelium. Subsequently, the inflammation will influence larger parts of the endothelium and spread out as a result of the local release of cytokinines, growth factors, free radicals, and adverse cell–cell interactions that cause derangements of cellular metabolism (24). Some members of the *cytokin* family, the so-called pro-inflammatory group, comprised of, among others, tumor necrosis factor-alpha (TNF-α), interleukin (IL)-1β, IL-6, and interferon induce expression of CAMs in healthy endothelial cells and activate leukocytes. Other members of the cytokine family, among others, IL-2, and IL-10 can modulate this response in order to reduce a spreading of the infection. In addition, the activated leukocytes will create an environment that supports occlusion of the vessel. When injured, the endothelium initiates repair mechanisms that include antiocclusive aspects. In inflammatory processes, cytokines such as IL-1β and TNF enhance the production of the "free radical" nitric oxide (NO) in the endothelium, the smooth-muscle cells, the macrophages, the platelets, and the brain. NO is a potent vasodilator, it inhibits adhesion of platelets and monocytes to the vessel wall and impairs vascular smooth-muscle proliferation (25). The response of the smooth-muscle cells to NO decrease, however, during progression of the atherosclerotic process and NO is inactivated by, among others, (dose-dependent), endothelin, superoxide anions, and tromboxane A_2.

How an infection interacts with the coronary endothelium is unknown. The injurious trigger, initiating a chronic and local inflammation, might be either a previous gram-negative bacterial infection with *Chlamydia pneumoniae*, *Heliobacter pylori*, or an infection with either cytomegalovirus (CMV), or herpes virus (26). Only recently have Chlamydia infections been recognized to be associated with atherosclerosis. *Heliobacter pylori* infections can induce an autoimmune reaction against endothelial antigen heat-shock protein (HSP). Subsequently, HSP may facilitate the slow process of atherogenesis *(27)*. However, for *H. pylori*, no associations has been found with other vascular risk factors *(28)*; therefore, the demonstration of *H. pylori* may be considered a by-stander phenomenon.

Conditions in which the energy requirements of the heart are not met by aerobic processes cause acidosis. This "unfavorable" intracellular condition triggers a selective activation of, among others, a group of stress proteins that participate in various cardioprotective mechanisms such as enhanced thermal stress resulting from increased work load. Jeopardized heart cells synthesize within minutes after the onset of the stressful condition, heat-shock proteins (HSP). HSP induction in vitro by short pre-exposure to sublethal temperatures protected cultured cells to survive lethal temperatures for a brief period of time. The temperature rise associated with inflammatory responses induces HSPs that contribute to stabilization of the cellular membranes and encapsulation of proteins with functions vital to cellular physiology *(29)*. Since the first reports of a thermotolerance effect of HSPs, it has been reported that many other stressors, such as pain, alcohol, endotoxins, amphetamines, and heavy metals *(30)*, can induce HSP expression. Therefore, today, HSPs are generally considered "stress proteins." Induction of HSPs synthesis increases, for example, the antioxidant barrier by improving the activity of the free-radical scavenger enzyme superoxide dismutase *(31)*.

Cytomegaloviruses, contained in contaminated monocytes that are recruited at the site of vascular injury, become reactivated after contact with elements of endothelial cells, smooth-muscle cells, and oxydized low-density lipoproteins (oxLDL). A cytomegalovirus infection, which causes immediate early gene expression, increases the uptake of oxLDL and stimulates the class A scavenger receptor gene *(32)*. Because oxLDL is thought to play an important role in atherogenesis, this compound provides a link between infection and atherosclerosis. One of the elements of the vessel wall that can activate the cytomegalovirus is the major immediate–early promotor (MIEP), controlling immediate–early gene expression and, thereby, viral replication (33). The activated cytomegalovirus may subsequently infect neighboring endothelial cells inducing a cascade of events predisposing the development of atherosclerosis.

Following infiltration of monocytes and T lymphocytes, adhesion receptors such as integrins mediate the atherosclerotic process (see above) (34). In addition, macrophage class A scavenger receptors (MRS-A) are able to modify the receptor-mediated uptake of LDL, yielding to both pathological deposition of cholesterol and an increased susceptibility to infection with herpes virus of the arterial vascular cells (35). Herpes virus infections alter cholesterol trafficking through the modulation of protein kinase activity (36).

Within atherosclerotic lesions, multipotent mediators of inflammation and immunity have been demonstrated (Fig. 2). Protein mediators of inflammation, such as growth factors, have been emerged as candidate monitor substances for alterations in cell function during the atherogenetic process. In addition, mediators of immunity, such as cytokines (tumor necrosis factor [TNF-α and TNF-β), interferon-γ [INF], interleukin [IL]), initially thought to exchange signals among leukocytes, have been found to also affect the function of vascular endothelial and smooth-muscle cells. The impairment of the function and integrity of the arterial wall through cytokines has been associated with the induction of selective enzymes, such as metalloproteinases. These enzymes induce a cascade of events that start with the degradation of constituents of the arterial matrix. Moreover, cytokines inhibit the proliferation of smooth-muscle cells (37). Although collagen and elastin usually have resistance to breakdown, their de novo synthesis can be inhibited by the metalloproteinases, which makes the cap of the plaque vulnerable to rupture.

In atheromata, a major portion of the cell population at sites of advanced atherosclerotic plaques have been identified as chronically activated T lymphocytes (38). These activated T lymphocytes release cytokines, such as TNF-α, that

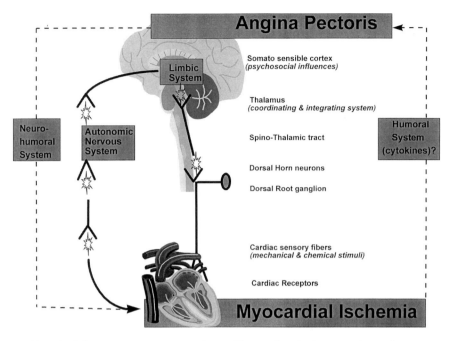

Fig. 2. Schematic representation of heart–brain interactions showing afferent (pain) pathways activated during myocardial ischemia and efferent (sympathetic) pathways conveying (mainly limbic) output from nervous circuitry involved in cardiovascular regulation. The efferent pathways are comprised of a nervous and a neuroendocrine (hypothalamo–pituitary–adrenal) system. We suggest a double-feedback system comprised of sensory afferent nerves and additional afferent humoral pathways. Activation of the latter system during myocardial infarction may be associated with adverse effects in the forebrain that could explain the occurrence of mood disorders and increased risk of sudden death in a group of patients. (See text for details.)

subsequently impair regulating functions of both smooth-muscle cells and macrophages. Also, acute-phase proteins like ferritine *(39)*, fibrinogen *(40)*, or compounds behaving like acute-phase reactants, such as lipoprotein-A [Lp(a)] have been associated with increased atheromatous events *(41)*. Lp(a) can be considered an interface between atherosclerosis and thrombosis. Lp(a) is found to employ antifibrinolytic effects in both chronic and acute thrombotic processes by impairing the binding of plasminogen to platelets, mononuclear cells, endothelial cells, and fibrin. In addition, Lp(a) weakens the binding of tissue plasminogen activator to fibrin and endothelial cells (42).

5. Mediators of Inflammation as Means of Communication in Coronary Artery Disease

Following an ischemic accident of the heart, we "feel" the anginal pain in the brain. The anginal pain pathways have been studied intensively. However, these pain pathways cannot sufficiently provide an answer for the coincidenced psychological changes that often accompanied an acute myocardial ischemic event. It has been well established that after a myocardial infarction, changes in the emotional state, like depressive feelings, are more pronounced. In particular, this altered mental state has also been noted after bypass surgery (43,44). The substrate through which an ischemic event in one organ (the heart) can induce changes in another organ (the brain) that lead to increased emotional states has not yet been clarified. A very fundamental question is whether this altered emotional processing in patients with CAD is solely disease related (i.e., to the recognition of life's finiteness) or to "hardware" defects resulting from neurodegenerative and/or neurochemical alterations in the emotional brain circuitry. We have provided a hypothesis for hardware defects in the emotional brain that particularly involve the anterior cingulate cortex.

Molecular messengers that are released from the ischemic myocardium or atherosclerotic lesions can convey signals from the heart to other organs like the brain (Fig. 3). For example, the cytokines fulfill a role in communication between sites of inflammation and the central nervous system structures that regulate body temperature to induce fever (45). Our hypothesis derived from the assumption that coronary atherosclerosis leading to an acute myocardial event is associated with immune activation (see Subheading 4). In addition to the pain signal resulting from myocardial nociceptor activation, cytokines and other mediators of inflam-

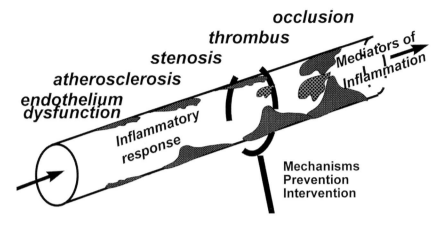

Fig. 3. Schematic drawing of a coronary artery with from the left (inflammatory triggers) to the right side, sequential development of the atherosclerotic process, resulting in occlusion of a coronary artery and release of mediators of inflammation. For the understanding of the ultimate result, Virchov's triad is useful. This includes changes in the vascular wall (endothelium), changes in blood flow (reduction through plaque formation), and alterations in composition of the different vaso-active and rheologic blood compounds.

mation and tissue damage are released into the circulation, to convey information to the central nervous structures for the neurohumoral responses. One of these cytokines, of which the release peaks early after an acute myocardial infarction is TNF-α *(46,47)*. However, alterations in plasma levels of other interleukins were found also *(48)*. It has been reported that TNF-α disrupts the integrity of the endothelial cell lining in various organs *(49)*. In the brain, circulating TNF-α increased the permeability of the blood-brain barrier. This latter effect was found to be selective, affecting only a very limited number of structures in the central nervous system *(50,51)*. As measured by deposition of IgG into selective brain regions after bolus injections of recombinant TNF-α in the rat, the anterior cingulate gyrus was the most heavily affected structure. Regional endothelial leakage in this structure of the visceral brain may have a role in physiological responses that are needed to cope with a "life-threatening" event. The anterior cingulate gyrus is anatomically connected with various structures of the limbic system that control cardiovascular activity and autonomic functions in general *(52)*.

Moreover, the anterior cingulate gyrus has been demonstrated to attribute to the occurrence of emotional responses to visceral pain *(53)*. Alternatively, however, increased permeability of the blood-brain barrier may be associated with neurodegenerative and/or neurochemical alterations triggered by infiltration of blood-borne components for which the brain is otherwise sealed off, including other mediators of inflammation. This "damage" would generate long-term defects in the functioning of the emotional circuitry, which can present itself in the form of emotional disorders as anxiety and/or depression. A consistent finding in patients who have experienced a myocardial infarction is that about 15–20% of them will develop a major depression and that this mood disorder is associated with a significant increased risk of mortality *(54)*. We hypothesize that TNF-α-induced cerebral endothelial leakage fulfills both the physiological and pathophysiological role after myocardial infarction (MI), rendering a subpopulation of patients vulnerable for occurrence of mood disorders *(55)*. A genetic predisposition for mood disorders may determine this vulnerability. Essential for our hypothesis is the role attributed to the anterior cingulate gyrus in limbic circuitry and mood disorders. Most likely, this area is superimposed upon nervous circuitry for cardiovascular regulation (Chapter 2), as cardiovascular effects triggered with electrical and chemical stimulations of the area in experimental animals involve participation of the hypothalamus. Arrhythmias or acute cardiac arrest incidentally accompanied interventions at the level of the limbic forebrain *(56)*. Dysfunction of the cingulate gyrus expanding throughout the limbic forebrain therefore could be a possible explanation for increased risk of mortality in depressed post-MI patients. The role of the anterior cingulate gyrus in mood disorders has gained interest lately. Responses of patients to antidepressant therapy could be correlated to alterations of regional metabolic activity in the anterior cingulate gyrus, as assessed with in vivo neuro-imaging *(57)*. Many previous neuro-imaging studies, in mood-disorder patients, have identified aberrant metabolic activity patterns in the anterior cingulate gyrus, implicating the region in the pathogenesis of the disease (Chapter 2).

6. Therapeutical Strategies and Putative Therapies for Angina and Myocardial Ischemia

Atherosclerosis and thrombogenesis are closely related. Therefore, analogous to the triad of Virchow for the pathogenesis of thrombosis, in general three components are thought to determine the progression of coronary artery disease. These three factors are interference with blood flow, modification of blood constituents, and alteration of (the function of) the vessel wall (Fig. 2).

To date, the majority of patients suffering from ischemic heart disease can be treated adequately with drugs (which influence one or more of the three components of Virchow's triad) and revascularization procedures (which alters the coronary blood flow). Anti-ischemic and, subsequently, antianginal drugs, such as β-blocking agents, calcium channel blockers, and long-acting nitrates, either reduce the myocardial oxygen demand or increase the oxygen supply to the myocardium by vasodilatation. In addition, many drugs have been developed with reference to secondary prevention. They are meant to reduce risk factors for coronary artery disease and thereby improve the prognosis of these patients, through, for instance, lipid lowering (statins), inhibition of platelet aggregation (aspirins and the glycoprotein IIa-3b inhibitors), or inhibition of either angiotensin-converting enzyme (ACE) or angiotensin II (ATII). In the presence of an acute myocardial infarction, both intravenous application of thrombolytic agents (streptokinase, recombinant plasminogen activators [rTPA]) and acute (primary or rescue) revascularization are the therapies of choice in conjunction to the standard therapies (heparin, nitroglycerine, pain-reducing drugs, β-blocking agents, oxygen, etc). Revascularization procedures, such as percutaneous transluminal coronary angioplasty (PTCA) or coronary artery bypass grafting (CABG), are meant to increase the oxygen supply to the heart and are mainly used to relieve complaints of stable angina. Finally, for patients suffering severe angina pectoris, despite optimal medication, in whom revascularization is not an option, newer therapies such as spinal cord stimulation (SCS) *(58)*, transmyocardial laser (TML), and intermittent urokinase administration have been suggested *(59)*. Of these therapies, SCS seems to be the most successful treatment *(60)*.

Because traditional risk factors, such as smoking, diabetes, hypertension, hypercholesterolemia, and so forth cannot fully explain the different manifestations of coronary artery disease, it is likely that alternatives for the conventional strategies will be administrated and developed. When considering atherosclerosis as an inflammatory response, new putative therapies emerge. The severity of inflammation, for instance, expressed either as C-reactive protein (CRP) *(61)*, troponin *(62)*, or serum ferritin *(63)* elevation, is clinical relevant to determine the risk of a subsequent myocardial event. In addition, immune activation appears to extend the size of the myocardial infarction. Subsequently, drugs to either treat or prevent atherosclerotic disease will come into sight when ongoing investigations gradually unravel the inflammatory mechanisms. Examples of preventive therapies may be manipulation of selective gene expression with sense or antisense mRNAs or viral transgene probes. Options for anti-inflammatory treatment are application of antibiotics like roxithromycin and azithromycin *(64)*, antibodies to limit myocardial infarction size, risk group loading with antibodies, or administration of x-ICAM.

7. Conclusions

In addition to classic risk factors influencing atherogenesis, the postulated mechanisms to link coronary artery disease with infection comprises aspects of both a systemic and a local inflammatory response to either a systemic infection or an autoimmune reaction. Because the inflammatory response may just be an epiphenomenon, the cause of atherosclerosis may not be an infection. The ultimate proof will probably be demonstrated in a laboratory setup. In conclusion, although atherosclerosis is associated with (alteration in parameters of) infection, the proof that an bacterial or viral agent induces atherosclerosis has not been provided yet.

It is postulated that cytokines as mediators of altered cellular functions trigger new molecular programs during atherogenesis *(65)*. Hypothetically, limitation of the inflammatory response might enhance plaque stabilization. The beneficial results of lipid lowering therapies may partly be explained by reduction of inflammation.

References

1. Heberden, W. (1772) Some account of a disorder of the breast. *Med. Trans. Coll. Physicians (London)* **2**, 59.
2. Mathews, M. B. and Julian D. G. (1985) Angina pectoris: definition and description, in *Angina Pectoris* (Julian, D. G., ed.), Churchill Livingstone, New York, p. 2.
3. Cohn, P. F. (1983) Seminar on asymptomatic coronary disease. *J. Am. Coll. Cardiol.* **1**, 922.
4. Feinleb, M., Kannel, W. B., Tedeschi, C. G., Landau, T. K., and Garrison, R. J. (1979) The relation of antemortem characteristics to cardiovascular findings at necropsy—The Framingham study. *Atherosclerosis* **34**, 145–152.
5. Borow, K. M., Alpert, J. S., and Cohn, P. F. (1978) The natural history and treatment of coronary artery disease; a perspective. *J. Cardiovasc. Med.* **3**, 87.
6. Maseri, A. (1997) *Ischemic Heart Disease.* Blackwell, New York.
7. Loeb, H. S., Saudye, A., Croke, R. P., Talano, J. V., Klodnycky, M. L., and Gunnar, R. M. (1978) Effects of pharmacologically-induced hypertension on myocardial ischemia and coronary hemodynamics in patients with fixed coronary obstruction. *Circulation* **57**, 41–46.
8. Sigwart, U., Grbic, M., Payot, M., Goy, J. J., Essinger, A., and Fisher, A. (1984) Appearance of events during transient coronary occlusion. Silent myocardial ischemia, in (Rutishauser, W. and Roskamm, H., eds.), *Silent Myocardial Ischemia.* Springer-Verlag, Berlin.
9. Holdright, D. R., Rosano, G. M. C., Sarrel, P. M., and Poole-Wilson, P. A. (1992) The ST segment, the herald of ischaemia, the siren of misdiagnosis, or syndrome X? *Int. J. Cardiol.* **35**, 293–301.

10. Lam, H. G. Th., Dekker, W., Kan, G., Breedijk, M., Smout, A. J. P. M. (1992) Acute non-cardiac chest pain in a coronary care unit: evaluation by 24 hour pressure and pH recording of the esophagus. *Gastroenterology* **102**, 453–464.
11. Rahimotoola, S. H. (1985) A perspective on the three large multicenter randomized clinical trials of coronary bypass surgery for chronic stable angina. *Circulation* **72**, 125–135.
12. Braunwald, E. and Kloner, R. A. (1982) The stunned myocardium: prolonged, postischemic ventricular dysfunction. *Circulation* **66**, 1146–1149.
13. Trevi, G. P. and Sheiban, I. (1991) Chronic ischemic ('hibernating') and postischaemic ('stunned') dysfunctional but viable myocardium. *Eur. Heart J.* **12(Suppl.)**, 20–26.
14. Murray, C. E., Jennings, R. B., and Reimer, K. A. (1986) Preconditioning with ischemia: a delay of lethal cell injury in ischemic myocardium. *Circulation* **74**, 1124–1136.
15. Yellon, D. M. and Baxter, G. F. (1995) A 'second window of protection' or delayed preconditioning phenomenon.: Future horizons for myocardial protection. *J. Mol. Cell. Cardiol.* **27**, 1023–1034.
16. Murry, C. E., Jennings, R. B., and Reimer, K. A. (1991) New insights into potential mechanisms of ischemic preconditioning. *Circulation* **84**, 350–356.
17. Meller, S. T. and Gebhart, G. F. (1992) A critical review of the afferent pathways and the potential chemical mediators involved in cardiac pain. *Neuroscience* **48**, 501–524.
18. TerHorst, G. J. (1998) Myocardial ischemia and pain, in *Advanced Imaging in Coronary Artery Disease* (VanderWall, E. E., Blanksma, P. K., Niemeyer, M. G., Vaalburg, W., and Crijns, H. J. G. M., eds.), Kluwer, Dordrecht, pp. 121–136.
19. Libby, P. (1996) Atheroma: more than mush. *Lancet* **348(Suppl. I)**, s4–s6.
20. Rekhter, M., Zang, K., Narayanan, A., Phan, S., Schork, M., and Gordon, D. (1993) Type I Collagen Gene Expression in human atherosclerosis. Localization to specific plaque regions. *Am. J. Pathol.* **143**, 1643–1648.
21. Maseri, A. (1995) in *Chronic Stable Ischemic Heart Disease* (Maseri, A., ed.), Churchill Livingstone, New York, pp. 271–278.
22. Harker, L. A., Schwartz, S. M., and Ross, R. (1981) Endothelium and atherosclerosis. *Clin. Haematol.* **10**, 283–287.
23. Hillis, G. S. and Flapan, A. D. (1998) Cell adhesion molecules in cardiovascular disease: a clinical perspective. *Heart* **79**, 429–431.
24. Jang. Y., Lincoff, A. M., Plow, E. F., and Topol, E. J. (1994) Cell adhesion molecules in coronary artery disease. *J. Am. Coll. Cardiol.* **24**, 1591–1601.
25. Lüscher, T. F. and Noll, G. (1995) The endothelium in coronary vascular control, in *Heart Disease Update* (Braunwald, E., ed.), W.B. Saunders, Baltimore, pp. 1–10.

26. Danesh, J., Collins, R., and Peto, R. (1997) Chronic infections and coronary heart disease: is there a link. *Lancet* **350**, 430–436.
27. Xu, Q. and Wick, G. (1996) The role of heat shock proteins in protection and pathophysiology of the arterial wall. *Mol. Med. Today* **2**, 372–379.
28. Yarnell, J. and Evans, A. (1997) Chlamydia infection and coronary heart disease. *Eur. Heart J.* **17**, 650–651.
29. Yellon, D. M., Pasini, E., Cargoni, A., Marber, M. S., Lachman, D. S., and Ferrari, R. (1992) The protective role of heat stress in ischemic and reperfused rat myocardium. *J. Mol. Cell. Cardiol.* **24**, 895–907.
30. Lindquist, S. and Graig, E. A. (1988) The heat shock proteins. *Annu. Rev. Biochem.* **22**, 631–677.
31. Maulik, N., Engelman, R. M., and Wei, Z. (1995) Drug-induced heat shock preconditioning improves postischemic recovery after cardiopulmonary bypass. *Circulation* **92(Supp. II)**, II-381–II-388.
32. Zhou, Y. F., Guetta, E., Yu, Z. X., Finkel, T., and Epstein, S. E. (1996) Human cytomegalo virus increases modified low density lipoprotein uptake and scavenger receptor mRNA expression in vascular smooth muscle cells. *J. Clin. Invest.* **98**, 2129–2138.
33. Guetta, E., Guetta, V., Shibutani, T., and Epstein, S. E. (1997) Monocytes harboring cytomegalo virus: interactions with endothelial cells, smooth muscle cells, and oxidized low-density lipoprotein. Possible mechanisms for activating virus delivered by monocytes to sites of vascular injury. *Circ. Res.* **81**, 8–16.
34. Hills, G. S. and MacLeod, A. M. (1996) Integrins in disease. *Clin. Sci.* **91**, 639–650.
35. Suzuki, H., Kurihara, Y., Takeya, M., Kamada, N., Kataoka, M., Jishage, K., et al. (1997) A role for macrophage scavenger receptors in atherosclerosis and susceptibility to infection. *Nature* **386**, 292–296.
36. Hsu, H. Y., Nicholson, A. C., Pomerantz, K. B., Kaner, R. J., and Hajjar, D. P. (1995) Altered cholesterol trafficking in herpes virus infected arterial cells. Evidence for viral protein kinase-mediated cholesterol accumulation. *J. Biol. Chem.* **270**, 19,630–19,637.
37. Davies, M. J., Richardson, P. D., Woolf, N., Katz, D. R., and Mann, J. (1993) Risk of thrombosis in human atherosclerosic plaques: role of extracellular lipid, macrophage, and smooth muscle cell content. *Br. Heart J.* **69**, 377–381.
38. Stemme, S., Holm, J., and Hansson, G. K. (1992) T Lymphocytes in human atherosclerotic plaques are memory cells expressing CD45RO and the integrin VLA-1. *Arterioscler. Thromb.* **12**, 206–211.
39. Halle, M., Konig, D., Berg, A., Keul, J., and Baumstrak, M. W. (1997) Relationship of serum ferritin concentrations with metabolic cardiovascular risk factors in men without evidence for coronary artery disease. *Atherosclerosis* **128**, 235–240.
40. Halle, M., Berg, A., Keul, J., and Baumstark, M. W. (1996) Association between serum fibrinogen concentrations and HDL and LDL

subfraction phenotypes in healthy men. *Atheroscler. Thromb. Vasc. Biol.* **16,** 144–148.

41. Constans, J., Wendling, G., Peuchant, E., Camilleri, G., and Conri, C. (1996) Lipoprotein A in 505 hospitalized patients with various pathological states: correlation's with cardiovascular diseases and therapies. *Int. Angiogr.* **15,** 1–5.

42. Loscalzo, J. and Simon, D. I. (1995) Lipoprotein (a): a risk factor for atherothrombotic disease, in *Heart Disease. A Textbook of Cardiovascular Medicine, Update #16* (Braunwald, E., ed.), W.B. Saunders, Philadelphia, pp. 368–375.

43. Shaw, P. J., Bates, D., and Cartlidge, N. E. F. (1985) Early neurological complications of coronary bypass surgery. *Br. Med. J.* **291,** 1384–1387.

44. Mills, S. A. (1993) Cerebral injury and cardiac operations. *Ann. Thorac. Surg.* **56,** 586–591.

45. Saper, C. B. and Bader, C. D. (1994) The neurologic basis of fever. *N. Engl. J. Med.* **330,** 1880–1886.

46. Basaran, Y., Basaran, M. M., Babacan, K. F., Ener, B., Okay, T., Gok, H., et al. (1993) Serum tumor necrosis factor levels in acute myocardial infarction and unstable angina pectoris. *Angiology* **44,** 332–337.

47. Lissoni, P., Pelizzoni, F., Mauri, O., Perego, M., Pittalis, S., and Barni, S. (1992) Enhanced secretion of tumour necrosis factor in patients with myocardial infarction. *Eur. J. Med.* **1,** 277–280.

48. Guillen, B., Blanes, M., Gomez-Lechon, M. J., and Castell, J. V. (1995) Cytokines signalling during myocardial infarction; sequential appearance of IL-1 beta and IL-6. *Am. J. Physiol.* **269,** R229–R235.

49. Worall, N. K., Chang, K., Lejeune, W. S., Misko, T. P., Sullivan, P. M., Ferguson, T. B., et al. (1997) TNFα causes a reversible in vivo systemic vascular barrier dysfunction via NO-dependent and -independent mechanisms. *Am. J. Physiol.* **271,** H2565–H2574.

50. Van der Werf, Y. D., DeJongste, M. J. L., and Ter Horst, G. J. (1995) The immune system mediates blood brain barrier damage: possible implications for pathophysiology of neuropsychiatric illnesses. *Acta Neuropsychiat.* **7,** 114–121.

51. ter Horst, G. J., Nagel, J. G., DeJongste, M. J. L., and Van der Werf, Y. D. (1997) Selective blood brain barrier dysfunction after intravenous injections of TNFa in the rat, in *Neurochemistry: Cellular, Molecular and Clinical Aspects* (Teelken, A. and Korf, J., eds.), Plenum, New York, pp. 141–146.

52. ter Horst, G. J., Hautvast, R. W. M., DeJongste, M. J. L., and Korf, J. (1996) Neuroanatomy of cardiac activity regulating circuitry: a transneuronal retrograde viral labelling study in the rat. *Eur. J. Neurosci.* **8,** 2029–2041.

53. Devinsky, O., Morrell, M. J., and Vogt, B. A. (1995) Contribution of the anterior cingulate gyrus to behaviour. *Brain* **118,** 279–306.

54. Glassman, A. H. and Shapiro, P. A. (1998) Depression and the course of coronary artery disease. *Am. J. Psychiatry* **155**, 4–11.
55. ter Horst, G. J. (1998) TNFa-induced selective cerebral endothelial leakage and increased mortality risk in post-myocardial infarction depression, *Am. J. Physiol.* **275**, H1910–H1911.
56. Oppenheimer, S. M., Wilson, J. X., Guiraudon, C., and Cechetto, D. F. (1991) Insular cortex stimulation produces lethal cardiac arrhythmias: a mechanism of sudden death? *Brain Res.* **550**, 115–121.
57. Mayberg, H. S., Brannan, S. K., Mahurin, R. K., Jerabek, P. A., Brickman, J. S., Tekell, J. L., et al. (1997) Cingulate function in depression: a potential predictor of treatment response. *NeuroReport* **8**, 1057–1061.
58. DeJongste, M. J. L., Hautvast, R. W. M., Ruiters, M. H. J., and ter Horst, G. J. (1998) Spinal cord stimulation and the induction of c-fos and heat shock protein 72 in the central nervous system of rats. *Neuromodulation* **2**, 73–84.
59. Schoebel, F. C., Frazier, O. H., Jessurun, G. A. J., DeJongste, M. J. L., Kadipasaoglue, K. A., Jax, T. W., et al. (1997) Refractory angina pectoris in end-stage coronary artery disease: evolving therapeutic concepts. *Am. Heart J.* **134**, 587–602.
60. Mulcahy, D., Knight, C., Stables, R., and Fox, K. (1994) Lasers, burns, cuts, tingles and pumps: a consideration of alternative treatments for intractable angina. *Br. Heart J.* **71**, 406–407.
61. Ridker, P. M., Cushman, M., Stampfer, M. J., Russell, P. T., and Hennekens, C. H. (1997) Inflammation, aspirin, and the risk of cardiovascular disease in apparently healthy men. *N. Engl. J. Med.* **336**, 973–979.
62. Muller-Bardorff, M., Hallermayer, K., and Schroder, A. (1997) Improved Troponin T ELISA specific for cardiac troponin isoform: assay development and analytical and clinical validation. *Clin. Chem.* **43**, 458–466.
63. Halle, M., Konig, D., Berg, J., and Baumstark, M. W. (1997) Relationship of serum ferritin concentration with metabolic cardiovascular risk factors in men without evidence for coronary artery disease. *Atherosclerosis* **128**, 235–240.
64. Lip, G. Y. H. and Beevers, D. G. (1997) Can we treat coronary artery disease with antibiotics? *Lancet* **350**, 378–379.
65. Libby, P. and Lee, R. T. (1995) *Heart Disease. Update #28* (Braunwald, E., ed.), W.B. Saunders, Philadelphia.

PART V

Heart Disease
and Brain Dysfunction

CHAPTER 13

Heart Disease and Cognitive/ Neuropsychiatric Disorders

Dorien M. Tulner and Hans. A. den Boer

1. Introduction

Neuropsychiatry is the discipline concerned with the diagnosis and treatment of psychiatric disorders from the perspective of their neurological basis and neurological disorders with concomitant behavioral and mood disorders *(1)*.

There is a certain neuropsychiatric perspective on each psychiatric or neurological disorder because no aspect of human behavior is independent of its physical underpinnings *(2)*. Yet, for some diseases, neuropsychiatric insights are of much greater heuristic value than others. Ideas about the neurological basis of behavior have existed for a long time and have changed dramatically in response to political, cultural, and scientific developments *(1)*. Nowadays, neuropsychiatry receives a great deal of attention. One of the youngest subspecialties in this field concerns the heart–brain interaction.

This chapter aims to give a limited overview of selected psychiatric and cardiac diseases whose connection can be discussed from a neuropsychiatric or sometimes purely biological perspective.

1.1. Historical Notes

There has always been a certain creative tension in Western medical science between psychological and neuro-

From: *The Nervous System and the Heart*
Ed: G. J. Ter Horst © Humana Press Inc.

491

logical/biological theories of behavior and emotional disturbances. For instance, before the 18th century, Satan and the
black bile were exponents of two different hypotheses with
respect to the cause of melancholia *(1)*. Toward the end of
the 18th century, different visions became more integrated,
and the first neuropsychiatric period emerged. Medicine,
itself, was struggling to find a place for rationalism within
its own discourse. At that time, neurology and psychiatry
were virtually indistinguishable *(1)*.

The first era of neuropsychiatry ended more or less with
the development of psychoanalysis, which, for the first time,
provided a coherent psychological theory by which mental
illness could be understood *(1)*. The discovery of psychopharmaca during the 1950s played a role with the beginning
of the second era of neuropsychiatry. Under the influence of
the cultural and sexual revolution in the sixties, the biologi-
cal/neurological causes of psychiatric disorders were mostly
rejected. This resulted in a period of "antipsychiatry," in
which the leading hypothesis was that the environment was
one of the most important factors in the pathogenesis of psychopathology. The second era of neuropsychiatry truly
started during the eighties, after people became more aware
of the limitations of this theory and the limited effect of psy-
chotherapy for several psychiatric diseases.

History shows the continuous switch in emphasizing the
importance of neurobiological and psychological theories
about the origin of psychopathology. This reflects the urge
which is felt in Western medicine (society) to differentiate
between disturbances of the mind (social sanction: negative)
and disturbances from the body (social sanction: positive).
This differentiation has its roots in the mind–body dichotomy
introduced by Descartes. This philosophy assumes that there
is a more or less strict boundary between the mind and the body.

Limitations of this still widespread model resulted in the
concept of psychosomatic diseases, whereby mental deviance
is transformed to and experienced in the physical domain. It
is only in recent decades that there has been renewed interest in the interaction between mind and body and reducing

this gap in a more causal way than merely creating a category of psychosomatic illnesses. One of the results is the scientific research concerning the connection between heart disease and psychopathology.

1.2. Symbolic and Cultural Significance of the Heart

The link between heart and soul is an old one. In ancient times, it was believed that the soul resided in the heart *(3)*. This belief faded away in Western culture, but our language still contains many expressions in which the heart is used in somatic metaphors to express emotion, which shows its continuing importance. In Western culture, the central place in emotional life is no longer the heart but the brain, with psychologization as a result. It is generally thought that when people feel discomfort, they ought to express this in psychological terms such as I feel sad, anxious, or frustrated. When they do this by means of somatic complaints, it is called somatization, which is judged as pathological. Scientific transcultural research, however, shows that psychologization is a way of expressing inner feelings only used by the intellectual upper class of the world (about 10% of the world's population).

Linguists have demonstrated that several non-Western societies even lack an extensive vocabulary to convey emotion in a psychological way and that emotions are expressed in another way. This can be done using facial expressions or bodily positions and actions but also by using a somatic metaphor. The central place of the heart in expressing emotional life is still apparent in these societies. For instance, in the Yoruba, a Nigerian language, an equivalent for depression is "the heart is weak," and for anxiety, "the heart is not at rest" *(4)*. In China, depression is also frequently expressed somatically as "it is uncomfortable inside my heart" *(5)*.

Both examples illustrate that diseases have somatic, psychological, and social components that can be emphasized depending on circumstances. In Western medicine, this frequently leads to a clinical dilemma for cardiologists and liaison psychiatrists, for instance, as they have to decide whether complaints are psychic or somatic. The heart takes a prominent place in this dilemma, as it is innervated abundantly and reacts with arousal of the central nervous system, which frequently accompanies psychiatric illness.

In this chapter, this dilemma of differential diagnosis will frequently recur and we shall return to it in our conclusion and make some suggestions for further research.

2. Depression and Cardiac Disease

2.1. The Concept of Depression

Nowadays, there are two leading psychiatric classification systems, the International Classification of Diseases (ICD) and the Diagnostic and Statistical Manual of Mental Disorders (DSM). The ICD was developed by the World Health Organization, and the sixth edition for the first time included a section on mental disorders. This part was heavily influenced by the Veterans Administration of the U.S. Army and primarily developed for research. The American Psychiatric Association Committee on Nomenclature and Statistics developed a variant on the ICD-6 that was published in 1952 as the first edition of the DSM. DSM 1 contained a glossary of descriptions of the diagnostic categories and was the first official manual of mental disorders to focus on clinical utility. Modifications were made on several occasions (resulting in DSM 2, DSM 3, and DSM 3-R), and the fourth and most recent edition (DSM 4) was published in 1994. As the DSM is worldwide and is the most frequently used classification system, a description of the relevant diagnostic categories will be given in accordance with DSM 4 *(6)*. (*See* Table 1.)

As we can see, this classification system contains psychological, somatic, and social criteria without describing etiology. However, to some extent the type of symptoms that occur show cultural differences. Transcultural research shows unequivocally that it is not clear which signs and symptoms are essential for the definition of depression *(4,5)*. This problem with diagnostic validity is not only a problem in

Table 1

Criteria for a Major Depressive Episode and a Minor Depressive Disorder

Criteria for Major Depressive Episode

A. Five (or more) of the following symptoms have been present during the same 2-wk period and represent a change from previous function; at least one of the symptoms is either (1) depressed mood or (2) loss of interest or pleasure.

Note: Do not include symptoms that are clearly the result of a general medical condition, mood-incongruent delusions, or hallucinations.

(1) Depressed mood most of the day, nearly every day, as indicated by either subjective report (e.g., feels sad or empty) or observation made by others (e.g., appears tearful). **Note:** In children and adolescents, this can be an irritable mood.

(2) Markedly diminished interest or pleasure in all, or almost all, activities most of the day, nearly every day (as indicated by either subjective account or observations made by others).

(3) Significant weight loss when not dieting or weight gain (e.g., a change of more than 5% of body weight in a month), or decrease or increase in appetite nearly every day. **Note:** As children have a weight gain during normal growth, an absence of weight gain might be a signal of lost appetite (depressive sympton). *Weight loss* is not a necessary symptom in children whereas it is in adults.

(4) Insomnia or hypersomnia nearly every day.

(5) Psychomotor agitation or retardation nearly every day (observable by others, not merely subjective feelings of restlessness or being slowed down).

(6) Fatigue or loss of energy nearly every day.

(7) Feelings of worthlessness or excessive or inappropriate guilt (which may be delusional) nearly every day (not merely self-reproach or guilt about being sick).

(8) Diminished ability to think or concentrate, or indecisiveness, nearly every day (either by subjective account or as observed by others).

(9) Recurrent thoughts of death (not just fear of dying), recurrent suicidal ideation without a specific plan, or a suicide attempt or a specific plan for committing suicide.

B. The symptoms do not meet criteria for a mixed episode (mixed episode = a period of time in which the criteria are met for a manic episode and a depressive episode nearly every day).

C. The symptoms cause clinically significant distress or impairment in social, occupational, or other important areas of functioning.

D. The symptoms are not due to the direct physiological effects of a substance (e.g., a drug of abuse, a medication) or a general medical condition (e.g., hypothyroidism).

E. The symptoms are not better accounted for by bereavement (i.e., after the loss of a loved one, the symptoms persist for longer than 2 mo or are characterized by marked functional impairment, morbid preoccupation with worthlessness, suicidal ideation, psychotic symptoms, or psychomotor retardation.

Criteria for Minor Depressive Disorder

The essential feature is one or more periods of depressive symptoms that are identical to Major Depressive Episodes in duration but that involve fewer symptoms and less impairment.

transcultural research but also in research that has as its subject the connection between depression and organic comorbidity.

2.2. Differential Diagnostic Problems in Cardiac Patients

A number of affective and behavioral changes can accompany illness and/or hospitalization *(7)*, but there is no consensus regarding their classification or their relationship with primary somatic and/ or psychiatric illness.

2.2.1. Hospitalization

Symptoms resembling depression can develop as a consequence of lying in bed all day and, in that case, it can be difficult to decide whether or not there is depression. To clarify this matter, Lesperance et al. *(7)*, compared symptoms in hospitalized post-myocardial-infarction (post-MI) patients who met DSM-3R criteria for depression with post-MI patients who were not depressed. Three major conclusions emerged from these comparisons: First, although sadness was very frequent and highly specific to the depressed group (depressed and nondepressed, 80% and 7%, respectively), only 48% of the depressed complained about loss of pleasure or interest. Second, fatigue was mainly a symptom of the depressed group (depressed and nondepressed, 77.1% and 7%, respectively) and was not related to cardiac dysfunction. Third, sleep and appetite disturbances were common in both the depressed and nondepressed groups (sleep: depressed and nondepressed, 65.7% and 49.6%, respectively; appetite:depressed and nondepressed, 80% and 71.1%, respectively). When sleep and appetite disturbances were eliminated from the criteria for depression and the number of symptom clusters needed to define depression was reduced from five to four, including sadness or lack of interest, 31 of the 35 patients originally classified as depressed continued to meet the criteria for depression *(7)*. It, therefore, seems that one can differentiate between depression and effects of hospitalization.

2.2.2. Cardiac Symptoms

Dysfunction of the heart can lead to a broad spectrum of signs and symptoms, whether or not specific. Excess fatigue, hopelessness, listlessness, loss of libido, increased irritability, and problems with sleep are complaints frequently reported by men in the months prior to their first myocardial infarction *(8,9)*. They can, therefore, be judged as early symptoms of serious cardiovascular disease. These symptoms together were called "the vital exhaustion syndrome." A retrospective study reported that these symptoms were present in 82% of the patients prior to MI *(10)*. In order to investigate the predictive value of this syndrome, a prospective study was conducted by van Diest and Appels *(11)*. A cohort of 3210 middle-aged men initially free of coronary heart disease were followed up over an average of 4.2 yr. A relative risk of 2.28 for having a myocardial infarction was found for those patients with complaints of vital exhaustion. The risk associated with vital exhaustion is highest in the first few months after assessment and decreases over time *(12)*.

The similarity in symptomatology between depressive disorders and "vital exhaustion" on the one hand, and the possible role of depression in coronary heart disease (CHD), on the other, which will be discussed later in this chapter, caused the same investigators to question whether men who were exhausted were suffering from depression. For this purpose, they selected a group of exhausted and nonexhausted men. Both groups were investigated through self-monitoring by means of the Profile of Mood States (POMS) *(13)* and the Beck Depression Inventory (BDI) *(14)*. They concluded, among other things, that "a state of vital exhaustion" was characterized more by excess fatigue and loss of vigor than by depressed mood. However, the total severity score of the BDI was significantly higher than in the nonexhausted group and the investigators judged these patients as mildly depressive. The BDI scores were not only heightened because of somatic complaints *(11)*.

A major problem with respect to the concept of vital exhaustion concerns the possibility that the symptoms of this syndrome are simply the physical sequelae of impaired myocardial function prior to MI *(9)*, although, in one study, no decrease of exhaustion was found by restoring the blood flow with percutaneous coronary angioplasty (PTCA) (15), which suggests that exhaustion is not only a consequence of impaired blood flow. As mentioned earlier, in the study on hospitalization, exhaustion was found among those patients with depression and barely among those without depression.

The results of the study on vital exhaustion have to be interpreted with caution. First, the BDI was not developed to assess depression. It is only suitable for quantifying the number of symptoms of depression when diagnosis is made clinically (14). Second, because no psychiatric investigation was performed, it was not possible to diagnose (what was called in the earlier days) a masked depression. This notion is important because research into the elderly has revealed that depression can manifest itself mainly by somatic complaints (16). Despite the observed differences, it remains a question of whether vital exhaustion and depression are separate disease entities. It is possible that the two syndromes share a common organic etiologic factor. An argument supporting this hypothesis is given by the fact that tiredness and exhaustion in the year before the MI had the strongest correlation with the incidence of depression the year after MI (17).

3. Cardiac Disease in Depressed Patients

3.1. Epidemiology

The first observation that mortality in depressed patients is higher than in the general population dates from the thirties. The higher rate was caused by unnatural (suicide, accidents) and natural deaths. Among the latter, cardiovascular causes played an important role. The first scientific research to establish a relation between depression and heart disease was done by Malzberg in 1937 (18). He compared the death rate of patients who were institutionalized with an "involutional melancholia" (an old name for depression in the elderly) with age- and sex-matched controls living in the same area. The death rate in the group of patients was six to seven times higher than in the controls. Cardiac death rate accounted for almost 40% of all the deaths in the patients with melancholia. This death rate was eight times the corresponding rate for cardiac death in the age group and general population at that time (the thirties). This study is unique in that none of the patients had ever used antidepressive medication. However, the study conspicuously confounded the influence of involutional depression with chronic institutionalization *(19)*. The results of Malzberg have been confirmed in part or completely by several studies. An association of depression and greater risk of short-term *(20)* and long-term mortality *(21–23)* has been found, whereas other studies have found no association *(24,25)*. (*See* Table 2.)

The heightened risk of CHD in patients with major depressive disorder (MDD) is often explained by the hypothesis that people with psychiatric diseases generally have other risk factors for the development of CHD. However, this hypothesis could not be confirmed for all kinds of psychopathology. To assess the relative risk of mortality in nine psychiatric disorders, 3560 men and women from the general community were followed over a 9-yr period and the relative risks differed significantly *(30)*. The baseline psychiatric diagnosis (recent and past) were major depression, chronic dysthymia, manic–depressive disorder, panic disorder, phobia, obsessive–compulsive disorder, alcohol abuse or dependence, drug abuse or dependence, and schizophrenia or schizophreniform disorder. MDD, alcohol abuse, and schizophrenia were the disorders with a heightened mortality. Respondents with a recent depression were two times more likely to die during the follow-up period than those without a recent depression. A significant interaction between recent depression and sex indicated that although depression was associated with mortality for both sexes, the effect was stronger for men than for women. Past depressions were not associated with mortality as a main effect for men or for women. There was no greater risk of mortality associated with dysthymia (a chronic mildly depressive mood state). No evidence was found that the effect of depression on mortality could be explained by somatic comorbidity. This result diminishes the chance of the existence of a common risk factor of mortality in psychiatric patients.

Table 2
Epidemiological Studies: Cardiac Mortality in Depressed Patients

	Author								
	Malzberg 1937 (18)	Weeke 1987 (26)	Murphy 1987 (21)	Carney 1988 (27)	Zilber 1989 (25)	Aromaa 1994 (23)	Sharma 1994 (28)	Bruce 1994 (20)	Barefoot 1996 (29)
Target population	Psychiatric institutionalized	Depressive and bipolar	General community	Depressive patients with coronary artery disease (CAD)	Psychiatric hospitalized patients	General community	Bipolar patients	General community	Birth cohort born in 1914
Number of patients ± controls	?	3795	1003	52	16,147	5355	472	356	975
Age	?	>15 yr	?	<70 yr	10–70 yr	>40 yr	?	>40 yr	All born in 1914
Gender	Male and female	Male	Male and female	Male	Male and female	Male and female	Male and female	Male and female	Male and female
Comorbid disease	?	All death registered	All deaths registered	CAD	Register of all natural and unnatural causes	All deaths registered; detailed cardiovascular st.	All deaths registered	All deaths registered	No specific
Diagnostic instruments	Clinical judgment	Part ICD-8 part clinical judgment	DPAX computer program	DIS, DSM-3	ICD-9	GHQ, PSE*CATE-GO computer program	DSM-3	DIS, DSM-3	MMPI Dscale OBD subscale

Control group design	Mortality rate depressives versus controls	Death from cardiovascular disease	Death from cancer
Age-controlled community sample	6X	8X higher	No excess
Age and sex controlled	Higher: 1.96–2.53X	Higher	Unrelated in men, higher in women
Nondepressive CAD patients	Higher	Higher	No excess
Age, sex, ethnicity	Lower	Lower	No excess
	Higher	2X higher	Not specified
Age, sex, and psychopharmaca controlled	Higher	Higher	No excess; excess of respiratory syndrome
Age and sex controlled; community sample	Higher (recent depression), lower as for past depression & dysthymia	Not investigated	Not investigated
Age and sex controlled community sample	Higher	Higher	Higher

Nearly all of the studies of the last decade, as listed in Table 2, document increased cardiovascular morbidity and mortality despite their difference in methodology, such as dissimilar research population, different diagnostic instrument, use of (psycho)pharmaca, and different specification of heart disease.

Table 2 shows that there is an unequivocal association between depression and cardiovascular disease and mortality. The nature of this relationship is not clear and several hypotheses have been suggested. Possible causes that have been mentioned include stress, use of psychopharmaca, changes in immune system, and smoking. These factors will be reviewed.

3.2. Neurobiology and Stress

A large number of studies shows biological abnormalities in depressive illness such as neuroanatomical, neurochemical, and neuroendocrine changes. Currently, the most prevalent idea about the nature of depression is that it involves a functional deficiency of serotonin (5-HT) *(31)* as well as catecholamines *(32)* (noradrenaline and, to a lesser extent, dopamine). The central role of catecholamines in maintaining the central mood state and the mechanism of action of many antidepressants have been validated; the exact mechanism has not.

3.2.1. Catecholamines

The major noradrenergic nucleus in the brain is the locus coeruleus (LC), which receives inputs from other neurotransmitter systems such as the serotonin (5-HT), opioid, gamma aminobutyric acid (GABA), dopamine (DA), and the glutamate system. The LC is very sensitive to external environmental stimuli and internal homeostasis *(32)*. The LC output is involved in flight-and-fight responses and regulates the level of arousal, the responses of the sympathetic nervous system, including pulse rate and blood pressure, and the signaling of the danger signal for the organism.

The LC may play a role in pathophysiological alterations that contribute to the increased vulnerability of depressed patients to CHD, as it is part of the hypothalamic–pituitary–adrenocortical axis, which is one component of the fight–flight stress reaction; the other component is the sympathoadrenal system (sympathetic nervous system and adrenal medulla) *(33)*. In response to stress, the hypothalamic neurons, containing corticotropin-releasing factor (CRF), increase synthesis and release of, for example, β-endorphin and ACTH. In medication-free depressed patients, evidence of a disturbed hypothalamic–pituitary–adrenocortical axis can be found [e.g., hypercortisolemia, blunting of the ACTH response to CRF administration, a disturbed dexamethason suppression test (nonsuppressing of cortisol secretion after dexamethason administration), and enlargement of pituitary and adrenal gland] *(34)*. Corticosteroids can induce hypercholesterolemia, hypertriglyceridemia, hypertension, and injury to blood vessels (endothelium and intima) *(35)*. Insulin resistance, which can be found more frequently in depression *(36)* could also contribute to atherosclerosis *(37)*.

As mentioned, hypothalamic neurons provide stimulatory input in the regulation of other sympathoadrenal systems also. Physiological and pathological conditions causing sympathoadrenal activation are physical activity, coronary ischemia, heart failure, and mental stress *(33,38)*. Among many patients with depression dysregulation, hyperactivity of the sympathoadrenal system can also be found, reflected by elevated plasma norepinephrine (NE) and NE metabolites. Sympathoadrenal hyperactivity contributes to the development of CHD through effects of catecholamines on the heart, blood vessels (contractility and endothelial leakage), *(39)* increased platelet aggregation *(40)*, and/or electric instability *(41)*. Although myocardial ischemia is the most significant factor in ventricular instability, central nervous system activity can also significantly affect electrophysiological properties of the heart so as to decrease the threshold for ventricular fibrillation (VF). In animals, the threshold for VF could be lowered by stimulation of the posterior hypothalamus, even in the absence of myocardial ischemia *(41)*. Psychological stress in humans with CHD increases the risk for ectopic ventricular beats and increases the risk for VF *(42)*. In animals, the same mechanism was demonstrated, but, interestingly, whereas the onset of increased vulnerability in response to stress is rapid, the return to normal electropysiologic status after the removal of stress is rather prolonged *(43–46)*. The mechanism of VF is relevant for the connection between major depression and CHD *(38,47–49)* because sudden death is almost always the result of VF *(50)*. In the study of Frasure-Smith et al. *(51)*, the excess of post-MI death with depression was almost exclusively the result of sudden death. However, the results of a study of autopsy cases demonstrated that in 90% of apparently healthy persons who suddenly died after a period of psychological stress, a cardiac disease was the underlying factor *(52,53)*.

3.2.2. Serotonin

Recent research has demonstrated that serotonin plays a role in coronary vasoconstriction and thrombogenesis and, therefore, in platelet aggregation *(54)*. Musselman and co-workers discovered that depressed patients exhibited enhanced baseline platelet activation and responsiveness and elevated platelet excretion products, which points to heightened susceptibility to platelet activation and secretion *(55)*. This finding could not be replicated in nondepressed CHD patients. Several studies demonstrate increases in platelet 5-HT2 binding density in depressed patients. These changes seem to be state dependent because the density decreased with clinical recovery *(32)*. As mentioned, the role of serotonin in depression has already been known for a long time. There is evidence from neuroendocrine studies that brain 5-HT neurotransmission at the level of the postsynaptic 5-HT 1a receptor in the brain is decreased in MDD and is restored to normal upon clinical recovery *(56)*. There is also evidence that persistent lowering of brain 5-HT function is related to a (lifelong) irritable mood and aggressive behavior, which, at worst, can result in automutilation, homicide, or suicide. In general, 5-HT pathways are especially involved in organizing the response of the organism to stress and adversity.

MDD can be judged as a maladaptive form of coping with stress. These studies therefore offer a hypothesis that links MDD, hostile personality traits, and cardiovascular disease. From a clinical point of view, there is evidence for this type of connection (depression after MI, in particular, is characterized by hostility), which could be clinically relevant if treatment of depression and/or hostility decreases the risk of adverse cardiac events *(56)*.

Laghrissi-Thode et al. *(57)* demonstrated in a comparative investigation with the serotonin reuptake inhibitor (SSRI) prozac versus nortryptiline (tricyclic antidepressant, TCA) that prozac lowered the platelet activation and clotting. It also lowered platelet factor 4 and B thromboglobulin (platelet-secretion products). Nortriptilin did not influence these factors. As far as the authors know, comparative long-term investigations of this kind are lacking.

Several mechanisms can contribute to higher cardiac fatalities among depressive patients. One likely possibility is that the central and /or autonomic nervous system events mediate the increase in morbidity and mortality. In the long term, there are the hormonal disturbances and presumed changes in the clotting system. For patients that already have CHD, the heightened risk for VF may contribute to heightened mortality. Anatomical regions in the brain implicated in "higher control" of the heart include the frontal–parietal and insular cortices, hypothalamus, and the limbic system (especially the amygdala). Several of these regions are also involved in the pathogenesis of depression *(58,59)*. This raises the question of whether one cerebral lesion or disturbance can lead to depression and cardiovascular morbidity at the same time, instead of the presumed cause–effect relation (depression contributes to the pathogenesis of CHD). Ter Horst and co-workers *(60)* found evidence for this hypothesis (*see* Chapter 12). They demonstrated that MI in rats induced immune activation, which led to leakage of the blood-brain barrier. This happened in certain cortical, subcortical, and hindbrain areas in discrete patches. Among the afflicted areas were the enthorhinal cortex, cingulair cortex, and the frontal cortex.

These areas are probably connected with neuropsychiatric disorders. Other afflicted areas were the hypothalamus and brainstem, which are involved in autonomic regulation of the heart, for instance (*see* Chapter 2).

3.3. Heart Rate Variability

Changes in autonomic nervous system activity, as demonstrated by reduced heart rate variability (HRV), represents another potential mechanism contributing to the higher than expected cardiac death rate in depressed patients. Central generation and control of the heart rate is regulated by the hypothalamus, the brainstem, and the limbic system.

The central nervous system exerts its influence on the heart through the sympathetic and the parasympathetic nervous system. Heart rate variability is the standard deviation of two successive R-to-R intervals in sinus rhythm and reflects the interplay and balance between sympathetic and parasympathetic input on the cardiac pacemaker. A high degree of HRV is observed in well-functioning hearts, whereas restricted HRV can be seen in patients with severe CHD *(61)*. It was found that a restricted heart rate variability emerged as an important predictor of mortality post-MI *(62)* and this restricted HRV in post-MI patients was caused by decreased parasympathetic activity *(63)*. In general, increased sympathetic input lowers the threshold for ventricular fibrillation, whereas a decrease augments the risk. Roose and Dalack *(61)* investigated HRV in depressed patients. He found that the overall HRV in depressed patients did not differ from controls. More detailed research, such as the power spectral analysis measurement of HRV, consists of the use of different frequency bands of the heart period power spectrum. The low-frequency variability reflects modulation of sympathetic and vagal tone by baroreceptor-reflex activity. The high-frequency variability reflects modulation of vagal tone by respiratory frequency and depth (parasympathetically mediated sinus arrythmia) *(61)* and this "beat-to-beat" or high-frequency variability did show differences in subgroups of depressed patients, but not in all *(64)*. Especially in depressed patients with CHD, significant differences were found *(65)*. This implies that some of the depressed patients have decreased parasympathetic activity that might contribute to a lowering of the threshold for ventricular fibrillation. As mentioned previously, the death rate in depressed patients is most probably caused by ventricular fibrillation leading to sudden death and myocardial infarction. However, the results of post-MI research indicate that very low-frequency power is most strongly associated with death secondary to arrhythmia *(32,66)*.

It is reported that treatment with antidepressants can normalize reduced HRV *(33,67)*. On the other hand, some antidepressants possibly cause restriction of HRV. The danger of restricting HRV was also pointed out by the Cardiac Arrhythmia Suppression Trial (CAST) *(68)*. The available data from this study demonstrated, unexpectedly, that drugs with class 1 antiarrhythmic action (i.e., suppression of ventricular arrhythmias) increased the mortality risk in patients with asymptomatic or minimally symptomatic ventricular arrhythmia following MI. TCAs, for that matter, also have class I antiarrhythmic properties and could, for that reason, contribute to an excess of sudden death.

3.4. Mental Stress

It seems reasonable to assume a causal relation among depression, increased cardiac mortality, and stress. It is known that the first depressive episode is mostly elicited by a stressful event or period. Later episodes can develop more spontaneously. Depression can be considered as a state of prolonged negative arousal or mental stress. Different studies have demonstrated that mental stress in patients with CHD was associated with significantly higher fatal and nonfatal cardiac events *(38,49,50,52)*. Severe stress can lead to histopathologic alterations in the normal heart. Whether this happens depends on the activation of stress limiting systems, namely the opioidergic, GABAergic, cholinergic, adenosinergic, and other systems *(38)*. Conversely, genetically determined or acquired dysfunction of these systems predispose to severe arrhythmias and sudden death *(38)*. In a study correlating cardiac resistance to physical and stress loads in persons with stressful occupations (pilots), arrhythmias occurred only in 11% in the standard test with bicycle load. However, during "almost breakdown" situations in the flight simulator, arrhythmias occurred in almost 60% *(49)*. Psychological stress predisposes to abnormal ventricular activity by lowering the vulnerable ventricular period threshold even to the point of fibrillation. Stress exerts its effect through sympathetic activity. Parasympathetic (vagal) activity has a protective effect on myocardial electric instability induced by increased sympathetic activity.

Another potential mechanism contributing to the diminished cardiac survival of depressed patients is the preventricular contractions (PVC). It was demonstrated that the risk of sudden cardiac death was highest in those depressed patients who had 10 or more PVCs in 1 h *(51)*. Depression without PVC and PVC without depression were significantly less at risk. One study demonstrated that reduction of PVCs alone did not reduce mortality, which was partly caused by the fact that the antiarrythmic drugs used caused reduced HRV *(69)*. Depression and (acute) stress, therefore, have some resemblance in the way they sometimes reduce the threshold for ventricular fibrillation. Another factor that may connect depression and stress are possible deficiencies in the stress-limiting systems mentioned, during depressive periods or perhaps even during the times that depression is in remission.

3.5. Smoking

In addition to the presumed influence of depression on cardiovascular disease, other factors may also contribute to the development of cardiovascular disease. Among these, smoking has been shown to be a major risk factor. The most extensive investigation on the relationship among nicotine, depression, and cardiovascular disease was done by Glassmann et al. *(70)*. They found that a history of major depression increased the chance that this subject would be a smoker *(70)*.

This relationship was not only found for patients who had sought help not only for their depressive illness but also for those with a lifetime diagnosis of major depression and had never sought treatment. It also turned out that cessation of smoking very commonly caused depressive symptoms and even a recurrence of MDD in those with a history of MDD *(71,72)*. This strong relation between depression and the use of nicotine seems, at first glance, a good explanation for the excess of cardiac death.

However, in the meantime, several epidemiological studies have been done to investigate this relationship *(22,23,73)*. Also, when controlling for smoking, the predictive power of depression on cardiovascular events continued to be present. Smoking, although a well-known risk factor, is therefore not the essential link between depression and cardiovascular disease.

3.6. Psychotropic Drugs

As signs of heightened mortality emerged as a result of cardiovascular diseases among depressive patients, attention was focused on the use of tricyclic antidepressants (TCA) as a cause of cardiac death. They were suspected because of their effect on heart rate, blood pressure, conduction in therapeutic dose, and the fact that they are fatal in overdose. As a consequence, treatment with tricyclics is avoided or done with great caution, especially in the elderly patients with cardiovascular disease. However, no studies were conducted that compared the effects and side effects of the use of tricyclic antidepressives with placebo in the cardiovascular compromised patients. For that reason Roose et al. extracted data from the current literature *(46)*. These studies had the same inclusion criteria and the same design, which made it possible to compare them. The dropout rate secondary to medical events in the group treated with placebo, imipramine, nortriptyline, and doxepine was 10.6%, 60%, 21.8%, and 46.2%, respectively. The mortality rate was 2.4%, 1.7%, 2.6%, and 2.6%, respectively. Regarding these results, the short-term risk of the use of TCAs on mortality is not striking. Regarding the long-term risk, conflicting results have been reported. A few epidemiological studies have reported an association between MI and use of psychotropic drugs *(74,75)*. In a Finnish epidemiological study with a cohort of 3127 male farmers with a follow-up of 12 yr, the most pronounced risk for MI was found among users of antidepressants. A heightened risk of mortality is registered also with the use of lithium *(74)*. Several others found a tendency in the opposite direction. *See* Table 3.

3.6.1. Retrospective Studies

The only study from the "preantidepressants area" published in 1937 by Malzberg *(18)* demonstrates indefinitely that excess mortality cannot be accounted for only on behalf of the use of TCAs, as the mortality rate of patients with involutional melancholia (an old name for depression in middle-aged and elderly perons) was six to seven times greater than in the general population. Weeke *(26)* is another investigator who compared mortality among users of TCAs and depressed patients who never could have used TCAs. In a retrospective study, she investigated a cohort from the pre-TCA era by using the data in the Danish Central Register. The pre-TCA era stands for those depressed patients who lived and received treatment in the time period prior to the introduction of TCAs. All these patients were discharged between 1950 and 1956 with the diagnosis of manic–depressive or involutional depression. She compared these data with data from the TCA era. This cohort lived in the time period (the fifties) when TCAs were available and was, therefore, probably treated with it. The total mortality in the pre-TCA-era cohort was 2.53 times the mortality in the total Danish population during the fifties. The total mortality during the TCA era was 1.96 higher than in the general population at that time. Both groups showed an excess mortality with cardiac disease and suicide as main causes. Thus, the depressed patient of the TCA era has a heightened risk of cardiovascular death, but the cardiovascular mortality in the pre-TCA era tended to be even higher, although less spectacular, than in the Malzberg study from 1937 *(18)*.

Baseline characteristics	According to Norris Prognostic Index	• History of previous MI • LVEF • Killip class • PVCs • β-blockade	Not specified in detail • Ventricular fibrillation • Dobutamine use • Dyspnea • Late potential	• History of previous MI • LVEF • Killip class • PVCs • Thrombolytic treatment • β-blockades Aspirins Sodium-warfarin • ACE inhibitors	Not specified in detail
Characteristics of depression vs nondepression	Depression disappeared spontaneously	Not specified	Depression signs related to: • Duration of anginal pain • Occurrence of ventricular fibrillation • Dyspnea No relation to infarction size	Depressives used more warfarin, female>male	Characteristic of depressives: hostility
Mortality, depressed	N.S.	N.S.	N.S.	16% at 6 mo	No deaths
Mortality of nondepressed	N.S.	N.S.	N.S.	3% at 6 mo	No deaths

(continued)

Table 5 (continued)

Author	Lloyd 1983 (88)[a]	Ahern 1990 (84)	Ladwig 1992/1994 (17,87)	Frasure-Smith 1993/1995 (51,90)	Honing 1997 (98)
Depression independent predictor for cardiac mortality	N.S.	Yes (BDI score)	N.S.	Yes	
Outcome measures associated with mortality	N.S.	LVEF Previous MI PVC No use of β-blockade Digitalis transmurality Bortner-B BDI level		LVEF Killip class PVCs Previous MIS Warfarin at discharge	

[a]Numbers in parentheses are reference numbers. N.S. = Not specified. DSM = Diagnostic and Statistical Manual of Mental Disorders; POMS = Profile of Mood States; BDI = Beck Depression Inventory; MDD = major depressive disorder; PVC = preventricular contraction; ICD = International Clarification of Diseases; LVEF = left ventricular ejection fraction; SSIAM = Scaled and Structured Interview for the Assessment of Maladjustment; SPI = standard psychiatric interview; EPQ = Eysenck Personality Questionnaire; STAI = State-Trate Anxiety Inventory; AES = Anger Expression Scale; MCS = Marlowe–Crowne Scale.

Table 6
Killip Classification of Patients
with Acute Myocardial Infarction (*see* ref. *90a*)

Class	Definition
1	Absence of rales over the lung fields and absence of S3
2	Rales over 50% or less of the lung fields or the presence of an S3
3	Rales over more than 50% of the lung fields (frequently pulmonary edema)
4	Shock

before MI *(89)*. As mentioned earlier, exhaustion before MI may point to the presence of a subclinical depression *(7,11)*. Besides the transient affective symptomatology post-MI, more persistent depressive disorders are found. The incidence is about 15–29% in the year post-MI, repeatedly associated with heightened cardiac mortality *(51,84,90)*.

4.3. Risk Analysis of Mortality

4.3.1. Cardiovascular Risk Factors

The first prospective study in this field has demonstrated that about a third of the patients became depressed after an MI *(89)*. Patients who met the modified DSM-3R criteria for MDD following an MI were at significantly greater risk to die from cardiac causes during the subsequent 6 mo than the nondepressed, 17% and 3%, respectively *(90)*. This risk remained significant after controlling for other risk factors such as severity of cardiac disease. MDD can, therefore, be considered an independent risk factor for mortality. In further exploring the mechanisms linking depression and post-MI, the prognostic importance of the Beck Diagnostic Instrument (BDI) was examined in a follow-up investigation covering 6–18 mo. The BDI is not a diagnostic instrument *per se* but is a self-report scale that quantifies the depressive symptoms when the diagnosis MDD has already been assessed. Elevated BDI scores (cutoff score >10) were increased among people living alone, women (Killip class > 2 [Table 6] and among people who did not receive thrombolysis.

There was no increased BDI score that correlated with, for example, smoking status, previous MI, left ventricular ejection fraction, or preventricular beats (PVCs). An important finding was that the users of β-blockers were less likely to have elevated BDI scores. This is relevant because it is a general belief that β-blockers (especially lipophylic) may cause depression.

One of the most important findings was that elevated BDI scores were related to the mortality 6–18 mo post-MI, independent of the traditional post-MI risk factors *(51)*. The patients who were most likely to die were the ones who had a combination of elevated BDI, PVCs, and impaired left ventricular ejection fractions The impact of the BDI scores remained over time, in contrast to the impact of the presence of MDD, which occurred primarily in the first 6 mo. This is somewhat in accordance with the finding that hopelessness as a single symptom and without the existence of a MDD is a strong predictor of adverse health outcome, independent of the existence of depression *(91)*. High levels of hopelessness predicted incident MI, and moderate hopelessness was associated with incident cancer *(73)*. The usefulness of the BDI as a significant predictor is also demonstrated in other studies *(84)*.

4.3.2. Psychological Factors

Many researchers made efforts to identify specific personality attributes causing or predisposing to certain physical illness that was for cardiology type A behavior (ambitious, overengaged persons) for a long time the most relevant *(89,92–94)*. However, in the cardiac arrhythmia pilot study, heightened mortality post-MI was associated with depression, lower pulse rate reactivity, and the Bortner type B behavior pattern (*see* Table 7) *(84)*. This is in contrast with the long-standing hypothesis that a type A behavior pattern predisposes for MI. Similar results are described *(95,96)*.

Taken together, it seems that it is not the ambitious, overengaged persons who are vulnerable to an MI, but exactly the opposite, namely those who have withdrawn from life's challenges and opportunities *(84)*. A certain non-type-A

Table 7
Psychosomatic Personality Type

Personality type	Description
Type A behavior pattern	Defined as scoring above a certain cutoff score on the Bortner scale Hard driving Work involved Expressive hostility Antagonistic interactions Cynicism Hostile affect
Type B behavior pattern	A relative absence of type-A response style Defined as scoring beneath a certain cut off score on the Bortner scale
Type D behavior pattern	Negative affectivity Tends to worry Often feels unhappy or irritated Negative sociability Tends to keep others at a distance Inhibits expression of true feelings

behavior pattern associated with higher mortality risk was also noticed by Denolet et al. (97). They defined a "new personality," type D (distressed). This type is characterized by the chronic suppression of negative emotions. The existence of negative emotions (hostility) in this subgroup (post-MI depression) of depressed patients was confirmed by Honig et al *(98)*. Concerning the phenomology, they found that depression after MI is not so much characterized by a depressed mood and feelings of guilt, but more by listlessness and significantly increased hostility. Feelings of guilt developed only after several months, when a premorbid level of functioning could not be reached. The remaining clinical features of post-MI depression were globally the same as in a matched sample of depressed inpatients without a cardiac history.

According to a 10-yr follow-up study among 303 patients with angiographically documented CHD, this type D personality was an independent predictor of both cardiac and noncardiac mortality *(97)*. Again, depression was also related to mortality, but according to Denolet et al., it did not add to the predictive power of type D, which means that the predictive power of the type D personality is not the result of an increased frequency of MDD in this group. Ladwig et al. *(87)* described a high-risk group with comparable features.

A possible special role of hostility and anxiety as part of certain subtypes of depression in the pathogenesis of CHD was also demonstrated by Fava et al. *(99).* They hypothesized that only certain symptom patterns would be associated with cardiovascular risk factors. Indeed, it was demonstrated that patients with higher-state anxiety levels and/or anger attacks had higher cholesterol levels. In the depressive group as a whole, cholesterol was not elevated, which is consistent with previous studies. The anxiety subtype was also associated with prolonged QT lengthening, whereas anger was not, to a significant extent. A possible explanation for this finding could be that anxiety usually lasts longer and, therefore, reflects continuous arousal, whereas anger attacks reflect more episodic arousal. Kawachi and co-workers demonstrated in a prospective epidemiological study the existence of a dose-response relation between level of anger and overall CHD risk *(100).*

4.3.4. Protective Factors

Identifying psychological factors that protect against or induce vulnerability to post-MI depression, it was found that denial and optimism were positively correlated with a low depression score *(87).* In a study that focused primarily on two coping strategies (attention and avoidance) for reducing anxiety after MI, it was demonstrated that denial is a more effective strategy than causal search, which is an attention strategy *(101).*

4.4. Treatment

It is apparent that there are many reasons to diagnose and treat depression in patients with cardiac disease. At this moment, there is probably undertreatment because depression in patients with CHD is rarely diagnosed by primary care physicians and cardiologists. One of the causes of this phenomenon is probably the fact that depression in CHD presents in an atypical manner *(98)*. Besides the diagnostic problem, there is the clinical dilemma in choosing the right antidepressant, which is necessary as stress management or behavioral counseling programs reported no benefit for the patients *(102,103)*.

There is no extensive literature with regard to antidepressants and heart disease, as, by far, the most clinical trials with antidepressants are done with somatically healthy persons. These systematic studies documented a number of cardiovascular effects, most notably (1) increase in heart rate, (2) orthostatic hypotension, (3) slowing of intraventricular cardiac conduction, and (4) type 1a antiarrhythmic activity *(104,105)*. Although tricyclic antidepressants are effective, their use requires caution, especially in cardiac patients. Whether tricyclic antidepressants can be described depends on the kind of cardiac disease. The tricyclic antidepressants doxepine, imipramine, and nortrilen were evaluated in congestive heart failure with radionuclide angiography. The vast majority of patients did not experience negative inotropic effects, but one patient did. This was reversible after discontinuing the drug *(104,105)*. In arrhythmias, TCAs may act as a 1A antiarrhythmic, which until recently was considered a beneficial effect. However, since the report of heightened mortality among users of 1A antiarrhythmic is possibly a result of restricted HRV, the use of TCAs is disputed in this subgroup of CHD. In patients with pre-existing bundle-branch block, there are no safe tricyclic antidepressants *(61)*. Treatment with TCA of several other cardiovascular diseases are also discussed by Roose and co-workers *(61)*.

Because of their fewer potential side effects on the cardiovascular system, selective serotonin reuptake inhibitors (SSRI) and noradrenaline and serotonin reuptake inhibitors (NSRIs) might be given an important place in the treatment of CHD. However, again, one cannot extrapolate the results from medication studies with healthy persons to patients with CHD. In other words, the safety of SSRIs in healthy people

must yet be determined in those with CHD. The only currently known side effect of SSRIs is a sinus slowing, which
occurs rarely *(105)*. Another consideration is efficacy. There
is evidence that the newer generation of antidepressants as
SSRIs are as effective in the mild–moderate MDD, but that
the effectiveness of TCAs is significantly greater in the most
severe MDD *(106)*. If future test results demonstrate that cardiac mortality in depressed patients decreases only after a
full remission, this will be an important consideration in the
risk–benefit analysis. The effect of the different antidepressants on platelet function or HRV is another topic for future
research.

5. Anxiety Disorders and Cardiac Disease

As mentioned earlier, several studies reported an association between anxiety as a symptom and CHD. With respect
to the relation between anxiety disorders (as syndrome) and
cardiac diseases, the findings are very different and sometimes contradictory. Research and literature on anxiety and
CHD is neither extensive nor as sophisticated as on depression *(19)*. A special problem in determining the mutual
influence of CHD and anxiety is the fact that anxiety and
MDD often coexist. For instance, lifetime prevalence of 2%
for panic disorder is reported. After reviewing the literature,
Griez and co-workers *(106a)* conclude that 50–75% of panic-
disorder patients have a lifetime comorbid depression,
whereas the reverse is less frequent as only 10–30% of mood-
disorder patients have a lifetime panic disorder. Controlling
for comorbidity is, therefore, essential in determining the
effect of anxiety on CHD.

Psychiatric classification recognizes a broad spectrum
of anxiety disorders. The ones associated most frequently
with cardiac disease are panic disorder, agoraphobia, and
generalized anxiety disorder. Other relevant categories are
adjustment disorder with anxiety and posttraumatic stress
disorder, although research results concerning these subjects
are scarce. The relevant subjects will be reviewed successively.

5.1. Panic Disorder and Cardiac Disease

Panic disorder is a common condition that shares many nonspecific symptoms with several medical conditions such as chest pain, palpitations, dyspnea, and presyncope (*See* Table 8). Because of this similarity, patients with panic disorder are high users of medical services *(107)*. Panic disorder has a special symptom overlap with angina pectoris and arrhythmia, and several investigators suggest that there is an above-normal frequency of panic disorder in mitral valve prolapse (MVP) and idiopathic cardiomyopathy. The relation to CHD in general is more conflicting. These disorders will be reviewed successively.

5.1.1. Chest Pain

Chest pain is one of the prominent and alarming symptoms of panic disorder and, therefore, an important reason for seeking medical attention. For cardiologists, it remains difficult to differentiate severe anxiety from cardiac disease.

One investigator reported that 30% of individuals who undergo cardiac catherization are found to have no significant coronary artery disease (NCA). Panic disorder (PD) occurs in 33–46% of the NCA group and in 5% of those with abnormal coronary angiography *(108)*. The NCA group has a good prognosis with regard to long-term survival, although half or more of patients after catherization continue to report problems such as chest pain or lowered capacity to perform work or daily activities *(108)*. When examining the NCA group more closely, it was demonstrated that patients with PD in this group had significantly more chest pain in common, both in rest and sleep (67% and 30%, respectively). It was striking that only 22% sought psychiatric treatment and only 30% were treated with benzodiazepines and/or antidepressants.

Chest pain is also mentioned in relation to mitral valve prolapse (MVP). The description of chest pain differs in both disorders. Chest pain in PD is usually characterized as atypical angina pectoris, whereas chest pain in MVP is highly variable *(108a)*.

Table 8
Criteria of Panic Disorder Without Agoraphobia

A. Both 1 and 2: To fulfill the criteria of a panic disorder a patient must have symptoms described in A1 and A2.

1. Recurrent unexpected Panic Attacks
   Panic Attack Criteria
   A discrete period of intense fear or discomfort, in which four (or more) of the following symptoms developed abruptly and reached a peak within 10 min:
   1. Palpitations
   2. Sweating
   3. Trembling or shaking
   4. Sensations of shortness of breath or smothering
   5. Feeling of choking
   6. Chest pain or discomfort
   7. Nausea or abdominal distress
   8. Feeling dizzy, unsteady, lightheaded, or faint
   9. Derealization (feelings of unreality) or depersonalization (being detached from oneself)
   10. Fear of losing control or going crazy
   11. Fear of dying
   12. Paresthesias
   13. Chills or hot flushes

2. At least one of the attacks has been followed by 1 mo (or more) of one (or more) of the following:
   1. Persistent concern about having additional attacks
   2. Worry about the implications of the attack or its consequences (e.g., losing control, having a heart attack, feeling of "going crazy")
   3. A significant change in behavior related to the attacks.

B. Absence of agoraphobia

C. The panic attacks are not due to the direct physiological effects of a substance (e.g., a drug of abuse, medication) or a general medical condition (e.g., hyperthyroidism).

D. The panic attacks are not better accounted for by another mental disorder, such as social phobia (e.g., occurring on exposure to feared social situations), specific phobia (e.g., on exposure to a specific phobic situation), obsessive-compulsive disorder (e.g., on exposure to dirt in someone with an obsession about contamination), posttraumatic stress disorder (e.g., in response to stimuli associated with a severe stressor), or separation anxiety disorder (e.g., in response to being away from home or relatives).

5.1.2. Mitral Valve Prolapse

This is a common cardiac disorder (5–21% in normal population) that can easily be diagnosed by auscultation and echocardiographic examination *(109)*. An exact classification of the MVP, however, is problematic. There is no consensus about the minimum extent to which the leaflets of the mitral valve may sag toward the left atrial chamber during the left ventricular systole. Besides this, abnormalities of the leaflets can be placed on a continuum. At one end, one can find only an abnormal movement, which is principally only an echocardiographic finding; on the other end, one finds MVPs with a complete clinical syndrome *(107)*.

A review of the literature demonstrates that MVP and panic disorder often co-occur *(107)*. This led to the hypothesis that there might be a cause–effect relationship between the two disorders that has never been proven up to now *(109,110)*. In both disorders, autonomic disorders do occur but the patterns of abnormality differ *(111,112)*. In a Greek study, it was demonstrated that during normal daily activities, patients with MVP have a significant deviation in tone produced by the autonomic nervous system *(111)*. In the spectral heart rate variability analysis, there appeared to be a predominance of the sympathetic nervous system, which is also found in depressed patients

As already mentioned, several studies have found that the prevalence of MVP in patients with panic attacks is higher than in the general population. Percentages of 24–35% MVP are mentioned *(113)*. However, it also appeared that panic attacks occurred more often in patients with mitral valve prolapse when compared with normal controls *(109)*. When cardiology patients were used as the control group, no significant difference was found. In several other studies, these high percentages could not be confirmed as resulting panic attacks in 0–8% of patients with mitral valve prolapse *(109)*.

5.1.3. Idiopathic Cardiomyopathy

In a sample ($n = 35$) of idiopathic cardiomyopathy derived from a prescreening program for cardiac transplantation, 51% met DSM-3 criteria for panic disorder and 31% had probable panic disorder. In a group of 25 patients with end-stage cardiac failure resulting from another disease, "only" 16% had a panic disorder, a highly significant difference *(114)*. This difference makes it clear that the panic attacks are not just a psychological reaction to a life-threatening disease. Kahn et al. *(114)* suggest several mechanisms that link panic disorder with cardiomyopathy. Patients with pheochromocytoma can have cardiac pathology, which resembles idiopathic cardiomyopathy. This suggests catecholaminergic involvement in etiology, although the catecholamine surges do not cause panic attacks. It might also be possible that idiopathic cardiomyopathy induces panic attacks such as congestive heart failure that are associated with elevated catecholamine levels, which might trigger panic attacks *(114)*.

5.1.4. Coronary Heart Disease

An excess of cardiovascular and cerebrovascular mortality was found in small retrospective studies *(115,116)* among patients who apparently met DSM-3 criteria for panic disorder *(112)*. The expected and observed deaths from circulatory system disease were in women with panic disorder, respectively 1.4 and 3, and in men 6.0 and 12, respectively. All the patients came from psychiatric, cardiac, or primary care clinics, which may cause a selection bias and exaggerate the association between panic disorder and cardiovascular and cerebrovascular events *(112)*. However, results from a (small) community survey demonstrate that the risk of stroke in persons with a lifetime diagnosis of PD was over twice that in persons without PD. An association among the presence of any psychiatric disorder (including PD), hypertension, and heart attacks was found, supporting the hypothesis that mental stress can induce silent myocardial ischemia *(117)*. One investigator analyzed acute psychological disturbances in the 24 h preceding a life-threatening ventricular fibrillation and revealed that 20% experienced acute emotional disturbances. In 70%, anger was the most predominant affect *(118)*. Bearing this in mind, it seems reasonable that comorbidity of panic disorder and cardiac disease may form a dangerous interaction, such as panic attacks producing angina through sympaticus activation and myocardial ischemia, whereas angina may produce panic attacks in susceptible patients. However, the 9-yr community survey of Bruce and co-workers revealed that only a past history of panic disorder had a significant association with mortality, as a recent history of panic disorder did not *(30)*.

5.2. Phobic Anxiety

Three prospective studies examined the association of anxiety with the risk of coronary heart disease *(119–121)*. The Health Professional Follow-up Study *(119)* is a longitudinal study of risk factors for cardiovascular disease and cancer. It consists of 51, 529 male medical professionals aged 46–75 yr in 1986. It was demonstrated that in men with phobic symptoms, the prevalence of smoking, hypertension, hypercholesterolemia, and diabetes mellitus was higher than in comparable age groups. Even when controlled for this and the use of medication, a strong association was found between phobic anxiety (Table 9) and fatal CHD. This increase was particularly because of an excess sudden death, whereas no association was found with nonfatal MI. These findings were consistent with the Normative Aging Study *(120)*, a longitudinal study with a cohort of 2280 men. The Northwick Park Heart Study *(121)* also demonstrated a dose-response gradient in the association of phobic anxiety and fatal CHD, although in this study, no distinction was made between sudden death and nonsudden fatal death. High scores of phobic anxiety at baseline measurement predicted higher mortality several years later.

As an explanation for this association, several mechanisms are hypothesized. Anxiety can induce hyperventilation, which can lead to coronary artery spasm *(122,123)*. Argentinean cardiologists found that hyperventilation could easily and reproducibly induce myocardial ischemia in patients with Prinzmetal's (variant) angina *(123)*. This kind of angina is associated with acute myocardial infarction,

Table 9
Criteria for a Specific Phobia

A. Marked and persistent fear that is excessive or unreasonable, cued by the presence or anticipation of a specific object or situation (e.g., flying, heights, animals, receiving an injection, seeing blood).

B. Exposure to the phobic stimulus almost invariably provokes an immediate anxiety response, which may take the form of a situation-bound or situation-predisposed panic attack. **Note:** In children, the anxiety may be expressed by crying, tantrums, freezing, or clinging.

C. The person recognizes that the fear is excessive or unreasonable. **Note:** In children, this feature may be absent.

D. The phobic situation is avoided or is endured with intense anxiety or distress.

E. The avoidance, anxious anticipation, or distress in the feared situation(s) interferes significantly with the person's normal routine, occupational (or academic) functioning, or social activities or relationships, or there is marked distress about having the phobia.

F. In individuals under 18 yr, the duration is at least 6 mo.

G. The anxiety, panic attacks, or phobic avoidance associated with the specific object or situation are not better accounted for by another mental disorder, such as obsessive–compulsive disorder (e.g., fear of dirt in someone with an obsession about contamination), post traumatic disorder (e.g., avoidance of social situations because of fear of embarrassment), separation anxiety disorder (e.g., avoidance of school), social phobia (e.g., avoidance of social situations because of fear of embarrassment), panic disorder with agoraphobia, or agoraphobia without history of panic disorder.

Specify type: Animal type, Natural environment type (storm, height), Blood, injection, Injury type, Situational type (Airplane, enclosed places), Other types.

---

severe cardiac arrhythmias, and sudden death *(124)*. Ischemia from such repeated episodes of spasm may have been responsible for the development of chronic cardiac damage. Reduced heart rate variability, which can be found in panic disorder patients, is also a known risk factor for sudden death *(112)*. Also, a heightened risk for thromboembolism is suggested *(112)*. These results must be cautiously interpreted because of the small numbers. In contrast with the mentioned results, Bruce and co-workers found no association of mortality with obsessive–compulsive disorder or phobia *(30)*. A possible explanation is that they use the full DSM 3 criteria and the other investigators used only symptoms, not the syndromes.

5.3. Generalized Anxiety and Posttraumatic Stress Disorder

As described in Subheadings 3 and 4, detailed examination revealed that the higher morbidity and mortality because of cardiac causes in depressive patients is probably (partly) the result of the coexisting anxiety symptoms. Most attention has been focused lately on myocardial infarction. This is a life-threatening event with considerable psychological effects. Anxiety is one of the most prominent ones. Several investigators have examined this effect, although thorough psychiatric investigations are rare, probably because anxiety after MI is a very understandable reaction. Most of the reports comprise the analysis of self-reporting questionnaires. Moser and co-workers *(125)* determined the effect of anxiety 48 h after MI on recovery and found more complications with higher levels of anxiety than with lower levels: 19.6% vs 6%. Complications were defined as reinfarction, new onset of ischemia, ventricular fibrillation, sustained ventricular tachycardia, or in-hospital death. A double-blind study with diazepam showed no decrease of symptoms of anxiety and cardiac dysregulation, although sedation was reached *(126,127)*. As for most people, an MI represents a life crisis, it is logical to assume that posttraumatic stress disorder (PTSD) may follow an MI. These symptoms include intrusive re-experiencing of the traumatic event, avoidance of stimuli associated with the event, numbing of responsiveness to the external world, and increased autonomic arousal. Patients with PTSD often experience extensive fear. Only a few reports document PTSD after MI *(127,128)*. In one study, 9% of the MI patients developed a PTSD between 6 and 12 mo post-MI. The group as a whole reported little distress *(127)*. However, this study has serious methodological limitations, as only men were included, diagnosis was based on self-reporting rating scales, and the number of patients was limited.

6. Cognitive Disturbances in Cardiac Patients

Little is known about the effect of cardiac dysfunction on cognitive performance. It seems logical to assume that severe cardiac dysfunction could influence cerebral function. The most serious cognitive disturbance is seen in delirium. However, delirium can be judged as a final common path of cerebral disturbance, because of a wide variety of somatic systemic disorders. This is illustrated by the fact that delirium is much more common after cardiac surgery (10–30%, 3–5 d postoperative) than after MI *(100,129)*. Other cardiac causes of delirium are low-output states, congestive heart failure, and shock *(130)*.

In several investigations among patients with cardiac disease, more subtle cognitive dysfunctions have been described. In these cases, mainly impairment in complex reasoning were found *(131)*. The problem with interpreting these results is that patients with cardiac diseases are mostly older and are also suffering from atherosclerosis *in cerebro*. Therefore, when one finds cognitive dysfunction, it is difficult to say whether this is the result of cardiac dysfunction or to perfusion disturbance caused by atherosclerosis in the brain itself. One way to resolve this question is to measure cognitive performance during cardiac dysfunction and after treating it. In two investigations, the effect of implantation of a pacemaker was measured *(131,132)*. The results were conflicting. Rockwood et al. did a prospective case control study among 19 elderly people (65+ yr) with dysrhythmias and found no improvement on psychological test after the implantation, although global function was improved *(133)*. Koide et al., on the contrary, did find improvement after implantation in his group of elderly people (mean age 75 yr) *(132)*. Verbal intelligence improved notably, which was the result of improved cerebral blood flow that was demonstrated. Cerebral blood flow was correlated with heart rate, not with cardiac output. Zuccala et al. *(131)*, on the other hand, found that cognitive dysfunction was independently associated with older age and left ventricular ejection fraction (VEF), when the VEF was below 30%.

Another cause of cognitive disturbance is the cardiovascular medication. The antihypertensive medications are described most extensively in this context and, to a lesser extent, diuretics and others. In short, they may cause mostly subtle cognitive disturbances, but it is important to realize that hypertension itself is also associated with neuropsychological changes *(134)*. However it is beyond the scope of the chapter to describe this in detail.

7. Summary

Of the neuropsychiatric and cognitive disorders associated with heart diseases, depressive disorders are the ones investigated most extensively and with the greatest sophistication. This is to a lesser extent the case with anxiety disorders. Research regarding cognitive disorders in heart patients is scarce.

There is convincing evidence that depression is associated with cardiovascular disease. This relation seems to be bilateral: Depression is associated with heightened cardiovascular disease and heightened cardiovascular disease with depression. The nature of this connection is unclear. It is even unclear whether the existence of certain symptoms of depression *per se* such as dysphoria, depressed affect, or anxiety are sufficient to raise the risk of CHD. There are signs that special symptoms such as anxiety and hostility alone place the patient with MDD at risk, whereas the patient without MDD but with feelings of hopelessness is also at risk.

Research studies point toward a cause–effect relationship with depression as a cause of cardiovascular disease. Features of the depressive disorder that makes it a risk factor for cardiovascular disease are neurohumoral disturbances, changes in the thrombotic system, changes in the autonomic nervous system demonstrated by a decreased heart rate variability, which probably predisposes to ventricular arrhythmias and bad habits such as smoking, and so forth.

Another mechanism through which depression may exert its effect is the fact that psychological stress can induce myocardial ischemia in the absence of coronary artery disease.

The influence of personality traits on the pathogenesis of CHD remains speculative. In contrast to earlier convictions, it is not the type-A behavior, with the overengaged workaholic as a representative risk factor, but especially the more depressive personalities that are prone to be at risk.

It is important to realize that an association is not the same as a causal relation. For instance, in the case of CHD and MDD, it might be possible that atherosclerosis is a cause of both depression and heart disease. It is also possible that a disturbance in certain brain areas induces both depression and a changed heart rate variability.

Anxiety disorders as a syndrome have been less extensively studied compared to depressive disorders and are, for that reason, only briefly summarized. Research was focused on anxiety primarily as a symptom and there is some evidence that there is a relation with higher cardiac mortality and a higher mortality because of cerebro vascular accidents. Anxiety as a syndrome received the most attention as a differential diagnostic problem in mitral valve prolapse and acute chest pain.

In addition to the etiologic and prognostic considerations, the most important question of whether treatment of MDD can prevent cardiovascular morbidity and mortality remain. Investigative strategies should include biological markers (associated with depression and relevant for heart disease) and the way they are influenced under the various treatments.

References

1. Schiffer, R. B. and Fogel, B. S. (1996) Evolution of neuropsychiatric ideas in the United States and United Kingdom 1800–2000, in *Neuropsychiatry* (Schiffer, R. B. and Fogel, B. S., eds.), Williams & Wilkins, Baltimore, pp. 1–10.
2. Cummings, J. L. (1995) Neuropsychiatry: clinical assessment and approach to diagnosis, in *Comprehensive Textbook of Psychiatry/4,*

6th ed. (Kaplan, H. I. and Sadock, B. J., eds.), vol 1, Williams & Wilkins, Baltimore, vol. 1, pp. 167–187.

3. Steinhart, M. J. (1991) Depression and chronic fatigue in the patient with heart disease. *Primary Care* **18(2)**, 309–325.

4. Leff, J. (ed.) (1988) *Psychiatry Around the Globe*. Gaskell, London.

5. Kleinman, A. and Kleinman, J. (1985) Somatization: the interconnections in Chinese Society among culture, depressive experiences and the meanings of pain, in *Culture and Depression* (Kleinman, A. and Good, B., eds.), University of California Press, Berkley, CA, pp. 429–491.

6. *Diagnostic and Statistical Manual of Mental Disorders*, 4th ed. American Psychiatric Association, Washington DC, 1994.

7. Lesperance, F., Frasure-Smith, N., and Talajic, M. (1996) Major depression before and after myocardial infarction: its nature and consequences. *Psychosom. Med.* **58,** 99–110.

8. Appels, A. (1990) Mental precursors of myocardial infarction. *Br. J. Psychiatry* **156,** 465–471.

9. Appels, A. and Schouten, E. (1991) Waking up exhausted as risk indicator of myocardial infarction. *Am. J. Cardiol.* **68(1),** 395–398.

10. Falger, P. R. J. (1989) Life-span development and myocardial infarction: an epidemiological study. Ph.D. thesis, Limburg University, The Netherlands.

11. van Diest, R. and Appels, A. (1991) Vital exhaustion and depression: a conceptual study. *J. Psychosom. Res.* **35(4/5),** 535–544.

12. Appels, A. and Otten, F. (1992) Exhaustion as precursor for cardiac death. *Br. J. Clin. Psychol.* **31,** 351–356.

13. Wald, F. D. M. and Mellenbergh, G. J. (1990) The short version of the Dutch translation of the Profile of Mood States (POMS), *Ned. Tijdschr. Psychol.* **45,** 86–90.

14. Beck, A. T., Rush A. J., Shaw B. F., and Emery G. (1979) *Cognitive Therapy of Depression*. Wiley, New York.

15. Kop, W. J., Appels, A. P. W. M., Mendes de Leon, C. F., and Bar, F. W. H. M. (1996) The relationship between severity of coronary artery disease and vital exhaustion. *J. Psychosom. Res.* **40(4),** 397–405.

16. Verhey, F. R. J. and Honig A. (1997) Depression in the elderly, in *Depression: Neurobiological, Psychopathological and Therapeutic Advances* (Honig, A. and van Praag, H. M., eds.), Wiley, Chichester, pp. 59–83.

17. Ladwig, K. H., R'll, G., Breithardt, G., Budde, T., and Borggrefe, M. (1994) Post-infarction depression and incomplete recovery 6 months after acute myocardial infarction. *Lancet* **343,** 20–23.

18. Malzberg, B. (1937) Mortality among patients with involutional melancholia. *Am. J. Psychiatry* **93,** 1231–1238.

19. Glassmann, A. H. and Shapiro, P. A. (1998) Depression and the course of coronary artery disease. *Am. J. Psychiatry* **155,** 4–11.

20. Bruce, M. L. (1989) Psychiatric disorders and 15 month mortality in a community sample of older adults. *Am. J. Public Health* **79,** 727–730.
21. Murphy, J. M., Monson, R. R., Oliver, D. C., Sobol, A. M., and Leighton, A. H. (1987) Affective disorders and mortality, a general population study. *Arch. Gen. Psychiatry* **44,** 473–480.
22. Barefoot, J. C. and Schroll, M. (1996) Symptoms of depression, acute myocardial infarction, and total mortality in a community sample. *Circulation* **93,** 1976–1980.
23. Aroma, A., Raitasalo, R., Reunanen, A., Impivaara, O., Heliovaara, M., Knekt, P., et al. (1994) Depression and cardiovascular diseases. *Acta Psychiatr. Scand.* **377(Suppl.),** 77–82.
24. Fredman L., Schoenbach V. J., Kaplan B. H., Blazer D. G., James S. A., Kleinbaum D. G., et al. (1989) The association between depressive symptoms and mortality among older participants in the Epidemiologic Catchment Area–Piedmont Health Survey. *J. Gerontol.* **44(4),** S149–S156.
25. Zilber, N. Schufman, N., and Lerner, Y. (1989) Mortality among psychiatric patients—the group at risk. *Acta Psychiatr. Scand.* **79,** 248–256.
26. Weeke, A., Juel, K., and Veath, M. (1987) Cardiovascular death and manic–depressive psychosis. *J. Affect. Dis.* **13,** 287–292.
27. Carney, R. M., Rich, M. W., Freedland, K. E., Saini, J., TeVelde, A., Simeone, C., et al. (1988) Major depressive disorder predicts cardiac events in patients with coronary artery disease. *Psychosom. Med.* **50,** 627–633.
28. Sharma, R. and Markar, H. R. (1994) Mortality in affective disorder. *J. Affect. Dis.* **31,** 91–96.
29. Barefoot, J. C., Helms, M. J., Mark, D. B., Blumenthal, J. A., Califf, R. M., Haney, T. L., et al. (1996) Depression and long-term mortality risk in patients with coronary artery disease. *Am. J. Cardiol.* **78,** 613–617.
30. Bruce, M. L., Leaf, P. J., Rozal, G. P. M., Florio, L., and Hoff, R. A. (1994) Psychiatric status and 9-year mortality data in the New Haven epidemiologic catchment area study. *Am. J. Psychiatry* **151,** 716–721.
31. Smith, K. A. and Cowen, P. J. (1997) Serotonin and depression, in *Depression: Neurobiological, Psychopathological and Therapeutic Advances* (Honig, A. and van Praag, H. M., eds.), Wiley, Chichester, pp. 129–147.
32. Anand, A. and Charney, D. S. (1997) Catecholamines in depression, in *Depression: Neurobiological, Psychopathological and Therapeutic Advances* (Honig, A. and van Praag, H. M., eds.), Wiley, Chichester, pp. 147–179.
33. Musselman, D. L., Evans, D. L., and Nemeroff, C. B. (1998) The relationship of depression to cardiovascular disease. *Arch. Gen. Psychiatry* **55,** 580–592.

34. Ansseau, M. (1997) Hormonal disturbances in depression, in *Depression: Neurobiological, Psychopathological and Therapeutic Advances* (Honig, A. and van Praag, H. M., eds.), Wiley, Chichester, pp. 235–251.

35. Haft, J. L. (1974) Cardiovascular injury induced by sympathetic catecholamines. *Prog. Cardiovasc. Dis.* **17,** 73–86.

36. Winokur, A., Maislin G., Philips J. L., and Amsterdam J. D. (1988) Insulin resistance after oral glucose tolerance testing in patients with major depression. *Am. J. Psychiatry* **145,** 325–330.

37. Stout, R. W. (1990) Insulin and atheroma: 20-year perspective. *Diabetes Care* **13,** 631–654.

38. Meerson, L. Z. (1994) Stress-induced arrhythmic disease of the heart—part I. *Clin. Cardiol.* **17,** 362–371.

39. Gerritsen M. E. (1996) Physiological and pathophysiological roles of eicoanoids in the microcirculation. *Cardiovasc. Res.* **32,** 720–732.

40. Anfossi G. and Trovati M. (1996) Role of catecholamines in platelet function: pathophysiological and clinical significance. *Eur. J. Clin. Invest.* **26,** 353–370.

41. Verrier, R. L., Calvert A., and Lown, B. (1975) Effect of posterior hypothalamic stimulation on ventricular fibrillation threshold. *Am. J. Physiol.* **228,** 923–927.

42. Tavazzi, L., Zotti, A. M., and Rondanelli, R. (1986) The role of psychologic stress in the genesis of lethal arrhythmias in patients with coronary artery disease. *Eur. J. Heart* **7(Suppl. A),** 99–106.

43. Lown, B. and Verrrier, R. L. (1976) Neural activity and ventricular fibrillation. *N. Engl. J. Med.* **294,** 1165–1170.

44. Lown, B., DeSilva, R. A., Reich, P. (1980) Psychophysiologic factors in sudden cardiac death. *Am. J. Psychiatry* **137,** 1325–1335.

45. Follick, M. J., Ahern, D. K., Gorkin, L., Niaura, R. S., Herd, J. A., Ewart, C., et al. (1990) Relation of psychosocial and stress reactivity variables to ventricular arrhythmias in the cardiac arrhythmia pilot study (CAPS). *Am. J. Cardiol.* **66,** 63–67.

46. Roose, S. P., Dalack, G. W., and Woodring, S. (1991) Death, depression and heart disease. *J. Clin. Psychiatry* **52(Suppl. 6),** 34–39.

47. Goldberg, A. D., Becker, L. C., Bonsal, R., Cohen, J. D., Ketterer, M. W., Kaufman, P. G., et al. (1996) Ischemic, hemodynamic, and neurohormonal responses to mental and exercise stress, experience from the psychophysical investigations of myocardial ischemia study (PIMI). *Circulation* **94,** 2402–2409.

48. McCarthy, R. and Gold, P. E. (1996) Catecholamines, stress and disease: a psychobiological perspective. *Psychosom. Med.* **58,** 590–597.

49. Meerson, L. Z. (1994) Stress-induced arrhythmic disease of the heart—part II, *Clin. Cardiol.* **17,** 422–426.

50. Davis, A. M. and Natelson, B. H. (1993) Brain–heart interactions, the neurology of arrhythmia and sudden cardiac death. *Texas Heart Inst. J.* **20**, 158–169.
51. Frasure-Smith, N., Lesperance, F., and Talajic, M. (1995) Depression and 18-month prognosis after myocardial infarction. *Circulation* **91(4),** 999–1005.
52. Lecomte, D., Fornes, P., and Nicolas, G. (1996) Stressful events as a trigger of sudden death: a study of 43 medico-legal autopsy cases. *Forensic Sci. Int.* **79,** 1–10.
53. Ruschena, D., Mullen, P. E., Burgess, P., Cordner, S. M., Barry-Walsch, J., Drummer, O. J., et al. (1998) Sudden death in psychiatric patients. *Br. J. Psychiatry* **172,** 331–336.
54. Vanhoutte, P. M. (1991) Platelet-derived serotonin, the endothelium, and cardiovascular disease. *J. Cardiovasc. Pharmacol.* **17(Suppl. 5),** S6–S12.
55. Musselman, D. L., Tomer, A., Manatunga, A. K., Knight, B. T., Porter, M. R., Kasey, S., et al. (1996) Exaggerated platelet reactivity in major depression. *Am. J. Psychiatry* **153,** 1313–1317.
56. Smith, K. A. and Cowen, P. J. (1997) Serotonin and depression, in *Depression: Neurobiological, Psychopathological and therapeutic Advances* (Honig, A. and van Praag, H. M., eds.), Wiley, Chichester, pp. 235–251.
57. Laghrissi-Thode, F., Wagner, W. R., Pollock, B. G., Johnson, P. C., and Finkel, M. S. (1997) Elevated platelet factor 4 and beta-thromboglobulin plasma levels in depressed patients with ischemic heart disease. *Biol. Psychiatry* **42,** 290–295.
58. Cameron, O. (1996) Depression increases post-MI mortality: how? *Psychosom. Med.* **58,** 111–112 (editorial).
59. Kojima, K., Ogomori, K., Mori, Y., Hirata, K., Kinukawa, N., and Tashiro, N. (1996) Relationship of emotional behaviors induced by electrical stimulation of the hypothalamus to changes in EKG, heart, stomach, adrenal glands and thymus, *Psychosom. Med.* **58,** 383–391.
60. ter Horst, G. J. (1998) TNF α induced selective cerebral endothelial leakage and increased mortality risk in postmyocardial infarction depression. *Am. J. Physiol.* **275** 1910–1911.
61. Roose, S. P. and Dalack, G. W. (1992) Treating the depressed patient with cardiovascular problems. *J. Clin. Psychiatry* **53(Suppl. 9),** 25–31.
62. Kleiger, R. E., Miller, J. P., and Bigger, J. T. (1987) Decreased heart rate variability and its association with increased mortality after acute myocardial infarction. *Am. J. Cardiol.* **59,** 256–262.
63. Bigger, J. T., Kleiger R. E., Fleiss J. L., Rolnitzky, L. M., Steinman, R. C., and Miller, J. P. (1988) Components of heart rate variability measured during healing of acute myocardial infarction. *Am. J. Cardiol.* **61** 208–215.

64. Rechlin, T., Weis, M., and Claus, D. (1994) Heart rate variability in depressed patients and differential effects of paroxetine and amitryptiline on cardiovascular autonomic functions. *Pharmacopsychiatry* **27,** 124–128.

65. Carney, R. M., Saunders, R. D., Freedland, K. E., Stein, P., Rich, M. W., and Jaffe, A. S. (1995) Association of depression with reduced heart rate variability in coronary artery disease. *Am. J. Cardiol.* **76,** 562–564.

66. Bigger, J. T., Jr., Fleiss, J. L., Steinman, R. C., Rolnitzky, L. M., Kleiger, R. E., Rottman, J. N. (1992) Frequency domain measures of heart period variability and mortality after myocardial infarction. *Circulation* **85,** 164–171.

67. Balogh, S., Fitzpatrick, D. F., Hendricks S. E., Paige, S. R. (1993) Increases in heart rate variability with successful treatment in patients with major depressive disorder, *Psychopharmacol. Bull.* **29,** 201–206.

68. Roose, S. P. and Glassman, A. H. (1994) Antidepressant choice in the patient with cardiac disease: lessons from the cardiac arrythmia suppression trial (CAST studies). *J. Clin. Psychiatry* **55(Suppl. A),** 83–87.

69. Echt, D. S., Liebson, P. R., Mitchell, L. B., Peters, R. W., Obias-Manno, D., Baker, A., et al. (1991) Mortality and morbidity in patients receiving ecainide, flecainide or placebo: the Cardiac Arrhythmia Suppression Trial. *N. Engl. J. Med.* **324,** 643–668.

70. Glassman, A. H., Stetner, F., Walsh, B. T., Raizman, P. S., Fleiss, J. L., Cooper, T. B., et al. (1988) Heavy smokers, smoking cessation, and clonidine: results of a double blind, randomized trial. *JAMA* **259,** 2863–2866.

71. Glassman, A. H., Helzer, J. E., Covey, L. S., Cottle, L. B., Stetner, F., Tipp, J. E., et al. (1990) Smoking, smoking cessation, and major depression. *JAMA* **264(12),** 1546–1549.

72. Anda, R. F., Williamson, D. F., Escobedo, L. G., Mast, E., Giovino, G. A., and Remington, P. L. (1990) Depression and the dynamics of smoking; a national perspective. *JAMA* **264,** 1541–1545.

73. Everson, S. A., Goldberg, D. E., Kaplan, G. A., Cohen, R. D., Pukkala, E., Tuomilehto, J., et al. (1996) Hopelessness and risk of mortality and incidence of myocardial infarction and cancer. *Psychosom. Med.* **58,** 113–121.

74. Penttinen, J. and Valonen, P. (1996) Use of psychotropic drugs and risk of myocardial infarction: a case-control study in Finnish farmers. *Int. J. Epidemiology* **25(4),** 760–762.

75. Thorogood, M., Cowen, P., Mann, J., Murphy, M., and Vessey, M. (1992) Fatal myocardial infarction and the use of psychotropic drugs in young women. *Lancet* **340,** 1067–1068.

76. Avery, D. and Winokur, G. (1976) Mortality in depressed patients treated with electroconvulsive therapy and antidepressants, *Arch. Gen. Psychiatry* **33,** 1029–1037.

77. Norton, B. and Whalley, L. W. (1984) Mortality of a lithium-treated population. *Br. J. Psychiatry* **145,** 277–282.

78. Weeke, A. and Veath, M. (1986) Excess mortality of bipolar and unipolar manic-depressive patients, *J. Affect. Dis.* **11,** 227–234.

79. Vestergaard, P. and Aagaard, J. (1991) Five-year mortality in lithium-treated manic–depressive patients. *J. Affect. Dis.* **21,** 33–38.

80. Muller-Oerlinghausen, B., Ahrens, B., Grof, E., Grof, P., Lenz, G., Schou, M., et al. (1992) The effect of long-term lithium treatment on the mortality of patients with manic–depressive and schizoaffective illness. *Acta Pscychiatr. Scand.* **86** 218–222.

81. Nilsson, A. (1995) Mortality in recurrent mood disorders during periods on and off lithium, a complete population study in 362 patients. *Pharmacopsychiatry* **28,** 8–13.

82. Pratt, L. A., Ford, D. E., Crum, R. M., Armenian, H. K., Gallo, J. J., and Eaton, W. W. (1996) Depression, psychotropic medication, and risk of myocardial infarction, prospective data from the Baltimore ECA follow-up. *Circulation* **94,** 3123–3129.

83. Coppen, A., Standish-Barry, H., Bailey, J., Houston, G., Silcocks, P., and Hermon, C. (1990) Long-term lithium and mortality. *Lancet* **335,** 1347–1357.

84. Ahern, D. K., Gorkin, L., Anderson, J. L., Tierney, C., Hallstrom, A., Ewart, C., et al. (1990) Biobehavioral variables and mortality of cardiac arrest in the cardiac arryhythmia pilot study (CAPS). *Am. J. Cardiol.* **66,** 59–62.

85. Kessler, R. C., McGonagle, K. A., Zhao, S., Nelson, C. B., Hughes, M., Eshleman, S., et al. (1994) Lifetime and twelve month prevalence of DSM-3-R psychiatric disorders in the United States: results from the National Comorbidity Survey. *Arch Gen Psychiatry* **51,** 8–19.

86. Havik, O. E. and Maelands, J. G. (1990) Patterns of emotional reactions after a myocardial infarction. *J. Psychosom. Res.* **34(3),** 271–285.

87. Ladwig, K. H., Lehmacher, W., Roth, R., Breithardt, G., Budde, Th., and Borgrefe, M. (1992) Factors which provoke post-infarction depression: results from the post-infarction late potential study (PILP). *J. Psychom. Res.* **36(8),** 723–729.

88. Lloyd, G. G. and Cawley, R. H. (1983) Distress or illness? A study of psychological symptoms after myocardial infarction. *Br. J. Psychiatry* **142,** 120–125.

89. Matthews, K. A. (1988) Coronary heart disease and type A behaviors: update on and alternative to the Booth-Kewly and Friedman (1987) quantitative review. *Psychol. Bull.* **104,** 373–380.

90. Frasure-Smith, N., Lesperance, F., and Talajic, M. (1993) Depression following myocardial infarction. Impact on 6-month survival. *JAMA* **270(15)**, 1819–1825.

90a. Killip, T. and Kimball, J. T. (1967) Treatment of myocardial infarction in a coronary care unit. Two-year experience with 250 patients. *Am. J. Cardiol.* **20,** 457–464.

91. Anda, R. F., Williamson, D. F., Jones, D., Macera, C., Eaker, E., Glassman, A. H., et al. (1993) Depressed affect, hopelessness, and the risk of ischemic heart disease in a cohort of US adults. *Epidemiology* **4,** 285–294.

92. Rosenman, R. H., Brand, R. J., Sholtz, R. I., and Friedman, M. (1976) Multivariate prediction of sudden cardiac death after healing of acute myocardial infarction. *Am. J. Cardiol.* **61,** 903–910.

93. Williams, R. B., Barefoot, J. C., Haney, T. L., Harrel, F. E., Blumenthal, J. E., Pryor, D. B., et al. (1988) Type A behavior and angiographycally documented atherosclerosis in a sample of 2,289 patients. Psychosom. Med. 50, 139–152.

94. Smith, D. F., Sterndorff, B., Ropcke, G., Gustavsen, E. M., and Hansen, J. K. (1996) Prevalence and severity of anxiety, depression and Type A behaviors in angina pectoris. *Scand. J. Psycholo.* **37,** 249–258.

95. Ragland, D. R. and Brand, R. J. (1988) Type A behavior and mortality from coronary heart disease. N. Engl. J. Med. 318, 65–69.

96. Schelleke, R. B., Gale, M., and Norusis, M. (1985) Type A score (Jenkins Activity Survey) and risk of recurrent coronary heart disease in the Aspirin Myocardial Infarction Study. Am. J. Cardiol. 56, 221–225.

97. Denollet, J., Stroobant, N., Rombouts, H., Gillebert, T. C., and Brutseart, D. L., Personality as independent predictor of long-term mortality in patients with coronary heart disease. *Lancet* **347,** 417–421.

98. Honig, A., Lousberg, R., Wojciechowski, F. L., Cheriex, E. C., Wellens, H. J. J. and van Praag, H. M. (1997) Depressie na een eerste hartinfarct, overeenkomsten en verschillen met "gewone" depressie. *Ned. Tijdschr. Gen.* **141,** 196–199.

99. Fava, M., Abraham, M., Pava, J., Shuster, J., and Rosenbaum, J. (1996) Cardiovascular risk factors in depression. The role of anxiety and anger. *Psychosomatics* **37,** 31–37.

100. Kawachi, I., Sparrow, D., Spiro, A., III, Vokonas, P., and Weiss, S. T. (1996) A prospective study of anger and coronary heart disease, the normative aging study. *Circulation* **94,** 2090–2095.

101. Lowery, B. J., Jacobsen, B. S., Cera, M. A., McIndoe, D., Klemann, M., and Menapace, F. (1992) Attention versus avoidance: attributional search and denial after myocardial infarction. *Heart and Lung* **21,** 523–528.

102. Jones, D. A. and West, R. R. (1996) Psychological rehabilitation after myocardial infarction: multicentre randomised controlled trial. *Br. Med. J.* **313,** 1517–1521.

103. Taylor, C. B., Miller, N. H., Smith, P. M., and DeBusk, R. F. (1997) The effect of a home-based, case-managed, multifactorial risk-reduction program on reducing psychological distress in patients with cardiovascular disease. *J. Cardiopulm. Rehabil.* **17,** 157–162.

104. Roose, S. P. and Glassman, A. H. (1989) Cardiovascular effects of tricyclic antidepressants in depressed patients with and without heart disease. *J. Clin. Psychiatry* **50,** 1–18.

105. Roose, S. P., Glassman, A. H., Attia, E., Woodring, S., Giardina, E. G. V., and Bigger J. T. (1998) Cardiovascular effects of fluoxetine in depressed patients with heart disease. *Am. J. Psychiatry* **155,** 660–665.

106. Roose, S. P., Glassmann, A. H., Attia, E. A., and Woodring, S. (1994) Comparative efficacy of selective serotonin reuptake inhibitors and tricyclics in the treatment of melancholia. *Am. J. Psychiatry* **151,** 1735–1739.

106a. Griez, E. and Overbeek, Th. (1997) Comorbidity of depression and anxiety, in *Depression: Neurobiological, Psyhological and Therapeutic Advances* (Honig, A. and Van Praagh, N. M., eds.), Wiley, Chichester, pp. 41–59.

107. Katon, W., Sullivan, M., and Clark, M. (1995) Cardiovascular disorders, in *Comprehensive Textbook of Psychiatry* (Kaplan, H. I. and Saddock, B. J., eds.), Williams & Wilkins, Baltimore, pp. 1491–1501.

108. Beitman, B. D., Matt, G., Kushner, M. A., Basha, I., Lamberti, J., Mukerji, V., et al. (1991) Follow-up status of patients with angiographically normal arteries and panic disorder. *JAMA* **65,** 1545–1549.

108a. Alpert, M. A., Mukerji, V., Sabeti, M., Russell, J. L., and Beitman, B. D. (1991) Mitral valve prolapse, panic disorder, and chest pain. *Med. Clin. North. Am.* **75(5),** 1119–1133.

109. Bowen, R. C., D'Arcy, C., and Orchard, R. C. (1991) The prevalence of anxiety disorders among patients with mitral valve prolapse syndrome and chest pain. *Psychosomatics* **32(4),** 400–406.

110. Arfken, C. L., Lachman, A. S., McLaren, M. J., Schulman, P., Leach, C. N., and Farrish, G. C. M. (1990) Mitral valve prolapse: associations with symptoms and anxiety, *Pediatrics* **85(3),** 311–315.

111. Kochiadakis, G. E., Parthenakis, F. I., Zuridakis, E. G., Rombola, A. T., Chrysostomakis, S. I., and Vardas, P. E. (1996) Is there increased sympathetic activity in patients with mitral valve prolapse? *Pacing Clin. Electrophysiol.* **19,** 1872–1876.

112. Weissman, N. J., Shear, M. K., Kramer-Fox, R., and Deveraux, R. B. (1987) Contrasting patterns of autonomic dysfunction in

patients with mitral valve prolapse and panic attacks. *Am. J. Med.* **82,** 880–888.

113. Margraf, J., Ehlers, A., and Roth, W. T. (1988) Mitral valve prolaps and panic disorder: a review of their relationship. *Psychosom. Med.* **50,** 93–113.

114. Kahn, J. P., Drusin, R. E., and Klein, D. F. (1987) Idiopathic cardiomyopathy and panic disorder: clinical association in cardiac transplant candidates. *Am. J. Psychiatry* **10,** 1327–1330.

115. Coryell, W., Noyes, R., and Clancy, J. (1982) Excess mortality in panic disorder: a comparison with primary unipolar depression. *Arch. Gen. Psychiatry* **39,** 701–703.

116. Coryell, W., Noyes, R., and Hause, J. D. (1986) Mortality among outpatients with anxiety disorders. *Am. J. Psychiatry* **143,** 508–510.

117. Deanfield, J. E., Shea, M., Kensett, M., Horlock, P., Wilson, R. A., de Landsheere, C. M., et al. (1984) Silent myocardial ischemia due to mental stress. *Lancet* **2,** 1001–1005.

118. Reich, P. and Desilva, R. A. (1981) Acute psychological disturbances preceding life-threatening ventricular arrhythmias. *JAMA* **246,** 233–235.

119. Kawachi, I., Colditz, G. A., Ascherio, A., Rimm, E. B., Giovannucci, E., Stamfer, M. J., et al. (1994) Prospective study of phobic anxiety and risk of coronary heart disease in men. *Circulation* **89,** 1992–1997.

120. Kawachi, I., Sparrow, D., Vokonas, P. S., and Weiss, S. T. (1994) Symptoms of anxiety and risk of coronary heart disease: the normative aging study. *Circulation* **90,** 2225–2229.

121. Haines, A. P., Imeson, J. D., and Meade, T. W. (1987) Phobic anxiety and ischaemic heart disease. *Br. Med. J.* **295,** 297–299.

122. Freeman, L. J., and Nixon, P. G. F. (1985) Are coronary artery spasm and progressive damage to the heart associated with the hyperventilation syndrome? *Br. Med. J.* **291,** 851–852.

123. Girotti, L. A., Crossato, J. R., Messuti, H., Kaski, J. C., Dyszel, E., Rivas, C. A., et al. (1982) The hyperventilation test as a method for developing successful therapy in Prinzmetal angina. *Am. J. Cardiol.* **49,** 834–841.

124. Pasternak, R. C., Braunwald, E., and Sobel, B. E. (1988) Acute myocardial infarction, in *Heart Disease. A Textbook of Cardiovascular Medicine* (Braunwald, E., ed.), W. B. Saunders, Philadelphia, pp. 1222–1314.

125. Moser, D. K. and Dracup K. (1996) Is anxiety early after myocardial infarction associated with subsequent ischemic and arrhythmic events. *Psychosom. Med.* **58,** 395–401.

126. Crowe, J. M., Runions, J., Ebbesen, L. S., Oldridge, N. B., and Streiner, D. L. (1996) Anxiety and depression after acute myocardial infarction. *Heart Lung* **25,** 98–107.

127. Doerfler, L. A., Pbert, L., and DeCosimo, D. (1994) Symptoms of posttraumatic stress disorder following myocardial infarction and coronary artery bypass surgery. *Gen. Hosp. Psychiatry* **16,** 193–199.

128. Kutz, I., Garb, R., and David, D. (1988) Post-traumatic stress disorder following myocardial infarction. *Gen. Hosp. Psychiatry* **10,** 169–176.

129. Walzer, T., Herrmann, M., and Wallesch, C.-W. (1997) Neuropsychological disorders after coronary care bypass surgery. *J. Neurol. Neurosurg. Psychiatry* **62,** 644–648.

130. Lipowski, Z. J. (1990) Vascular diseases, in *Delirium: Acute Confusional States* (Lipowski, Z. J., ed.), Oxford University Press, New York, pp. 375–398.

131. Zuccala, B. G., Cattel, C., Manes-Gravina, E., Di Niro, M. G., Cocchi, A., and Bernabei, R. (1997) Left ventricular dysfunction: a clue to cognitive impairment in older patients with heart failure. *J. Neurol. Neurosurg. Psychiatry* **63,** 509–512.

132. Koide, H., Kobayashi, S., Kitani, M., Tsunematsu, T., and Nakazawa, Y. (1994) Improvement of cerebral blood flow and cognitive function following pacemaker implantation in patients with bradycardia. *Gerontology* **40(5),** 279–285.

133. Rockwood, K., Dobbs, A. R., Rule, B. G., Howlett S. E., and Black, W. R. (1992) The impact of pacemaker implantation on cognitive functioning in elderly patients. *J. Am. Geriatr. Soc.* **40(2),** 142–146.

134. Dimsdale, J. E. (1992) Reflections on the impact of antihypertensive medications on mood, sedation, and neuropsychologic functioning. *Arch. Intern. Med.* **152,** 35–39.

Index